Wash and Be Healed

The Water-Cure Movement and Women's Health

Health, Society, and Policy

A series edited by Sheryl Ruzek
and Irving Kenneth Zola

Wash and Be Healed

The Water-Cure Movement and Women's Health

Susan E. Cayleff

TEMPLE UNIVERSITY PRESS

PHILADELPHIA

Temple University Press, Philadelphia 19122
Copyright © 1987 by Temple University. All rights reserved
Published 1987
Printed in the United States of America

The paper used in this publication meets the minimum
requirements of American National Standard for Information
Sciences—Permanence of Paper for Printed Library Materials,
ANSI Z39.48-1984

Library of Congress Cataloging-in-Publication Data

Cayleff, Susan E., 1954–
  Wash and be healed.

  (Health, society, and policy)
  Bibliography: p. 229
  Includes index.
  1. Hydrotherapy—United States—History—
19th century. 2. Women—Health and hygiene—
United States—History—19th century. I. Title.
II. Series. [DNLM: 1. Balneology—history.
2. Therapeutic Cults—history. 3. Women.
WB 525 C385w]
RM811.C39   1987   615.8'53'0973   86-23027
ISBN 0-87722-462-5 (alk. paper)

For Nat and Fritzie

Contents

Acknowledgments   ix

Introduction
    The Rise of Medical Sectarianism   1
Chapter One
    Wash and Be Healed: The Hydropathic Alternative   17
Chapter Two
    Hydropathy, Woman's Physiology, and Her Role   49
Chapter Three
    Ideology in Practice: Water-Cure Establishments   75
Chapter Four
    Hydropathy and the Reform Movements   109
Chapter Five
    Women at the Cures: Rest for the Weary Activist   141
Conclusion
    Demise and Legacy of the Water-Cure Movement   159

Notes   177
An Essay on Sources   229
Index   237

Acknowledgments

My gratitude and indebtedness in completing *Wash and Be Healed* is myriad and heartfelt. I would like to thank Mari Jo Buhle of Brown University, who, as an academic mentor and friend gave me her tireless and incisive criticisms and support of this project from its inception in 1981. In my years at Sarah Lawrence I benefited tremendously from the scholarship of Gerda Lerner and Phyllis Vine, both of whose advice and guidance have continued to inform my work. And while a neophyte Women's Studies student at the University of Massachusetts at Amherst, Ann Ferguson illuminated the limitless dimensions of feminist scholarship.

For insightful readings of the manuscript in various stages I am indebted to Joan Scott and Lois Monteiro, both then of Brown University. More recently, Barbara Melosh of the Smithsonian Institution and George Mason University has provided me with invaluable readings of the manuscript, bolstering phone calls, and a comprehensive camaraderie that has helped me through many difficult junctures. Bill Waller's sterling comments clarified and eased the book's completion. My gratitude to Janet Francendese and Mary Capouya, my editors at Temple University Press, for their advice and counsel.

I would like to thank the staffs of the following libraries for their help in securing documents and facilitating my research: the Francis Countway Library of Medicine of Harvard; the Brown University Rockefeller Library; the Moody Medical Library at the University of Texas Medical Branch; the Department of Biomedical Communication at the University of Texas Medical Branch for providing slides for the illustrations; the Forbes Library in Northampton, Massachusetts; the Springfield, Worcester, Boston Public, and Easthampton libraries, all in Massachusetts; and the Dansville, Elmira, and Binghamton libraries in New York.

My gratitude for secretarial support is directed warmly and whole-heartedly toward Betty Herman of the Institute for the Medical Humanities at the University of Texas Medical Branch. Her skill, commitment, enthusiasm, genuine good humor, and supportiveness for the project—well beyond her professional role—are deeply and fondly appreciated. On earlier versions of the manuscript I benefited from the help of Jo Pope and Judy Follansbee.

Personally, I owe special gratitude to my parents, Nat and Fritzie Cayleff, for all that they have done to aid and ease this project. Their friendship and understanding, like the water cure itself, has been a source of strength, meaning, and sustenance. Similarly, Dorothy Pettigrew, Edie Pearlman, Barb Siegel, and Pat Rapson have, over the years, borne the trials and tribulations of this book, and my struggles with its progress.

While I have gained immeasurably from the tutelage, guidance, and support of all the people named herein, the ultimate strengths and short-comings of the book are mine alone. The journey was eased, however, by their presence, faith, community, and trust.

Wash and Be Healed

The Water-Cure Movement and Women's Health

Introduction

The Rise of
Medical Sectarianism

In the spring of 1857, being out of health and having read in the Water Cure Journal *articles on health by Dr. Jackson, it was thought best by my family that I put myself under his care. This was at considerable sacrifice on my husband's part, both as concerned the feelings and the purse, for it was a year of panic in the financial world, but I often heard him say afterward that he never made another investment that paid him so well.*

Dr. James C. Jackson was then at the height of his power to lift and carry his patients along the often difficult road to health and to impress them with his fresh thought. I was taken into his family as quite an intimate member and formed there the close friendship with Dr. Harriet N. Austin that lasted during her lifetime. I went to Dr. Jackson expecting to remain six weeks but I stayed six months and went home well, and I have been well ever since. Think of fifty years of unbroken health!—and this is the important part of my message—I learned my lesson and have taken care of myself. I have not taken doses or tonics; I have taken care.—Fanny B. Johnson, quoted in The Jackson Health Resort

Fanny B. Johnson, in her eighty-eighth year, delivered this message in 1907 at the fiftieth-anniversary celebration of the founding of the Dansville, New York, Water-Cure. As one of Jackson's earliest water-cure patients, she could well attest to the changes that the cure had brought about in her life: the restoration of health, the formation of

1

friendships that lasted a lifetime, and the assumption of responsibility for her own health care. Other women wrote similar accounts, glowingly recalling their stay at water-cure establishments and praising the hydropathic program of patient participation and eventual patient autonomy.

In addition to physiological remedies, the principles, therapeutics, and environment of these water-cure establishments offered their patients psychological relief. Women, whose ordained role in the nineteenth century demanded an unvarying round of domestic responsibilities and the nurturing of husband and family, especially found respite at the water cures; here, *their* needs were paramount. The cures addressed complaints ranging from organic ailments to nervous disorders, from "broken-down constitutions" to emotional malaise. While men were equally attracted to the cures—for their social vision as well as the therapeutics—and at times outnumbered women in attendance at the establishments, it is women's relationship to the movement that is the focus of this study.

Hydropathy was one of the most celebrated alternative forms of medical care in an age generally characterized by more dramatic therapeutics. Social historians have focused considerable attention on the allopathic ("regular") treatments, which included bloodletting and purging. These were aimed at calming the general or local fever that resulted from irritation or excitement and caused, so the theory held, the diseased condition. The goal of these treatments was to aid nature in evacuating the body of its "ill humors" and restore a balance of elements by removing putrid matter from the system. These therapeutics were employed when treating "female complaints" as well as other ailments.

Conventional medical tracts, asserting that women's disorders emanated from the womb, focused on the reproductive organs. These texts commonly portrayed women as impaired by menstrual difficulties and subject to an unpredictable physiology that rendered them unable to perform intellectual work.

Hydropathic theory, in contrast, maintained that allopathy weakened the female constitution and rendered women incapable of bearing and rearing children. Thus, hydropaths rejected dramatic therapeutics in managing women's diseases. They also challenged the allopathic view of women's physiology, redefining these processes as natural, not medical, and thus deemphasized doctors and drugs. Hydropathy's moderate, if not noninterventionist, procedures stressed ingesting water and the application of cold water to the body through wraps, sprays, and soaks to relieve local or general discomfort and illness. Changes in personal habits were also urged. These included more exposure to daylight and proper ventilation, simple food (preferably vegetarian) and nonstimulating drink, loose-fitting clothing of lightweight material, regular physical exercise, and moderate exposure to emotional and sexual stimulation. In rejecting the notion that women's physiology caused and even justified their social status, hydropaths provided an important impetus for American women to question both the conventional therapeutics they were receiving and the consequently constricting definitions of their physiology.

In a century in which numerous medical practitioners (approximately 20 percent of them were composed of alternative sectarians who, to varying degrees, disagreed with the allopaths' conventional use of drugs and evacuative therapeutics) were competing for patients, hydropathy was dubbed a cult or "quack" fad by allopathic physicians, who thought its therapeutics irresponsible and who, like all other practitioners, were themselves seeking popular support.[1] Despite charges of quackery, the water-cure movement enjoyed widespread acceptance among the American populace and was, for a few decades in the mid-nineteenth century, a staunch competitor of allopathic physicians and other health-reform sects. Especially prolific between 1840 and 1900, hydropathic establishments, or water cures, flourished primarily in New York, Massachusetts, New Jersey, and Pennsylvania. There were, by one historian's count, 213 water-cure establishments nationwide.[2] In addition, the *Water-Cure Journal*, which served as the primary literary organ of the movement, was published from 1843 until 1913 and saw its subscription list reach 100,000 in the 1850s.[3]

Our understanding of the social context and meaning of healing systems can benefit from exploring both the hydropathic movement in general and women's specific affinity for it. If the movement is viewed as a separate system that had internal coherence, popular appeal, and social and medical value in its own right, then the characterization, not uncommon in earlier medical writing, of hydropathy as just another short-lived sect competing unsuccessfully for clientele and influence against the allopaths will give way to a richer, more historically comprehensive analysis.

Hydropathy in Medical History

Before the 1970s, historiography often focused on the triumph of scientific methodology over experiential skills, of technological advances over lay knowledge, and of professionalism over folk healing. At times this interpretation reduced the history of medicine to charting the triumph of science over folkways. What emerged from this approach to medical history was a version of events and personalities that focused on the innovators, stressed scientific "breakthroughs," romanticized the contributions of the allopathic, or "regular," sect, and often viewed other, competing, sects as "irregular" cults. This interpretation blurred the historical reality of mid-nineteenth-century America and minimized the complex factors that combined to create science and health care as we know them today.[4]

These "March of Science" writings generally posited that "great men and their discoveries" should be used as the primary organizing principle for the history of medicine. The overriding assumption in these texts was that medical science (allopathy) was primarily, if not exclusively, responsible for innovative therapeutics and decreased mortality rates. This interpretation failed to consider, or minimized, factors or contributions beyond the allopathic sect; medical sectarianism was nearly always portrayed as a stumbling block on the way to true knowledge.

More recently, historians have moved away from the linear model of medical progress and adopted a social or cultural approach. These professional medical historians have rewritten medical history to stress the contribution and influence of nineteenth-century sects. One of their strategies has been to question the actual contribution of medical therapeutics to the decline of mortality rates and to expand the list of factors causing health and illness. This social approach asserts that broad improvements in sanitation, food quality, and shelter, not physicians' innovations and interventions, accounted for decreased mortality.[5]

By emphasizing the nonmedical causes of improved health, the recent historians reveal that medical science faltered considerably on its way to insight and that sects contributed significantly to solving medical problems (through urging personal habit reformation, diet, hygiene, bathing, and less drugging). The diminishment of a one-cause, one-cure theory of disease that advocated heroic therapeutics, which entailed dramatic physician and drug intervention, had brought allopathic physicians into an uncertain era, in which the sects' moderate remedies served to further medical knowledge.[6] This interpretation of reciprocity between alternative and regular healers points out the shared errors and advances of the sects, avoids portraying modern medical history in terms of scientists conquering disease, and alters earlier portrayals of the innovative pre-scientist leaving the stubborn lay or sectarian healer behind.[7]

Most recently, there has been a general resurrection of the claim that medical science contributed significantly to declining mortality rates and that "medicine" needs to be reasserted in medical history.[8] This claim reiterates the important advances gained through laboratory research, immunization, surgical techniques, and general technological innovations such as the X ray. The contributions of the alternative sects are heeded, but the emphasis lies on scientificism and its attendant accomplishments. While interpretations vary as to the origin of true innovations in healing, it seems reasonable to say that we can gain much by focusing attention on the complex regimens and systems of meaning that emerged from the various healing sects. This informs not only medical history but our understanding of what it means to feel well or sick, the needs and expectations people bring to medicine, and what constitutes good doctoring.

For these reasons, hydropathy can serve as a highly instructive healing system, not only as a contributor to the present-day treatment of fevers and to exercise therapy (its common depiction in contemporary medical articles),[9] but also as a health-reform philosophy and world view that operated effectively in mid-nineteenth-century America.

Despite the obvious interest in hydropathy as a case study, only two books have focused exclusively on it.[10] This may be, first, because hydropathy was not medicine in the traditional sense, although it was a healing system; it did not sanction drugs, physician control, or the radical manipulation of human physiology. Second, hydropathy may have been excluded from discussions of cults and fads because so much of it was later adopted into regular medical practice. Finally, since the cold-water cure (not to be confused with contemporary hydrotherapy), unlike homeopathy, chiropractic medicine, and hypnotism, has no direct present-day derivative (our fascination with pool exercises, spas, jacuzzis, and hot tubs notwithstanding), it may have been of less interest to modern historians.

There are notable exceptions to this general oversight on hydropathy. Scholarly attention has hitherto focused on the cold-water system for its emphasis on self-doctoring,[11] its panacea approach to illness and curing,[12] its similarities with other hygienic and reformist nineteenth-century sects,[13] and its significance in providing women with psychological havens while offering respites from repeated pregnancies.[14] Recent scholarship in women's history has considered the hydropathic movement and women's involvement in it as part of a long tradition of domestic self-help and as a means by which women participated and exercised control in an uncertain world.[15] Other authors are similarly aware of the opportunities hydropathy afforded women and of its appeal to them.[16] Still, a portion of this scholarship characterizes hydropathy as an amusing aberration, not as an internally coherent system with social and medical value in its own right.[17] In short, the water-cure's importance as a healing system, world view, and gender-conscious ideology and community that provided physiological retreats and varied life choices for women has yet to be sufficiently explored. This book attempts to show that the movement contributed significantly to reexamining attitudes about women's physiology and in so doing helped redefine their social capabilities. For its followers, hydropathy was a way of living; for the larger public, it offered an articulate critique of medical care and social relations.

The State of Nineteenth-Century Health Care

Nineteenth-century medical theory and treatment were an extremely uncertain business for all practitioners. No one sect had a secure base in scientific knowledge, yet practitioners in all the sects had to do something for patients in need. The different solutions and philosophies, each claiming efficacy and preeminence, tell us a great deal about the unevenness of cultural change and of the human need to create order and meaning through health-care "systems." Within the context of nineteenth-century America, health-care sects proposed competing models that offered social and cultural continuity. The sects provided a social function; they did not, despite their claims, provide truth and preeminence.

The nineteenth-century historical milieu in which hydropathy gained popularity and ascendance can best be understood as an era of conflict and competition among the sects. (I am considering allopathy, although numerically predominant, as one of the sects because of the competitive nature of nineteenth-century health care.) The various sects approached the theory of medicine with important commonalities, but their therapeutics differed significantly. Allopaths emphasized remedial drug intervention, whereas reform-oriented sects, operating out of a zealously guarded let-nature-take-its-course position, stressed (to varying degrees) preventive, patient-controlled, hygienic living principles, a different view of drugging, and, often, less intrusive therapeutics. By mid-century, however, allopaths were integrating aspects of the milder regimens of the sects; thus their emphasis increasingly stressed helping nature.

In nineteenth-century America the allopathic sect diagnosed and treated disease according to the "fever theory," which was the most popular explanation of disease: "[It] stated rather vaguely that disease is a result of irritation or excitement. Before rehabilitating a patient by various drugs, it was best to 'depress' or calm him. Despite variation in procedure in specific diseases, the general program was followed by a majority of the profession."[18]

Nineteenth-century medical practitioners and laypersons shared certain beliefs about the human body. They assumed that the body possessed a finite amount of "fixed energy," or "vital force." Physicians believed that health was achieved through an equitable distribution of this fixed quantity of life force. Consequently, illness resulted when one area of the body possessed too little or too much of the needed force. Further, all believed that every part of the body was interrelated with other parts, that the environment (climate and seasons) could affect the working harmony of these parts, that health or disease was the state of the entire system, that physiological turning points for both men and women were potentially dangerous because the body was trying to achieve a new balance, and that maintaining a balance of the body system constituted health. To accomplish this, all practitioners regulated and altered excretions and secretions through various agents.

In the early part of the century, regular practitioners sought to restore the system's balance through bloodletting, purgatives, emetics, and cathartics. As the century progressed, the more invasive therapeutics gave way to drugs and alcohol-based medications that produced somewhat less identifiable results. Thus, all healers judged the discharge of the body's putrid matter in perspiration, eruptions, urination, boils, blisters, etc., as efficacious and demonstrative of a reaction leading toward health. Both healer and patient could see these tangible results from treatment, and the visible effects sanctioned the physician's role—especially since the effects often coincided with alterations in the body's state. In essence, all healers sought to aid nature. Their agents and regimens varied, not their theoretical outlook.

Thus, regular practitioners and hydropaths shared significant elements: Both assumed an interventionist role that produced tangible physical results (via secretions and excretions); both sought to regulate and restore the body's expulsions when they went awry; both "prescribed" on an individual basis according to a patient's singular constitution; both viewed the body as a system struggling to achieve and maintain balance; both sought to relieve their patients' anxiety and discomfort through their therapies; both believed in the body's "vital power" and the necessity of keeping that power intact to aid healing; and both served clients who at times wanted even greater "proof" of healing, thus indulging in and insisting on therapeutic excesses themselves.

By the 1830s, conventional practitioners believed, as hydropaths did in the next decade, in the self-limiting nature of disease; thus they came to see the physician's role as somewhat less interventionist and more attuned to assisting nature. To this end, allopaths advocated rest and improved diet as well as mild cathartics. After 1850, evacuative bleeding was deemphasized, as were most depletive therapeutics; alcohol-based medications and others came into play, thus preserving the instrumentality appealing to physicians and patients alike. Moderation in frequency and dosage characterized this era, although bleeding was still used by some, and purgatives were widely employed.[19] Nevertheless, allopaths differed dramatically from hydropaths on the use of drugs; the former readily utilized them as their main healing agent, whereas hydropaths abhorred them.

These conventional therapeutics, while they actively sought to aid nature in counterattacking disease and ridding the body of its putrid matter, were not particularly conducive to securing a clientele for the allopathic practitioner because of their discomforting and often dangerous effects. This was one reason that, for several decades in the early nineteenth century (and going well back into the eighteenth century in the case of male midwifery), regular physicians were in a precarious position. The practice of heroic medicine itself, potentially life threatening in its effects, had, in fact, contributed to the popularity of the preventive hygienic doctrines of the alternative sects, called the Popular Health Movement.[20] Other factors contributing to the allopaths' low status were early attempts at professionalization and standardized education, which conflicted with the leveling effect so heralded during Jacksonian America, and a proliferation of questionable medical degrees, which rendered a diploma of little value.[21]

This is not to deny that allopathic medicine was sought out by large numbers of men and women. Its "cures" were unpleasant and largely inefficacious, but it did offer active intervention, a "Do something!" approach to health care that was (and still is) seen as the *only* measure of "good" doctoring by many patients. In fact, allopaths were not the only ones using harsh therapeutics; even folk medicine was harsh because people demanded it. In this regard, homeopathy and hydropathy, the least-harsh sects, are particularly instructive because their widespread adoption marked a turning away from this kind of medical care. Popular among "common folk," as well as those in the social and intellectual vanguard, the two milder systems signaled a move toward prevention, as opposed to remedial care and an emphasis on self-control through healthful living.

Contributing to the credibility of allopathic physicians was their appeal to the middle and upper classes through prescriptive literature. They understood and perhaps mostly shared those classes' views of men and women. As such, in mid- and late-nineteenth-century America they became the "true experts" and cultural spokesmen on women's physiology. Their literature, arguing that only through allopathic management of women's "diseases" could women's complex physiology be properly administered to,[22] stands as testimony to the role of physical and moral adjudicator that allopaths adopted. Thus, by employing an apprentice or university-trained physician instead of a less educated (and possibly less expensive) lay practitioner, a family signaled its social status.[23] It is also possible that middle-class women, removed as they were in their separate sphere from the rapid social changes wrought by industrialism, viewed the personal adoption of medical innovations and "scientific principles" as a way to experience the progress and change of nineteenth-century America.

In the larger sense, male management of female physiology was a new phenomenon. A female domain in seventeenth- and eighteenth-century America, healing was gradually becoming a male-dominated arena.[24] Simultaneously, what had previously been considered the natural sequence of women's physiology—puberty, menstruation, childbirth, and menopause—was now diagnosed as a series of potentially dangerous medical events because the system went out of balance while adjusting to the physiological changes. These junctures, physicians argued, were particularly critical for women, given their weaker constitution and the controlling influence of their reproductive organs on all of their physiology; thus, scientific understanding was needed, which only doctors could provide.[25] Hydropaths, conversely, did not adhere to this notion of life-cycle periodic frailty or to the extreme emphasis placed on women's reproductive organs as the controlling physiological force. Nor did they see themselves as the only appropriate intervenors in these events if they became complicated.

Male and Female "Nature"

Indeed, the changes in woman's social and familial roles between 1820 and 1860 served as both the justification for and the "proof" of these "scientifically based" perceptions of woman's physiology. During these decades a sharp division between male and female work roles relegated middle- and upper-class women almost exclusively to the domestic sphere and attributed to them a romantic and moral character as well as weaker physiology and intellect. Expectations of proper female behavior increasingly emphasized serving as a counterbalance to the competitive, individualist, and achievement-oriented world of public (i.e., male) pursuit.[26] The domestic realm was raised to the status of a familial and societal oasis amid rapid social growth and uncertainty.[27] Women within the home were to serve as regulators and protectors in the last realm where commitment to others and morality were reigning creeds. Relationships between women, based on mutual cooperation and nurturance,[28] formed an informal network focused in the private realm. This network contrasted dramatically with the male hierarchical organization of personal and work relationships that was gaining ascendancy in the public realm and that emphasized separation rather than connection.[29] These discrete spheres for women and men yielded rewards and limits for both sexes. The "innate" values attributed to women included a kind of physical and intellectual frailty that legitimized a near-total exclusion from the competitive economic realm but offered as a counterbalance a culturally constructed female "nature" that embodied all that was humane and nurturant. To offset women's nurturance and susceptibility to emotionalism, the male "nature" postured as the "social opposite": Men were rational, competitive individualists whose worth was largely measured in terms of economic achievement and social standing. While these views converged into complementary union for marriage purposes, it was generally acknowledged that each gender only truly understood its own. As such, a separate female "world" evolved where support, nurturance, and sorority bonded women to their female relatives, friends, and special "romantic friends."[30]

Any expansion of women's sphere into the public realm, therefore, depended on this belief in an innate moral and nurturant female nature.[31] As a result, numerous benevolent reform activities, including health, fell under women's purview.[32] In short, culturally constructed class and gender-specific behaviors that had been exaggerated to assuage societal upheaval became seen as innate characteristics that ought to determine familial and social roles and opportunities for both women and men.

Within this gender-based social context, the relationship between allopathic physician and female patient assumes particular importance. As mid-century approached, this portrayal of male and female characters was often presented as scientific or social truth. These cultural beliefs provided the physiological basis from which physicians prescribed and circumscribed woman's opportunities.

The implications of allopathic physicians adjudicating female physiology and sexuality were critical (as hydropaths emphasized repeatedly). In what has been called "the Age of the Womb,"[33] woman was seen as a being "built up around her uterus." Women thus became unalterably linked to their reproductive system and were duly prescribed a role that kept them tied to home and family.[34] In essence, doctors were, as two chroniclers of this era have characterized them, "also men of science, and this meant in the cultural framework which equated science with goodness and morality, that doctors saw themselves almost as moral reformers. It was the self-assigned duty of the medical profession to define 'her natural physical and mental constitution.'"[35]

These beliefs regarding women's physiology determined their procreative future, since, it was believed, birth control hastened not only the mother's mental and physical collapse but society's as well. Further, these beliefs fostered female passivity, which effectively removed women from the process of defining and controlling their own physiology. Finally, they explicated women's perceived intellectual (in)abilities.

Of particular importance is the idea that woman's mental capacities were impaired by her physiology. This idea had progressed so far that by the 1860s, Dr. Horatio Storer, a Boston gynecologist, charged that women were unfit to practice medicine because of their "menstrual difficulties." In 1873 this argument found support from the Harvard University overseer, Dr. Edward H. Clarke, whose book *Sex in Education; or a Fair Chance for the Girls*—a decided misnomer—became the definitive text for those opposed to women's education.[36]

Another recurring subject among physicians was the size of the female skull (and brain) and how this affected woman's physiology and social role. One physician, Alexander Walker, after measuring the skulls of twins, noted the lesser intellectual functions of woman (even at birth) and her greater powers of observation and sensitivity.[37] Walker's argument, interestingly, quickly expanded to include an opposition to woman's rights. In a similar vein, another physician argued that a woman's need to devote full attention to childbearing rendered her incapable of mental exertion. The young girl "commences life with an inheritance of a certain amount of nerve force which, if squandered in mental culture, will leave the physical growth defective at some point."[38]

This process of naming and taming female sexuality was accompanied by redefining women's physiological processes as medical events—if not sickness. No longer considered natural functions requiring little or no medical intervention, puberty, menstruation, childbirth, and menopause became crucial and even dangerous junctures in every woman's life. Again, this reflected the belief that her system was "out of balance":

> Woman's reproductive organs are pre-eminent. They exercise a controlling influence upon her entire system, and entail upon her many painful and dangerous diseases. They are the source of her peculiarities, the center of her sympathies, and the seat of her diseases. Everything that is peculiar to her, springs from her sexual organization.[39]

Woman's reproductive future was determined by the proper medical management of these physiological turning points.[40]

Whether these physicians' views about women's physiology were "punitive moralism," expressions of hostility toward women, or mechanisms of social control, as claimed by some, or whether they demonstrated the woefully inadequate state of scientific knowledge,[41] there certainly is evidence of gender ideologies that strongly informed both the rationale for the care dispensed and the ultimate goal of perpetuating a sharp distinction between the sexes. Further, whether physicians were intentionally contributing to women's subordination or whether, as a consequence of women's position in the class they wished to serve, they were simply doing nothing that indicated any critique of predominant gender relations, the *effect* was to reinforce women's subordination.

A History of Health-Reform Sects

Health-reform sects, offering a different therapeutic approach to disease management and often consciously appealing to a less-rigid sense of gender and class appropriateness and destiny, built on a rich tradition of hygienic reform. To varying degrees they stressed the ability of nature to heal when aided by changes in personal habits. Additionally, these sects shared an increasingly critical evaluation of the allopathic management of disease.

The literature on personal hygiene dates from the sixteenth century, when Luigi Coronaro published *Discourses on a Sober and Temperate Life* (1558), in which he pleaded for moderation and temperance.[42] Following Coronaro's tract, hygienic writings became increasingly popular. Sir John Sinclair's *Code of Health Longevity*, published in 1807 (four volumes), listed 1,878 books with health themes, among them 312 texts in English. Concurrently, numerous popular works emphasized moderation and self-care, and these, too, received a welcome response.[43]

Samuel Thomson, the premier nineteenth-century botanic physician, found his path primed by these accessible and easy-to-read texts. His own therapeutics, which he sold to the public in "kits" for home use, cannot be considered mild, however. While he opposed certain allopathic drugs, he strove to restore the balance among the four elements of earth, air, fire, and water, which he believed constituted the body; their imbalance, he claimed, diminished the body's heat and caused illness.[44] Thomson used native herbs in his patented medicines, said he had sold 100,000 copies of his book, and professed roughly three million followers.[45] The popularity of Thomsonianism, despite its harsh use of purgatives, can be explained in part by the appeal of home self-doctoring and the sense of self-determination it yielded, as well as the demonstrable physiological effects the therapeutics produced. In addition to attacking allopathic therapeutics, Thomson derided regular apothecaries and pharmacists, calling them "purveyor[s] of poisons."[46] The Thomsonian movement went on to found its own infirmaries and stores for making and selling the medications.[47] The full extent of the movement's popularity is reflected in the one hundred medical colleges that arose to promulgate its ideology.[48] Eclecticism, one of the offshoots of Thomsonianism, was composed of self-proclaimed reformers who welcomed women to the profession on an equal status with men.[49]

Following quickly in the favorable wake of Thomsonianism, Samuel Hahnemann's homeopathic philosophy, introduced in 1825, was well received by 1850. The system favored professional education and credentials, and Hahnemann's increasingly popular "law of cure" was based on the belief that like cures like. Believing that the cause of illness was *psora* (the itch), Hahnemann's *materia médica* represented a high point at the time in minimizing the use of drugs. (Hydropathic theory advocated abandoning the use of all drugs.)[50] Claiming a following of tens of thousands, the homeopathic movement produced numerous physicians to meet increasing demand.[51] Emphasizing self-care, minute doses of tinctures and powders, and a rational and moderate living regimen including fresh air, pure foods and water, and avoidance of overstimulation, the homeopathic doctrine followed in the tradition of moderation set by earlier hygienic systems. Like Thomsonianism, homeopathy had a distinct antiallopathic strain.[52] Hahnemann himself levied frequent brutal attacks on the allopaths.[53]

What is important is that homeopathy, like eclecticism before it, allowed a place for women in its practice and developed different views about the female anatomy and physiology that did not define women's illnesses as womb oriented. In fact, women's participation in these sects anticipated the formation of numerous Ladies' Physiological Institutes in the 1840s and 1850s. These clubs focused on female culture, personal and domestic health, and self-improvement through social crusading.[54]

Despite the dubious worth of the homeopathic medications, the movement yielded tangible results. Specifically,

Homeopathy, whether one accepted its theories or not, inevitably increased public doubts about the regular profession while it reinforced a belief in the curative powers of nature and lent strength to the view that abiding by the laws of nature was the best way to stay healthy. Such views . . . formed the basis of nineteenth century health reform.[55]

At the time that homeopathy was enjoying its greatest popularity, a significant proportion of the American populace was becoming concerned with personal hygiene, another trend that favored the introduction of hydropathy. The movement was personified in the moralistic enthusiasm of Sylvester Graham, the first hygienic "health crusader."[56] Originally a temperance lecturer in Philadelphia in 1830, Graham took to freelance lecturing in 1831. In addition to writing on hygiene, Graham, along with David Campbell, founded the *Graham Journal of Health and Longevity* in 1837. In his two-volume classic, *Lectures on the Science of Human Life*, which appeared in 1839, he argued for frequent bathing, fresh air, regular exercise, vegetarianism, dress reform, sunlight, and sex hygiene.[57]

Graham's activities provide an early, clear example of how various health-reform groups tended to coalesce around similar issues (such a network emerged as a central element of the hydropathic movement). Graham's disciples included Mary Gove Nichols (later a prominent hydropath) and Paulina Wright Davis, both of whom lectured to female audiences on hygiene and dress reform.[58] In fact, this overlapping concern with hygiene and women's sphere of influence was an integral part of the antebellum world view. Women health reformers linked their insistence on sexual restraint to family limitation, since, as one historian portrayed their argument, "excessive childbearing endangered female health while it drained most women of the energy needed to perform the duties of scientific motherhood."[59] Similarly, popular health journals were among the first to advocate birth control.[60] Like Thomsonians, eclectics, and homeopaths, Graham was opposed to drugs and doctors, and saw right living as the certain way to health.

William Andrus Alcott also joined the ranks of hygienic reformers, making a significant impact on the American consciousness. Alcott, like Graham, preached physical and moral salvation. He advocated public school instruction in physiology, and his general philosophy was similar to Graham's: He believed that only water and vegetables should be ingested.[61]

In addition to his private writings, Alcott's views were found in *The Moral Reformer and Teacher on the Human Constitution*, which he started in 1835.[62] Spurred on by the success of these early publications, Alcott enjoyed a long and varied writing career.[63]

In 1855 Alcott's *The Young Woman's Book of Health* appeared. In it he argued in favor of women's education, despite the controversy surrounding it: "Every young woman should have her mind well stored and disciplined were it only for the sake of improving her own health."[64] Thus, Alcott, like other reformers before him, urged a reconceptualization of women's social pursuits based on the perception of a healthy (i.e., natural) female physiology. Alcott wrote several more volumes, each urging moderation and hygienic living habits.

The combined effect of Graham and Alcott was powerful indeed. The American Physiological Society was formed in Boston in 1837, partially as a result of Graham's lectures. Alcott became the first president, and the neophyte organization sought to educate people to care for themselves while reforming the medical profession to emphasize preventive measures. Given the centrality of mothers in treating family health, women as well as men were admitted to the society.[65] Through Alcott, as through Graham, varied reform activities found a common meeting ground. Alcott, quite possibly influenced by his female colleagues, embraced a women's issue when he urged the founding of anticorset societies, whose members "signed the pledge" not to wear them.[66]

One other early-nineteenth-century sect deserves mention for the challenges it posed, the popularity it garnered, and the influence it had on hydropathy. Phrenology held that the brain was divided into sections, each having a separate mental faculty, "and that the development of each faculty could be judged by the shape of the skull over it."[67] Originated by Franz Joseph Gall in Germany, the concept gained widespread popularity in America through the energies of Orson Squire Fowler.[68] The role of his brother, Lorenzo N. Fowler, is discussed in Chapter Four.

Orson Squire Fowler wholeheartedly believed that humanity could be improved by phrenology. After "reading a head" by its contours, he made recommendations for rectifying shortcomings by identifying areas needing further development. To meet the demands for his publications Fowler bought a publishing house. The *American Phrenological Journal*, which he took over in 1842, had articles and departments on the money system, diet, housing, physiology, hypnotism, and the modern woman.[69] Like the health-reform sects before it, phrenology linked arms with other reform movements of the day. Since phrenology, with its expertise on mental constitution, denied women's mental inferiority, "as early as 1833 Mrs. Sarah J. Hale, editor of Boston's *Ladies Magazine* wrote that 'excepting Christianity, phrenology will do more to elevate women than any other system has ever done. It gives her a participation in the labors of the mind.'"[70] Slavery, like woman's rights, preoccupied the public imagination. George Combe, another American popularizer of phrenology, was similarly unwilling to justify slavery on the ground that the skulls of black people were inferior to those of whites.[71]

Phrenology took the reformist stance on numerous other issues: temperance, exercise, fresh air, and reform dress. Once again, a reconceptualization of women's physiology opened the way for a critique of women's limited social sphere; there was no place for the invalid woman in a phrenological world view, which ridiculed "the equally silly fashion of appearing frail even to the point of invalidism, an affectation popular with women during this era of sentimentalism."[72] The phrenological movement aligned itself with vegetarianism, hydropathy, clairvoyance, animal magnetism (or mesmerism), and finally (to its detriment) with hypnotism.

Fowler, himself a strong advocate of the water cure, cited as one of its chief advantages that the curative agent was found everywhere.[73] Fowler experimented on himself first and then, despite Mrs. Fowler's objections, used the water cure on his family members for burns, fever, poison ivy, sores, and earaches. He was totally in favor of water for "taking up and carrying out of the system those noxious matters which obstruct the function of life, breed disease, and hasten death. . . . [F]or infusing new life throughout all its borders, water excels all other agents combined."[74]

The tradition of health reform begun with Coronaro's 1558 tract continued through the Thomsonians, eclectics, homeopaths, Graham, Alcott, and the phrenologists. Although they possessed extreme points of divergence (e.g., degree of professional education, methods of recruitment, rural vs. urban and working vs. middle-class supporters), they were not categorically different from hydropathy. The goal here is to survey the significant *commonalities* among these sects; these are the most instructive in understanding their precedent-setting role for hydropathy. The sects' common beliefs included a rejection of allopathic therapeutics and, in many instances (Thomsonians and eclectics the exceptions), an unswerving faith in hygienic principles. Although the sects had varied theories of disease, they agreed on nature's ability to aid in the curing of disease, critiqued the kinds and amounts of drugs, offered comparatively less dramatic—although interventionist—therapeutics, stressed healthful living as a prerequisite for a strong physical constitution, and, in some instances, offered women a vibrant participatory role as practitioners.

Hydropathy: A Special Case

Hydropathy followed in the path cleared by the earlier sects. I would argue, however, that hydropathic living represented a high point in its comprehensive world view and its extreme emphasis on self-sufficiency, two features that distinguish it from the other sects and warrant in-depth exploration. The immediate popularity that hydropathy achieved[75] on its introduction into America in the 1840s by proponents and practitioners of the system familiar with its European successes is best understood with the health-reform tradition and its attendant critique of allopathic disease management in mind. In *theory*, hydropathy proffered inclusive and flexible principles, as opposed to either nihilism or monism; in *therapeutics*, moderate remedies utilizing water and changes in personal habits, as opposed to vigorous drug and depletion therapeutics; in *medical philosophy*, an emphasis on cooperation with nature through preventive care, as opposed to a reactive posture that counterattacked disease through episodic crisis interventionism; in *doctor–patient relationships*, mutual responsibility and ultimate self-determination for the patient, as opposed to authoritarianism and secrecy; and in *social ideology*, a reformist, even progressive, stance, as opposed to conservatism and a perpetuation of a class- and gender-based status quo. Thus, its medical and ideological content were competitive with, and even more congenial than, the tenets of allopathy or the other reform sects. Hydropathy appealed to a cross-section of the American populace that was attracted by its drugless therapy, its eventual self-doctoring for patients, its staunch faith in nature's ability to heal, its economic accessibility, its efficacy through changes in personal habits and the medical encounter, and its allegiances with other reform movements.

Additionally, hydropathy's impact on gender issues was profound. This is not to argue that either the hydropathic leadership or patient populations at the cures were predominantly female. Cures were utilized by men in equal or greater numbers than women. Men sought relief from general health problems as well as sexual ones. With the dual appeal of hydropathy thus noted, this work explores how the movement's ideology and therapeutics affected women's lives. Because of the way hydropaths viewed disease (as a systemic disorder in which nature and external life conditions had gone awry), they did not counterattack by assigning the patient a passive role; instead, they chose to modify the life conditions of the ill person. This outlook served to expand women's control over their lives. Perhaps most important, because hydropaths were not seeking medically elite status and economic predominance and because they did not wish to foster the notion of a chronically infirm segment of the population (women), they were less *politically* motivated to construct culturally debilitating definitions of women's physiology. For women, then, the tenets of hydropathy offered the opportunity to redefine their physiological processes, control their medical care and, ultimately, expand their social roles and opportunities. No other nineteenth-century sect offered such an all-encompassing, accessible, and empowering medical and social ideology.

Chapter One

Wash and Be Healed
The Hydropathic Alternative

Water-cure philosophy as a medical regimen offered a simple set of therapeutics that entailed various applications of cold water. To this was added staunch advocacy of reforming personal habits of diet, dress, exercise, and ways of living. Adherents of hydropathy could participate in the system either through home self-care or under the tutelage of a water-cure physician at a site away from home. To place hydropathy within a larger framework before fully developing these themes, I first examine the significance and appeal of hydropathy as a societal vision within the nineteenth-century milieu. I then recall the significance of water as the ultimate healing agent, give a brief history of the medical use of cold water and the introduction of the practice in the United States, and discuss the influence of mineral spas.

Hydropathy as a Vision of Society

The water cure as a popular health system offered a consensual ideology that posited a harmonious universal vision. Informed by a millennial ideal of human perfectability, and consequent societal uplifting, hydropathy championed personal and social advancement through health. It instilled hope, provided a moral base, offered internal logic radiating from a central truth, and proffered inclusive answers for all of life's uncertainties.[1] Yet, amid this communal context, hydropathy offered autonomy and individuation. It appealed, therefore, not only to strains of individualism and personal advancement in American thought but also to gender-specific and culturally valued communal bonds, responsibility to others, and continuity in relationships; it offered a group context in which personal improvement could serve as a model for societal reformation.

17

As a medical system, hydropathy utilized basic psychosocial factors critical to the healing process. It mobilized the patient's natural healing powers, aroused hope and expectancy of cure, and reinforced ties with the social group and the cultural world view. It also placed primary importance on the healer–patient encounter for providing hope, relief of symptoms, communication, and therapeutic touch while instilling faith and trust.[2]

The water cure as a system and as a world view promoted a sense of meaning, ordering, power, and control. It provided autonomy without anarchy; personal improvement could be achieved without sacrificing the common good. As posited in the early mastheads of the *Journal*, one need only "Wash and Be Healed."[3] In fact, one of hydropathy's unique contributions among the sects was that it offered a vision of a good life unencumbered by theoretical uncertainty and provided the entire context in which to live it.

The hydropathic theory and management of human (particularly women's) physiology was the means through which personal change would inspire societal reformation. Since hydropaths refused to classify women as physically and intellectually hampered by their physiology, the redefinition of women's social role became a primary concern. By soliciting a female readership, rethinking the treatment of female diseases, urging women's active participation in home health care, and actively supporting the inclusion of female physicians, the water-cure movement appealed to women as the primary caretakers of others[4] and fostered an extension of woman's sphere of influence from the domestic into the informally political realm. Further, it evinced a feminist ideology (termed "emancipationist" in the literature) that stressed woman's right to increased choices, opportunities, and rewards, and her resultant obligation to care for her own and others' health.

Water as the Great Curative

Water, which has been used as a curative agent for thousands of years, was the medium charged with bringing about this cultural rebirth. Symbolically, water possesses potent powers. As a cleansing agent, its universality and value are unparalleled, not only as a remover of soil but also as a metaphoric purifier of souls. The religious and mystical significance of water can be seen in its use in Christian baptism, the Jewish *mikveh*, and the transferring out of bad spirits from an ailing person in folk healing. Water is also the primary life-giving substance on earth. Its necessity for human, animal, and vegetative survival prompted Native American cultures to worship gods imbued with the power to deliver it.[5] (Its power to destroy is equally undeniable: Floods, tides, and drownings have taxed human understanding and control.) When used topically, water is a soothing, cooling, relaxing, and stimulating agent; and it is employed in life-cycle rituals as diverse as birth, religious initiation, fertility, trials of adulthood, spiritual awakenings, sickness, death, and mourning.

The water cure, as it was popularized in the United States, directly utilized several key components of water's symbolic nature. Water's ability to cleanse, purify, facilitate the transfer of putrid matter, give renewed life, soothe, cool, relax, and stimulate were all articulated by hydropaths. The more nebulous qualities associated with water added an otherworldliness to the procedures, a sense that powers beyond human understanding were at work during a water cure. For while hydropaths did not lay claim to direct spiritual advancement or cosmic insight for their followers, neither did they disavow the unidentifiable attributes of healing with water. If symbolic and mystical powers accrued while taking the cure, no attempt was made to disassociate from them. This may account, in part, for the often mystical and pseudoreligious portrayal of water evidenced in the writings of hydropathic leaders and followers.

A History of Water Cures

Until the eighteenth century the curative power of water was thought to lie primarily in its minerals, its heat, or its mystical properties. American Indians, for example, used water in religious rituals long before it was thought to have hygienic properties. Numerous European and American explorers, among them Amerigo Vespucci (1497), William Penn (1683), Meriwether Lewis and William Clark (early nineteenth century), and the artist and ethnologist George Catlin (1841), noted the Indians' bathhouses and mud lodges and their use of sweating and plunging into cold baths.[6]

In Europe, "taking the cure" involved healing waters but included many other variations. It could be a "quest for healing waters; hot water, cold water, mineral waters, stinking waters or holy water. It was sometimes a quest for healing muds or gases."[7]

In these earliest sojourns for health, the cure was not ascribed "to the action of water itself, but to magic properties in it or to supernatural influences shed by nymphs and water gods. Hence well worship, as practiced in ancient Babylon and modern Derbyshire. Priests and oracles set themselves up beside springs or escapes of natural gases."[8] This emphasis on magic and faith healing shifted over the centuries to one of physical treatment. But not until the eighteenth century did the water cure experience a large-scale revival. Prompted by the increased popularity of European spas, medical observers began writing tracts that criticized both the medicinal value of mineral water and the nonhygienic practices that abounded at Europe's watering places. These critiques produced a spate of writing on the curative powers of cold water, or hydropathy.

John Floyer, an English physician, wrote *Psychrolusia, or History of Cold-Bathing*, which triggered the turn toward cold water. The tract appeared in London in 1702 and had gone through five editions by 1722.

In his works, which were reprinted in German and Latin, he discussed the subject historically and recounted illnesses cured with water.[9] Floyer's work was followed by American editions of John Smith's publications, *The Curiosities of Common Water* (1723) and *The Curiosities of Common Water, or the Advantages Thereof in Preventing Cholera* (1725).[10]

Floyer's and Smith's theses were followed by Tobias Smollett's *An Essay on the External Use of Water* (1752) in which he claimed:

> I can easily conceive how extraordinary cures may be performed by the mechanical effects of simple WATER upon the human Body; and I fully believe that in the use of BATHING and PUMPING, that Efficacy is often ascribed to the MINERAL PARTICLES, which properly belongs to the ELEMENT itself, exclusive of any foreign substance.[11]

Smollett also detailed the bad conditions existing at the baths in Bath, England, including their use by diseased persons, lack of protection from natural elements, shortage of attendants, lack of sex segregation, and inadequate dressing facilities.[12]

Floyer's, Smith's, and Smollett's path-breaking works were complemented by John Wesley's *Primitive Physic, or an Easy and Natural Method of Curing Most Diseases* (1747), which claimed that cold water, if skillfully administered, could cure nearly every disease. Similarly, James Currie's *Medical Reports on the Effects of Water, Cold and Warm, as a Remedy in Fever and Febrile Diseases* (1797) urged the exclusive use of cold water. Currie, the first to chronicle precisely the effects of cold bathing, recorded and followed the body's temperature in treating fever.[13] These medical texts and therapeutic innovations led many practitioners to adopt the use of cold water.

In the United States, Dr. Benjamin Rush of Philadelphia also recognized and advocated the use of cold bathing.[14] Its effect, he said, was "to wash off impurities from the skin, promote perspiration, drive the fluids from the surface to the internal parts of the body, brace the animal fibres, stimulate the nervous system, and prevent the 'diseases of warm weather.'"[15] Like Rush, John Bell, in *On Baths and Mineral Waters* (1831), discussed "the various bath forms [and] their effects and applications in cold, warm, hot and vapor baths."[16]

Despite this increased attention to the use of cold water and the notable improvements following its use, cold water as a therapeutic procedure was little utilized until Vincent Priessnitz advocated its use. As one historian has noted, "Others had used water as a method of treatment, Priessnitz made it a panacea."[17] Priessnitz, born in 1799 on a small farm in Silesia, first experimented with water as a curative agent after he sprained his wrist, holding it under the pump and wrapping it in cold bandages until the swelling went down. Later, he cured his father's feverish cow with water applications. But his "conversion" to cold water (a similar "personal revelation" would become a significant rite of passage for many hydropathic followers) occurred when his ribs were crushed in a wagon accident, and he was pronounced incurable. Refusing to accept this diagnosis, Priessnitz applied wet bandages and replaced his broken ribs by pressing his abdomen with great force against a chair and holding his breath to swell his chest. He ate little, remained quiet, was mobile in ten days, and was working in the fields within a year.[18]

Word of Priessnitz's successes spread, and his services gained popularity among his Silesian countrymen. He was the first to systematize the wetting and sweating procedures long advocated by Floyer, Smith, Wesley, Currie, and Smollett. His most significant therapeutic innovation was the wet sheet, which covered the entire body and was utilized when disease was not localized. He promoted the use of specific "baths" when the ailment was localized (head, eye, leg, and foot baths); to these regimens he added the douche, which entailed wet packing to induce perspiration, then sponging, then a plunge bath.[19]

Francis Graeter, one of Priessnitz's faithful chroniclers, wrote of his less-schooled mentor, who was not inclined to record his activities, that he believed water was the univeral nostrum, and thus he posited his theory of cure:

> All diseases, such only excepted as are produced by external lesions from foreign bodies, originate in bad humors, from which result either a general distemper, or maladies of single parts. Hence his whole method has for its aim to remove the bad [humors] out of the body, and to replace them by good ones. The means ... by which he employs for this purpose are, *Water, Air, Exercise and Diet*.[20]

In 1826 Priessnitz opened Grafenberg, affectionately called the "Water University," in the mountains of Silesia. Because the waters used at Grafenberg had no chemical distinction, his cure was not a spa. He called it a cold-water cure but did not use the term *hydropathy*. Priessnitz met with immediate success. Retrospectively, his success stemmed from removing patients from the stresses and excesses that had often induced their illnesses, providing a pleasant communal setting, implementing diet and exercise regimens that strengthened the body, ceasing heroic therapeutics, letting nature help right what was reversible, involving patients in their own cure through habit reformation, and applying the mystical healing powers attributed to Priessnitz personally.

Grafenberg opened with forty-nine patients, but by 1840 fifteen hundred to seventeen hundred people sought help each year. The guest list in 1839 included "one royal highness, one duke, one duchess, 22 princes and princesses, 149 counts and countesses, 88 barons and baronesses, 14 generals, 53 staff officers, 196 captains and subalterns, 104 high and low civil servants, 65 divines, 46 artists, and 87 physicians and apothecaries."[21] These illustrious patients' places of origin were equally varied: "In 1840 Prussia supplied over 500, Austria over 350, Russia about 100, and Hungary and Poland each over one hundred."[22] One patient was Elizabeth Blackwell, the first woman to graduate from an American allopathic (regular) medical school, who went to Grafenberg in 1850 after contracting opthalmia in 1849. Although her general health was strengthened through diet and exercise, her eye was very badly inflamed, and in June 1850 it was removed.[23]

In addition to the therapeutic innovations at Grafenberg, strictures on diet and habits were adopted. The food was coarse, heavy, and always cold, and no spices were allowed to those with bad stomachs. Patients were advised to drink twenty to thirty glasses of water daily to induce internal cleaning; water was the only permissible beverage. They were urged to exercise, behave temperately, and avoid flannel and cotton, since, it was claimed, those materials made people delicate and weakened the skin. No medicines were allowed, nor was reading, writing, or other intellectual effort. Similarly taboo were gambling and "immoral excitement."[24]

These demands to change personal habits are understandable when one considers the large percentage of Priessnitz's patients who suffered from overexposure to mercury ingested under allopathic instruction (half of his clientele) and liver and stomach disorders caused by dietary and alcoholic excesses. For these patients, Priessnitz counseled:

> The first means of strengthening a weakened stomach is to avoid all the causes that have contributed towards destroying its tone. Live temperately and simply. . . . At the same time you ought to wear constantly cold fomentations round your abdomen and the stomach; early in the morning you ought to sweat moderately, and after this take a cold bath; in the evening a seat-bath, constantly rubbing during both the latter, the afflicted parts with cold water. In drinking cold water, avoid excess. . . . Frequent exercise is to be added.[25]

Whether Priessnitz understood the mechanisms of his success is a matter for speculation. It could be simply fortuitous that he cured patients essentially by keeping them away from the rigors of heroic treatment and allowing the human body to heal itself. This is not to argue that Priessnitz did nothing. Like the water curers who modeled themselves after him, Priessnitz placed great importance on the medical encounter, on communication, and on touch. Given that Priessnitz treated seven thousand patients between 1831 and 1841, the thirty-eight deaths that occurred at Grafenberg stand as a credible record, although he rejected some prospective patients and others very likely left of their own choice. Despite this percentage, Priessnitz was haunted by his critics. Between

1821 and 1828, three neighboring physicians in the village of Friewaldau had him brought before the legal authorities to answer charges of unlawful practice of medicine. His acquittal (because he used only water, not medicine) brought him even greater fame.[26] Perhaps Priessnitz's strongest critic was Dr. Robert May Graham, who wrote *Graefenberg; or, a True Report of the Water-Cure, with an Account of Its Antiquity* (1844). Graham found the environment distasteful and the therapeutics too severe. As he pointed out, Priessnitz did not "discover" the water cure, but he advocated its use at a time when his contemporaries were receptive to it. In fact, water had been used in England before it was employed in Germany, and a Dr. John Sigmund Hahn, in a town near Grafenberg, used and wrote about the water cure before Priessnitz did. Hahn's *Observations on the Healing Virtue of Cold Water, Internally and Outwardly Applied as Proved by Experience* came out originally in 1739 and was reprinted as late as 1804.[27]

Priessnitz, as he was characterized in 1865, did *not* offer a demonstrable theory of the healing art or any philosophy of medical science. What he did originate was a collection of "certain facts which he embodied into a principle and made the basis of a new method for treating disease. [Untrained by regular medicine] he derived . . . the rules of his Healing Art from his own observations and experience."[28]

R. T. Claridge, writing in 1842 during his own stay as a recovering invalid, noted that Priessnitz did not detect disease in regular ways (e.g., by checking the pulse, looking at the tongue, or inquiring about the condition of his patients). His theory, which informed American hydropaths for decades to come, held the following: Health was a natural condition and disease an unnatural one. The body, let alone, would heal disease produced by external injuries except broken bones and needed surgery and invading foreign elements. Applications of water, by disrupting the foreign matter, stimulated a chronic condition to develop into an acute disease. All disease, theoretically, was acute, and manifested the body's desire to expel it through eruptions. This "crisis" took varying lengths of time to accomplish and yielded visible results such as boils, rashes, diarrhea, sores, sweating, and eruptions, which were indicative of the healing process. Regular therapeutics (drugging and bleeding) worsened all acute sickness, leading to the eventual ruin of the body's systems. Fever, although produced by the aforementioned diseased states, was not a disease in and of itself. Water was the one universal remedy that effectively dissolved the diseased matter and aided a sufficiently strong body in curing disease. The skin was the route through which disease would leave the body. Thus, applications of water, wraps, sweating, and applying pressure and friction cleansed and opened the pores, aided circulation, invigorated the skin, and drew the putrid matter out of the body.[29]

Claridge chronicled his accounts in case-study format and substantiated his voluminous observations with corroboration from other witnesses,[30] thus commencing a tradition of oral and written testimony to the efficacy of the system.

Like Claridge, Dr. John King, a regularly educated British physician and a sufferer from chronic rheumatism, resided at Grafenberg, was cured, and charted the recoveries of others. King noted with particular interest the improvement of people pronounced incurable by medicine.[31] Another contemporary devotee of Priessnitz's, John Gibbs, added his approving thoughts in his *Letters from Graefenberg, in the Years 1843, 1844, 1845, 1846*. Gibbs, an Irishman, recounted Priessnitz's ability to evaluate a body's health by the condition of the skin. In fact, Priessnitz's reputed ability to look into the body and see the disease—a talent not denied by him—added to the mystery and lure of the cure.[32]

Hydropathy Comes to America

Priessnitz's theories and practices were introduced in the United States in the 1840s, although American medical journals, familiar with his claims and following, had published accounts of his therapeutics for a decade. The tone of the medical authors was at times critical, as repeated attacks in the *Medical News* demonstrate. These and other articles pointed out dangers and shortcomings of the system.[33]

Much early *popular* response in the press was more positive, even evangelical; it was also accessible to average people. An excerpt from the *New York Observer*, in 1847 is demonstrative: "We have great confidence in the virtues of cold water, and we believe that the substitution thereof for stimulating drinks, together with pure air and regular exercise, has restored health to many invalids."[34] The editors of the newspaper concluded by promising that they would recommend the water cure to patients who consulted them, and they challenged critics to prove their charges. Not all popular responses were as positive, though, as a satire in the *Knickerbocker*, a monthly New York magazine, revealed.[35] Received with great enthusiasm in some quarters, despite condemnatory prose from others, hydropathy had, according to one historian of the movement, "soon gained an equal position among the other panaceas promising better health."[36]

Despite hydropathy's critics, mid-nineteenth-century America was hospitable ground for its philosophy and emphasis on self-care. By 1843–1844, Joel Shew and R. T. Trall, two of the founders of the hydropathic movement in America, had opened a water-cure establishment, based on many of Priessnitz's principles, in New York City. Shew, characterized by some as blessed with common sense but not with a philosophical mind, was a tireless health reformer who owned and operated numerous cures and was a consistent influence in the early years of the *Water-Cure Journal*. Shew, writing in *Hydropathy, Or, the Water-Cure* (1845), relied on cases observed at Grafenberg. To this he added theories on the significance of the water cure within the history of medicine. He asserted that among all theories of medicine, "the water-cure is the most natural and best system."[37]

Trall, Shew's colleague, is credited by some with developing hydropathy into a comprehensive healing philosophy, which he and his followers called the Philosophy of Medical Science and the system of Hygienic Medication. He based his theory of medical science and the healing art on the laws of nature; he explained the nature of disease, the effects of remedies, the doctrine of vitality, the purpose of hygienic medication, and the law or conditions of cure: He made the hygienic system, with water as the central element, a "universal application."[38]

American popularizers of hydropathy retained much of Priessnitz's theory and application, but, as demonstrated in Trall's *The Illustrated Hydropathic Encyclopedia* (1871) [revised from his *Hydropathic Encyclopedia . . . of* 1850], they integrated far more comprehensive information on anatomy, physiology, dietetics, surgical techniques, and the application of hydropathy to midwifery and the nursery. The properties now attributed to water as a curative included being the only substance able to carry nutrient matters to the blood, the only solvent of excrementitious matter, and the only material that circulates and penetrates all tissues of the body. Thus, water was ever present in the healthy organism, since the bulk of the body, including the brain, the blood, and colorless fluids and secretions, were water based.[39]

A diseased body, according to Trall, was suffering from impure blood, unhealthy secretions, vascular or capillary obstructions, unequal temperature, and/or excessive action (or deficient action) in some part of the organs. In other words, there was a loss of balance "in the circulation and action of the various parts of the vital machinery, producing great discord in some portion of it, and more or less disorder in all." The goal of American hydropathy, therefore, was to remove obstructions, dissolve and wash away impurities, supply nutriments, regulate temperature, and relax intensive action or intensify torpid action. All of this was to be done with water—and its supporting forces of air, light, food, and temperature.[40]

In February 1847 twenty-one cures were open in eight states; in 1848–1849 there were thirty water cures in nine states; and by November 1844 the *Water-Cure Journal* began publication, with Shew as editor and David Campbell (former publisher of the *Graham Journal*) as one of the proprietors.[41]

The *Water-Cure Journal* served as the primary source of information for the movement from its inception in 1844 through its last issue (under a different name) in 1913. It gained a healthy subscription under the management of the Fowlers and Wells publishing house in New York City (beginning April 1848), which was run by three staunch supporters of the movement, Orson Squire Fowler and Lorenzo N. Fowler and S. R.

Wells. The Fowlers are discussed in the Introduction and in Chapter Four. In 1849 Wells became the secretary of the short-lived American Hydropathic Society, also in New York, and by 1865 he was the sole editor of the *Phrenological Journal* and sole proprietor of the (formerly) Fowlers and Wells publishing house. He was not a prolific author but an astute businessman committed to the circulation of "good books for all."[42]

The journal's original cost was one dollar per year, with the subscriber receiving two issues a month. The journal's editors self-consciously charted their expansion and growing popularity and reported the number of subscribers as twenty-five thousand in June 1851, fifty thousand in December 1852, and a projected one hundred thousand by late 1860, totaling, they claimed, over a million readers.[43] The accuracy of the first two claims is fairly certain;[44] the projected figures are difficult to verify. But since the journal was the primary education and communication tool of the movement, these early claims are within reason—allowing for some self-congratulatory exaggeration. The editors claimed, plausibly enough, that every issue sold was "read" by ten people—this can be loosely translated to mean that in a household with several children, the mother and/or father read the journal and governed the family hydropathically. Similarly, lending the journal to friends and neighbors, giving it as a gift, receiving it free for securing a certain number of paid subscriptions, and receiving it as a charitable offering were all exhorted. As the front page of the July 1864 issue implored: "Every *Herald* we can circulate accelerates the time of this consummation [the total adoption of the Hygienic Medical System]. . . . Every person who sends us a name secures us a co-worker. Need we present any other consideration than this to induce our friends to send us ONE HUNDRED THOUSAND SUBSCRIBERS?"[45]

Hydropathy did not have "field agents," although each individual committed to the movement was exhorted to bring in new believers. Sharing the journal, and prostelytizing for it, was a common form of inducting converts into the fold, and to speed this task prizes were offered for securing new subscriptions.[46] Finally, correspondence in the journal reveals just what a critical role that publication played both in educating home self-doctorers and in maintaining the commitment of those who had frequented the cures first and later *became* self-doctorers. The movement prospered by word of mouth and written testimonials, and the journal was the central organ for fostering those processes. Its ongoing concerns included articles on the history of water-cure techniques, the successes of the cure, and the ever-expanding list of new water-cure physicians and their facilities.

The journal underwent a number of name changes, each of which reflected a shift in emphasis and priorities by the movement's leadership. Originally known as the *Water-Cure Journal,* the publication adopted the title *Water-Cure Journal and Herald of Reforms* in 1847. This gave way in 1862–1863 to *The Hygienic Teacher and Water-Cure Journal,* which lasted only until the title *Herald of Health* came into use from 1863 to 1865. This in turn was followed by *Herald of Health and Journal of Physical Culture,* which remained with the publication from 1865 to 1892. *Journal of Hygiene and Herald of Health* reigned from 1893 to 1897, and the final, cryptic title that ruled the publication until its demise in 1913 was, simply, *Health.*[47]

Despite the frequent changes, the journal enjoyed a relatively stable series of owners and editors. Campbell and Whitemarsh were proprietors of the original 1844 series; Fowlers and Wells was the publishing house from 1845 through March 1864; and during April through June of that last year R. T. Trall & Co. served as publishers. In July 1864 Miller and Browning became the publishers, and in November Miller and Wood assumed the helm until at least 1867.[48] These publishers had in common a belief in the hydropathic system and a commitment to societal reformation through hygienic living. The journal told little else of them, for they assumed their duties with essentially no editoral introduction. The editorship, meanwhile, traveled from Shew (accompanied briefly by F. D. Pierson) to Trall to M. L. Holbrook. It becomes increasingly difficult to trace the editorship and is not specifically mentioned in all instances.[49]

In the pages of the journal, American pioneers in hydropathy were ever-mindful of their debt to Priessnitz. In an 1865 article it was written of the Silesian peasant:

Vincent Priessnitz may be called the father of the Hydropathic system of treating disease, in the same sense that Hippocrates is regarded as the father of the Allopathic system, and Hahnemann the author of the Homeopathic system. That he possessed wonderful sagacity, a remarkable perceptive intellect, and sterling honesty, is conceded on all hands.[50]

In fact, Priessnitz's European hydropathic experience prophetically anticipated several patterns that were to be relived in the American movement. These included medicinal simplicity, major reforms in diet and personal habits, personal "conversion" experiences or a brush with death (which often precipitated adherence to hydropathic principles), and the ridicule of more established medical authorities. Even the death of Priessnitz at age fifty-two (considered premature by his contemporaries) from "dropsy of the chest"[51] had an American parallel in the early death of Joel Shew. The former's cardiac arrest was probably a result of overwork or congenital weakness; the latter's a result of exposure to toxic chemicals. Neither hydropath was cured by his system, thus potentially discrediting it.

Hydropathy and the Spas

Both Priessnitz's European water cure and its American descendant gained in popularity in an era characterized by ambivalence toward allopathic therapeutics and sympathy with the use of mineral springs. Although the popularity of spas[52] eased the way for American acceptance of the cold-water cure, the principles behind the two uses of water could not have been more different. To the emerging cold-water curers, spas represented the playground for exactly the life style they were so eager to eradicate. Demanding very little from the patient, spas promised cures through the properties of the water itself, not through the elements Priessnitz (and later Shew, Trall, and others) found so critical: water, air, exercise, and diet. As one chronicler of American spas observed:

> Touring the spas had become more a social than a therapeutic episode. . . . Significantly, for most of the travelers, the waters were only a pretext. What attracted them were not precisely medical problems, but the company of others, the multicolored world of a social life with promenades, clubs, cotillion, mask and other balls; races, hunting, sketching and later photographing; courting, serenades, romance, faro, price euchres, champagne suppers, and the marriage market. Health and water, the excuse of all, had importance for only a few.[53]

Hydropathic opposition to the spas focused not only on their social and culinary aspects but on the medicinal side as well. Classifying spas' mineral properties as drugs, the *Herald of Health* left little doubt as to their efficacy:

> The people have been so miseducated that they regard poison and medicine as synonymous terms, and imagine that, if any pool or stream can be found whose waters are so adulterated or impregnated with earthy, alkaline, saline or mineral ingredients that they are not fit to drink . . . it must of necessity be a grand article to swallow for medicial purposes. There was never a more irrational and absurd practice invented than that of running after sulphur, iodine, iron, and other drugged water for health purposes.[54]

In case the readers found that response lacking in verve, they could refer to Dr. A. L. Wood's column in 1866, two years later, which likened the drinking of mineral water to ingesting strychnine.[55]

American cold-water cures disdained the life style they associated with mineral springs because it emphasized indulgence and frivolity in lieu of restraint and commitment. Believers in the water-cure system, like other nineteenth-century healers, were searching to check the spread of contagious disease (they were not ahead of their contemporaries with scientific knowledge on this score, although hygienic living did help fore-stall the conditions most conducive to the spread of contagious disease), infant and maternal mortality, and nervous debility. To this end they embraced the harsher of the two water systems, hoping to find in its tenets solutions to national health concerns. Further, their system effec-tively embodied the American attraction for self-determination through self-doctoring, as well as the belief in moral commitment, medical and social purity and simplicity, and the hope of perfectibility for humanity through health reform.

American Hydropathy

Transplanted from its European origins, the cold-water cure—while it had several salient features in common with other reform sects—represented a unique voice in nineteenth-century America healing systems. Its distinc-tive characteristics were its emphasis on water as the primary curative agent, its abandonment of all drug medication, its extreme emphasis on the necessity for hygienic habit reformation and self-reliance, its social context, and its philosophy, which stressed a comprehensive approach to disease management that left no aspect of life unregulated.[56]

The differences and similarities between hydropathic and allopathic systems for management of disease are evident in several areas. Hydropaths sought to aid nature in its fight against disease, but they did not assume a passive posture as healers. Like allopathic therapeutics, water treatments constituted active intervention. Hydropaths used less-harsh *agents*, their prolonged attendance served to hearten or cheer the patient, and the treatment was more pleasant; allopaths employed drug medication to counterattack the disease, often inducing discomfort. As a result, hydrop-athy relieved suffering and offered comfort while striving to cure disease, whereas many contemporaries believed that allopathic therapeutics them-selves induced suffering and contributed to patients' fear.[57] But both sects operated out of a common ethos: Aid nature by restoring the natural balance of the elements. Hydropaths pursued this goal with water therapies and habit reformation; allopaths sought a cure through evacuative therapeutics and drugging aimed at depleting elements "out of balance." As subsequent chapters show, these therapeutic differences were par-ticularly notable in the management of women's diseases.

In addition to presenting an alternative to the allopathic sect, hydropathy offered a new concept of healthful living to those who had been patients of other sects. Based on an all-encompassing philosophy of health care, American hydropathic authors borrowed from Priessnitz and informed their writings with the principles espoused in early texts such as *The Water-Cure in Chronic Diseases* by Dr. James Manby Gully (1846). Texts arising out of this heritage that greatly influenced the new hydropathic practitioners included Shew's *Water-Cure Manual* (1847), Trall's *The*

Hydropathic Encyclopedia, a System of Hydropathy and Hygiene (1851), and *The Water-Cure in America: Two Hundred and Twenty Cases of Various Diseases Treated with Water, by Drs. Wesselhoeft, Shew, Bedortha, Schieferdecker, and Others, etc.*, edited by a water patient in 1848.[58]

The philosophy of health care taught to physicians through the hydropathic texts found a popular voice in James Caleb Jackson's article in the December 1847 issue of the *Water-Cure Journal*. Jackson (an active health reformer for several decades and water-cure physician at, first, the Glen Haven Water Cure and, later, the Dansville, New York, Water Cure) articulated the philosophy of the water cure as containing the following elements: a cessation of drugging, with water as the primary curative agent; therapeutics in the hands of a skillful physician; good nursing for patients; consumption of simple food only; fresh air, exercise, and freedom from high excitements; and, finally, pleasant associations and cheerful companions.[59]

Healthful living as prescribed by the hydropathic leadership could be attained through home self-doctoring or at a live-in cure establishment. Thus, two kinds of hydropathy, domestic and physicians', are discussed intermittently throughout hydropathic literature. As Shew acknowledged in his *Hydropathic Family Physician*, most people could not go to an establishment, and since it was the duty of water-cure physicians to teach the prevention of disease, there needed to be a reciprocity between the two water cures. His text, a manual for self-doctoring, demonstrates this dual approach with a lengthy section on "The Formation and Management of Water-Cure Establishments."[60]

Thus, Jackson's and Shew's advocacy of skillful doctoring and good nursing suggests a commitment to expert opinion, a kind of professional ideology, and an unself-conscious reliance on the medical encounter within a curing establishment or a physician–patient dyad. Invoking the truism that patients came to hydropaths seeking relief from discomfort and dysfunction, as one scholar of healing systems noted, like most satisfied patients, "They found what they sought and they honored the provider." The social dynamics of the medical encounter no doubt contributed significantly to the symptomatic relief, since, as this scholarly interpretation continues, "This bonus to medicine as craft . . . has been a plague to medicine as science. [Too often] the benefits patients obtained have been attributed to the procedures in fashion rather than the social dynamics of the medical encounter."[61] Hydropaths used contact, touch, attention, listening, faith, and trust as part of the healing process. This helps considerably in explaining the efficacy of water cure. In fact, "There is little doubt that much of the therapeutic success of the healing profession of the medicine man, and of the priest, as well as the modern practitioner, has been due to the undefined emotional rapport between physician and patient."[62] When considering the efficacy of these healing encounters, therefore, one cannot ignore the possibility that "many of these cases of healing have emotional rather than physiological etiologies. In such cases, even fraudulent healers could heal, in much the same way that placebos alleviate symptoms."[63] Similarly, other observers of "nonquantifiable" healing have noted that whether health is gained through manipulation (physical cure) or the attached suggestion (psychodynamics between healer and patient) is, essentially, irrelevant. What is important is that efficacy exists as a result of some combination of the two.[64] For those who doctored at home, different factors contributed to the water-cure's efficacy, and these are discussed shortly.

While it is difficult to specify the linkage, it is likely that hydropathy's efficacy benefited from the credibility given in late-nineteenth-century America to the faith cure, which legitimized the possibility of healings, or being healed, by faith.[65] Believers promoted, with scriptural backing, a concept of religious salvation that included health as an integral part of it. Similarly, the fairly widespread employment of "professional" spiritualist mediums also signified a willingness on the part of a significant number of Americans to believe in mystical channels of communication and non-quantifiable, yet tangible, results.[66] The popular credibility both of these practices achieved revealed an acceptance of mystical happenings, particularly as they affect health and illness. This belief in divine inspiration and interference, and the power attributed to the healer or medium to achieve spiritual and physical perfection, could only have benefited hydropathy, which, relying on the "mystical" powers of the healer–patient dyad and water, preached physical and moral "salvation" through hygienic living.

In 1853 Trall addressed himself to the matter of "clairvoyance" in healing. Asked in his "Professional Matters" column in the journal if the claims of two traveling clairvoyants that they could prescribe for diseases and locate precious metals were reasonable, Trall responded, "Our advice is, most decidedly, that the clairvoyants are humbugs." But he qualified his denouncement: "But that there is such a thing as clairvoyance, we have no manner of doubt. It is, however, sometimes difficult to distinguish the genuine article from a spurious imitation; and the application of the very best quality to the healing of diseases, and the discovery of gold mines, is exceedingly limited."[67] Effectively, Trall acknowledged clairvoyance, classed it as a gift, and deemed it a possible healing aid, although a rare commodity.

Philosophy

Yet, despite hydropathy's reliance on charismatic and expert healers and on mystical properties (i.e., unexplainable healing powers), its *articulated philosophy* was one of eventual patient autonomy that could be achieved through home self-doctoring. This paradoxical message yielded conflicting and fascinating results.

Water-cure philosophy was all encompassing and began, understandably, with an explanation of the cause of disease. According to hydropaths, disease stemmed from two sources. The first consisted "in a lack of nervous energy, or the presence of morbid matter in the system, or both combined. . . . The primary cause of disease is a hereditary lack of vitality either in the germ, the sperm, or in the combination of both."[68] Contrary to the teachings of other sects, hydropaths believed that disease was never a *positive entity* but always a *negative quality;* it was the absence of health. Therefore, the second cause of disease (although it was not a separate issue from the first) was a violation of hygienic laws. As Trall explained in the *Hydropathic Encyclopedia:* "In a general sense, diseases are produced by bad air, improper light, impure food and drink, excessive or defective alimentation, indolence or over-exertion, unregulated passions, in three words—unphysiological voluntary habits."[69]

Thus an 1856 article in the journal, "Water-Cure Catechism," delineated the ABCs of the water cure once again. In addition to those facets mentioned by Jackson nine years earlier, the author stated that diseases were cured by hygienic agencies, which include "light, air, food, water, temperature, clothing, exercise and passional influence."[70] This emphasis on "unphysiological voluntary habits" marked a more finely honed interpretation of the cause of disease, beyond Priessnitz's humoral theory. The lack of nervous energy, theorists pointed out, could be cured by hygienic living habits. Implicit in this idea was that patients must take responsibility for their own health. As Mrs. M. L. Shew, an author and the wife of Joel Shew, wrote in 1844:

> The writer believes in "temperance in all things." To understand how to be thus temperate, requires an amount of physiological knowledge possessed by few. . . . To do this people must learn to *think for themselves.* . . . By far too much, we have been in the habit of trusting our health to keepers whose profession and interest are not always most favorable. Physicians are employed to *cure,* not to *prevent* disease. . . . The writer, has seen, and *experienced,* too, the wonderful effects of water. Water-Cure is truly "a new world in the healing art." . . . Here is a difference between water-cure and drug systems—a most important one. Water-Cure rightly administered is *always safe and will do good.* Not so with poison drugs.[71]

These basic principles warrant reiteration: Hydropathy emphasized prevention through hygienic principles, moderation in living habits, an informed clientele, a deemphasis of the physician–patient relationship (in home self-doctoring; away-from-home cures operated more complexly), and drugless therapy. In direct contrast, the university-trained allopathic physician brought to the physician–patient relationship an aura of educa-

tionally derived omnipotence, harbored information with no philosophical obligation to explain and elaborate diagnosis and treatment, relied on
patient passivity (i.e., "receptivity"), and used a therapeutic dynamic that
did not encourage patient instrumentality. Water-cure philosophy, conversely, promoted the demystification of physiological processes and the
physician–patient relationship when discussing drugless treatment, home
health care, and patient responsibility.

Clearly, the principles of hygienic living were intended to usurp the
need for the drug and evacuative therapies, as well as to avoid the illness
and discomfort that resulted from allopathic therapeutics. Jackson, writing in *How to Treat the Sick Without Medicine* (1874), discredited drugging as unnatural and iatrogenic while heralding hygienic principles and
water as curative agents:

> There are two ways of treating human invalids; the one by means
> which are abnormal or unnatural, . . . [which], when used by per-
> sons in health,make them sick or *tend* to make them sick; the other,
> by means which are normal or natural . . . whose effect on the human
> body, in health, is to keep it in health. The former way I discard;
> the latter way I accept and follow.[72]

Jackson claimed he had never given a dose of medicine. Emphasizing
the standard hygienic principles, he wrote:

> I have used, in the treatment of the diseases of my patients, the
> following substances or instrumentalities: First, air; second, food;
> third, water; fourth, sunlight; fifth, dress; sixth, exercise; seventh,
> sleep; eighth, rest; ninth, social influences; tenth, mental and moral
> influences.[73]

Significantly, Jackson lists water as a curative agent third, thus revealing
his own ordering of priorities within the consensual system. Like Jackson,
Trall emphasized the total *in*compatability of hydropathy and drug
medications: "The person, be he layman or physician, who says that he
believes a great deal in Hygeio-Therapy, and yet believes that a little
medicine is necessary sometimes, is perfectly and profoundly ignorant of
the philosophy, the rationale, and even the fundamental premises of
hygienic medication."[74]

The *Water-Cure Journal* seized every available opportunity to reveal
the horrid nature and results of dramatic therapeutics and drug therapy.
In the January 1847 issue, the editors (at that time Shew and Dr. F. D.
Pierson) reprinted an article from the *London Lancet* entitled "Hemorrhage from Leech-Bites." In the article the attending physician, E. Gervis,
is called on to stop the hemorrhaging from a leech bite that cut through
the jugular vein of a woman being treated for an attack of cynanche

tonsillaris. Gervis applies lint and then alum to stop the bleeding. In another case of hemorrhage from leech bites, Gervis suggested that lint dipped in spirits of turpentine or smoking tobacco be used.[75] The hydropathic abhorrence of the use of leeches was highlighted three years later in a *Water-Cure Journal* article entitled "Swallowed a Leech." In this case, a leech was applied to the inside of each nostril of a man suffering from a head cold. One leech made its way up the nose and down the throat. Since it could not be dislodged, the man swallowed it. Numerous doctors came to his aid, one recommending the lancet and another suggesting that the patient swallow another leech. Finally it was decided he should receive emetics. Thus, ipecac, copper, zinc, and tartar emetic were used, vomiting was induced, but the leech never surfaced. It took the young man several weeks to be able to crawl about after his ordeal.[76]

In addition to rejecting the use of leeches, hydropaths disdained the practices of bleeding, blistering, cupping, and purging. In a tale of dismay, A.E.H. from Mississippi told of his treatment at the hands of allopaths for a "nervous sick headache, with constipation," from which he suffered for twenty-two years.[77] This man's problems were solved when he adopted water-cure principles and began to spread the teachings himself. In a similar article in 1851, Dr. E. Potter, in "Isn't It Murder?" recalled the case of a two-year-old child given calomel for dysentery. Shortly thereafter, the baby died.[78] In what becomes recognizable as the typical impassioned editorializing style of the *Water-Cure Journal*, Potter asked: "Oh! when shall these things cease to be? When will parents learn that poison is not MEDICINE? When will physicians act consistently, and give innocent remedies, or none—assisting nature when necessary, or do nothing?"[79]

Not all of the *Water-Cure Journal's* antiallopathic sentiments were directed at specific cases gone awry. Some were simply poems, witticisms, or anecdotes that emphasized the author's perception of the brutality of allopathic therapeutics and the sensible, natural alternative available in hydropathy. But regardless of the medium, these pieces all bore the same message: Allopathy was a dangerous and debilitating system that drained the body of its energy and promoted drug use and patient weakness. By using first-person accounts and the "conversion experiences" of former allopathic physicians who had embraced the water cure, hydropathic authors portrayed a grim and frightening portrait of allopathic medicine. One piece of doggerel, "On a Doctor," which appeared in April 1849, sardonically attacked the role of the allopathic physician:

> Pray heaven will be forgiving!
>   Such sin is on his head;
> For he cuts us down while living,
>   And cuts us up when dead![80]

A caustic one-liner in an 1850 volume remarked: "An extraordinary surgical operation was lately performed, which resulted in the complete removal—of the patient to another world. The physician is doing well."[81] All these gibes sought to convince the American public of the evils of allopathy and the preferable alternative available in hydropathy.

A corollary theme that received considerable attention in the *Water-Cure Journal* was patient autonomy, responsibility, and self-determination, readily achievable through home self-doctoring. Logically, since the philosophy of the water cure rejected drugging and stressed hygienic living, total patient cooperation was imperative. Hydropaths argued that all patients, especially women, were encouraged to surrender their judgment and their body to allopathic physicians. Water curers assumed a different posture, urging their followers to use skilled hydropaths as teachers while striving to become their own physicians. Numerous texts and journal articles urged patient responsibility, but none as clearly as "The Doctor's 'Occupation Gone'—A Healthy Country," in which the editors refused to commiserate with an upstate New York allopathic physician who had lamented the decline of his livelihood. The journal commentator followed the tale with: "We are sorry for the doctor, but can offer no consolation. The 'medicine business' will continue to decline till, finally, the good time coming shall usher in Universal Health."[82] Similarly, F. B. Perkins, in "Self-Government in Diet and Doctoring," reiterated the case for patient responsibility.[83] As Thomas Nichols, a prominent author and lecturer in the cause of hydropathy, so emphatically stated, prevention through living habits learned at home or at a cure (as opposed to physician-directed cures), was the goal of responsible doctoring and healing systems:

> How can diseases be prevented? Simply in two ways: by living, as far as possible, in accordance with all the conditions of health; and by avoiding, in like manner, every cause of disease. By keeping up the strength and purity of the system; by avoiding all excess, and every means of exhaustion; and by living in such a manner as to keep free from all matter of disease.[84]

Therapeutics

The hygienic laws of living were not alone in the battle against disease. Water, pure and simple (not standing or stagnant), was the chief remedial agent, which could—if circumstances and need allowed—be administered by a competent water-cure physician. Each therapy was designed according to a patient's "reactive power," and, similarly, the temperature of the water was adapted to the nature of the case and the constitution of the patient.[85]

The rise in the popularity and credibility of hydropathy both aided and was aided by the growing acceptance of bathing as a summer sport, and the use of water in public bathhouses, urban luxury hotels, and insane asylums.[86] In addition, home bathing among Americans was made easier by indoor plumbing, which was largely available for the well-to-do in the early decades of the nineteenth century through municipal water and sewage systems. Most people, however, were not hooked up to city services or were unable to afford indoor plumbing. This necessitated carrying water to fill basins and disposing of waste water by hand. This method was employed in most homes through the 1850s, and as advertisements in the journal as early as 1846 show, a variety of portable shower baths, bathing tubs, and sponge, seat, foot, and hip baths—which could be filled with half a dozen buckets of water—were available at very reasonable prices.[87] By the 1860s, home bathing equipment was affordable for the upper middle class as well as the wealthy, and architectural and ladies' magazines were advocating the inclusion of bathrooms in home designs.[88] This acceptance of frequent bathing echoed familiar strains of moral strengthening through self-improvement. As one chronicler of American bathing habits noted:

> Bathing advice . . . helped reconcile the new industrial attention to moral character with earlier concern over religious conversion or rebirth. . . . The truly moral and pure individual was noted for frequently bathing and immaculate personal hygiene. Cleanliness was indeed next to godliness.[89]

While nearly all agreed on the desirability of bathing, the use of soap was debated. Many opposed its use, believing that it would remove the skin's essential oils. Neither John Bell, an early author on water's usage, nor an 1850 filler in the *Journal* agreed. As "A Sermon on Cleanliness," asserted, "An habitually dirty man can hardly be religious. He is breaking one of the first of nature's laws. Cleanliness in person prepares for purity of heart, and for a reception of life-giving principles of the Gospel. FRESH AIR, PURE WATER AND GOOD SOAP FOREVER!"[90]

Aided by the availability and credibility of in-home bathing, nearly every hydropathic text contained a lengthy section on "Water-Cure Processes" in which the specific applications of water were delineated.[91] Mary Gove Nichols's outline of these therapeutics can serve well as a demonstrative text. Gove Nichols, hydropath, lecturer, author, and wife of T. L. Nichols, wrote her classic *Experience in Water-Cure* in 1850. In that valuable, slim volume, she described the use and application of water in various ailments. Water processes were to serve as conduits to remove putrid matter from the human system, internally and externally, and pave the way for rejuvenation.

Gove Nichols, familiar with current disclaimers, pointed out that bathing was often avoided on the ground that it was inconvenient. Dismissing this reasoning, she remarked: "Wherever a pail or even a pitcher of water can be obtained, a cleanly person will have a bath, by means of a towel, a sponge, or by standing in a tub, and pouring it over the person."[92] A pouring bath (not to be confused with a shower bath, which was never used in water-cure processes) was recommended for "persons in full health and strong reactive power, but is found too chilling for invalids." For the pouring bath, 60°F. was most often recommended, but not until two hours had elapsed after eating. A variation on the pouring bath found the patient, with already wet head and face, "crouch(ed) in a tub or any convenient place, while the attendant pours over him one or two pailsful of cold water."[93] This bath could also be given by patients themselves with the aid of a large sponge to release water on the back of the neck and the rest of the body.

This treatment was superseded by the plunge, the dripping sheet, or other processes, depending on the ailment and the patient's physical strength. The plunge bath was used for general daily ablutions and followed the wet sheet and blanket packings. As Gove Nichols prescribed it, "[Fill] the common bathing tub sufficiently to immerse the entire person. In this, as in all other cases, the head should be wet before immersing the body."[94] According to Gove Nichols, the dripping sheet was of particular service in the treatment of fevers. First, patients wet their head. Then the attendant dipped a common sheet in cold water, enveloped the standing patients, and rubbed them briskly all over with the sheet.[95]

The douche, used locally to treat tumors, rheumatic swellings, and spinal and nervous diseases, was another very popular therapy. It was an application aimed at exciting the nervous system and acted powerfully on the whole body:

> A stream of water, from half an inch to three inches in diameter, and falling from five to twenty feet, constitutes a more or less powerful douche. The head may be wet first, or the stream allowed to break over the hands, held above the head for a moment, but the full force of the douche should never fall upon the head, but upon the back and limbs.[96]

The sitz bath, prescribed in a variety of instances, was used for ten or fifteen minutes for "its stimulating and tonic effect upon the nerves of the bowels or pelvic viscera." But when it was used to lessen "inflammation of the head or chest, it is continued for half an hour, or even longer." In this simple, yet effective, procedure the patient sat in a common washing tub (roughly one-third full) with the feet remaining outside. The patient began with tepid water, with the goal being to make each sitz bath's water colder "so that at the end of the week it is the natural temperature."[97] Similar to the sitz bath was the shallow bath, or half bath, in which the patient sat in a tub with four or five inches of water and was rubbed by attendants. Valuable in fevers and congestion, the half bath could take the place of the plunge bath, following the wet sheet.[98]

Clearly the most universally applied water-cure process was the wet-sheet pack. Its efficacy, according to its advocates, was that it "cools febrile action, excites the action of the skin, equalizes the circulation, removes obstructions, brings out eruptive diseases, controls spasms, and relieves pain like a charm."[99] In short, it sought to restore balance to the system by inducing "crisis," thus affecting a cure while mitigating discomfort. Hydropathic leaders, including Trall and Shew, saw the process as a drawing out, and infusion of, bad and healthy elements:

> When the pure water of the wet sheet came into contact with the skin the impure water of the blood on the inside of the skin passed through the skin into the water of the wet sheet while pure water of the wet sheet passed through the skin to supply the place of the impure water. An interchange took place.[100]

Used in almost every form and stage of disease, the wet-sheet pack served as a conduit (one of the oldest forms of mystical power attributed to water) for the transference of sick and healthy elements. While the wet-sheet pack had an initial shock of cold, it quickly produced a feeling of physical well-being and often a sedated deep sleep. This procedure was performed by having the patient lie on the sheet, which had been dipped in cold water, wrung out, and placed on top of four blankets. The patient was wrapped first in the wet sheet and then in each blanket in turn. Every body part was covered except the face; the result was a mummylike encasement. On top of this the attendant laid either a small featherbed or more blankets—"enough to make a thick covering." If the patient was extremely chilly, hot water bottles could be put at the feet and armpits, although artificial heat was never encouraged. The patient remained in the pack "until warmth is fully established, and the whole skin is aglow, and just ready to burst into a perspiration."[101] Gove Nichols cautioned that a nervous and uneasy patient could be taken out at any time. On coming out of the wet-sheet pack, she warned, "The patient must go as quickly as possible into a plunge, pouring, or other cold or tepid bath. This rule is invariable, except when, in cases of high inflammation, one wet sheet follows another in quick succession."[102]

A derivative of the ever-popular wet-sheet pack, the blanket pack placed patients in dry blankets, where they remained until perspiration was excited. This treatment was followed by a cold bath. On emerging from any of these treatments, "the patient should be well rubbed with coarse towels, a brush, or the hand, or with all these; and sometimes which friction is necessary to excite the skin, quicken the circulation, and produce a healthy reaction."[103] Water-cure procedures also included hand baths, eye baths, foot baths, head baths, and so on, which allowed the ailing part direct and primary contact with water.

In addition to the hydropathic texts that elaborated these procedures, the *Water-Cure Journal* kept its reading public informed of the latest therapeutics; the journal's editors often featured these articles as the issue's lead story. Indicative of these is an 1849 article, "The Water-Cure Processes Illustrated." It described the purpose of the wet-sheet wrap as reducing the body's heat and forcing the circulation, as well as correcting morbid secretions and restoring healthy ones. The article also described the douche, the rubbing wet-sheet, the sitting bath, the foot bath, and local applications.[104] Other articles focused more directly on a single procedure, such as "The Wet Bandage," "Bathing" (which described the different effects of sitz and sitting baths), "A Rubber Sheet," "Fomentation" (the equivalent of a wet compress), and Dr. E. P. Miller's serialized article, "How to Bathe."[105]

Efficacy of Water-Cure Therapies

Clearly some forms of water treatments did produce tangible (i.e., medically quantifiable) results: the control of fevers, the reduction of inflammations, the healing of burns, and the inducing of sleep (wet packing was employed in mental institutions for this latter purpose well into the twentieth century). Treatments should ideally be measured not only by their curing of disease but also by their relief of suffering,[106] which came through diminution of pain and discomfort, touch, and communication. Particularly in an era when the therapeutics themselves held only minimal hope of curing disease, the symptomatic relief offered by water-cure therapies, because they emphasized the relief of suffering, was significant and accounts in large part for their efficacy.

In either an away-from-home cure or home use, numerous repetitions of bathings, wrappings, rubbings, and washings were, for many, a far more meaningful way of being cared for (or caring for oneself) than ingesting medicine or being the recipient of a one-time, unpleasant therapy. "Meaningful" in this context entails greater relief from suffering, more tactile stimulation, and a longer therapeutic encounter. Thus there was more time for the patient to be observed performing the therapy, thereby inducing conversation about and attention to the ailment and the healing process. This was important both in home self-doctoring, where water therapies would surely capture the family's notice, and in cure establishments, where discussion of one's ailment(s) served as a main topic of conversation. The efficacy of water-cure therapies, therefore, far exceeded quantifiable medical results. The basic components of the healing process were ritualistically and systematically reenacted, and they provided not only symptomatic relief but also psychosocial validation and communication within a communal context.

Narratives of Healing

Consider the case of Harriet Penfield, who after home self-doctoring (with the aid of her sister) entered Shew's Lebanon Springs (Ohio) Cure in 1846 because of the severity of her (unspecified) condition. Of special note is the fluid "crossing over" between the two kinds of water cure, domestic and physician-directed. Penfield recalls the value of the journey to Shew's Cure for her health and the "good opportunity of pursuing the treatment at our friends in different places."[107] Crediting both the time at Shew's Cure and her adoption of self-doctoring water therapies with reversing her life, Penfield wrote: "The treatment has worked wonders in my case, and I am sure I should not have lived, had I not obtained information in regard to it."[108] Penfield made her illness very much a communal experience by enlisting the aid of her sister, the cooperation and recognition of the friends in whose homes she performed her ablutions while on the way to and from Lebanon Springs, and the tutelage of Shew and his staff at the cure. Thus validated and nurtured within a communal context, Penfield expressed her readiness to spread the hydropathic word, promulgating the teachings from which she had so benefited.

While the hydropathic leaders recognized the persuasive power of the "healing narratives" of reformed patients, they were similarly aware that imaginative approaches to educating the unconverted were necessary so as not to alienate or overwhelm them with the "how-to's" of water cure. To this end, and to avoid boring those already-practicing followers of the system, the editors of the *Water-Cure Journal* made the good-natured decision to print poems such as "A Wet-Sheet Pack," written by Carrie May at the Saratoga Water-Cure around 1857. The poem gives a patient's view of some of the attendant pleasures of this treatment and, because of the inactivity required of the patient while wrapped, some of the attendant frustrations (in this case dripping water and a pesky fly).

A Wet-Sheet Pack

READER, did you ever
    Take a wet-sheet pack,
Rolled up like a mummy,
    Lying on its back;

Wet cloth on your forehead,
    Bottle at your feet?
You would truly find it
    A hydropathic treat. . . .

First, they wrap you closely
    In a dripping sheet,
A bottle of hot water
    Is then placed at your feet;

Blanket after blanket
    Wrap about your form,
Comfortables in plenty,
    Keep you nicely warm; . . .

Acting like an opiate,
    Easing all your pain,
Claming down your bounding pulse,
    Cooling off your brain—
Puts you in a slumber,
    Gives you dreams of bliss,
Naught is any "Treatment"
    Is so nice as this. . . .

If you're feeling nervous—
    Tired—and can not rest,
You'll surely fail to like them,
    Though you try your best. . . .

If you should make the effort
    To get into a doze,
First you know, a saucy fly
    Has lighted on your nose— . . .

Then perhaps the bottle,
    Tucked up with your feet,
Loses out the stopple,
    Water scalding heat. . . .

And scream perhaps until you're hoarse,
    To make some person hear,
For you're more than lucky,
    If anyone is near—

Unless it be some comrade
    In the self same plight,
Lying on another bed,
    And tucked up just as tight.

Still, with such exceptions,
    A pack is very fine—
If you never tried one,
    Reader it is time.[109]

The use of the wet-sheet pack and other water-cure procedures, if coupled with hygienic reforms, promised the patient a cure-all. The therapeutic application of water, Nichols asserted in *An Introduction to the Water-Cure*, was a universal nostrum "adapted to the human constitution in every condition of sickness and health; . . . promote[s] the cure of all curable diseases; . . . [and] gives relief in all cases, if rightly applied. It not only removes symptoms, but removes the causes upon which all disease depends."[110]

For hydropaths, each disease had a water-cure procedure and set of hygienic laws that served as "the prescription" to rid the patient of the disorder. An examination of some of the treatments for a specific ailment will illuminate the treatment a water-cure patient received at a water-cure establishment, in a hydropath's office, or under self-care at home.

Dyspepsia, or stomach troubles, plagued nineteenth-century Americans. Indeed, that time has been characterized as the era of the Great American Stomachache. In the more extreme instances, health reformers claimed, many Americans depended on pork, lard, gravies, rich soups, pies, cakes, salted and fried meats, candies, sweetmeats, spices, vinegar, grease, and an excess of salt, liquor, and bitter coffee as the mainstays of their diet.[111] Hydropaths gladly accepted the challenge of trying to reform America's eating habits because they believed that these habits were the cause of much ill health. As Trall wrote in *Digestion and Dyspepsia* (1873):

> We are a nation of dyspeptics; and . . . we are growing worse continually. . . . The public mind has been so long accustomed to rely on medicine to remove the penalties of transgression, when persistent disobedience to the laws of health has resulted in disease. . . . [This] delusion, however . . . is surely undermining the stamina of the American people.[112]

Trall and other reform-oriented hydropaths seized this opportunity to advocate the entire spectrum of hygienic principles. Dyspepsia, they argued, contraindicated the use of both tobacco and tight lacing, which strained and inflamed sensitive parts.[113] They also blamed tea, coffee, warm water, strong alcoholic liquors, spices, sour tasting foods, snuffs, excessive eating or drinking, rigid fasting, an indolent or sedentary life, habitual exhaustion from intense study, late hours, and, finally, "becoming a prey to the violent passions, and especially those of the depressing kind, as fear, grief, deep anxiety; immoderate libidinous indulgence, and a life of too great muscular exertions."[114]

In this instance, as in many others, hydropathic leaders seized the opportunity of disease management to advocate the adoption of complementary social reforms. They clearly overstepped the physician's usual sphere of influence by urging substantial changes in their patients' personal habits. Such forays into preventive and *socially* prescriptive therapeutics, while not new among medical practitioners, were extended by the hydropaths and were justified, they believed, by their all-inclusive definition of health and the rejuvenation and rebirth that their followers enjoyed.

What interested Trall, in the spirit of the true social reformer, was not the quick cure of dyspepsia, but its cause. In keeping with this concern, he prescribed appropriate food, drink, exercise, bathing, clothing, sleep, ventilation, light, temperature, mental influences, and occupation, all based on hygienic principles.[115] Other texts, including Trall's *The New Hydropathic Cook-book* (1856), Miller's *Dyspepsia* (1870), and Julia A. Pye's *Invalid Cookery* (1880), focused more directly on the specific diet for a dyspeptic and accompanying water-cure procedures.

While Trall begrudgingly admitted he allowed his patients animal food, he clearly considered vegetarianism "the true theory of diet,"[116] especially for the dyspeptic. Consequently, *The New Hydropathic Cookbook* has chapter headings such as "Bread and Bread Making," "Whole Grains and Seeds," "Roots and Vegetables," and "Prepared Fruits."[117]

Miller, who wrote the serialized article for the *Water-Cure Journal* entitled "How to Bathe," emphasized bathing as well as diet to correct dyspepsia. In *Dyspepsia*, Miller urged "a daily bath to cleanse the skin and improve the external circulation." This, he wrote, "should be the rule of all, except those who are too weak and feeble to secure a reaction."[118]

Pye's *Invalid Cookery* also was informed by hydropathic principles and emphasized the simplest diet possible. Indicative of the recipes in her 1880 volume are: wheat bread, graham gems, oatmeal, #2 flummeries, rice gruel flour, tapioca lemon jelly, and nutritive enemata.[119] Unlike Trall's book *Invalid Cookery*, which was not a doctrinaire hydropathic text, did not object to meat on principle.

That the hydropathic approach to dyspepsia had positive results is exemplified in the testimony of the Reverend Joseph Scott, a chronic dyspeptic, who at the urging of a friend visited Dr. Wellington's New York City Water-Cure Institution and wrote his tale in the *Water-Cure Journal* in 1852. Knowing nothing of hydropathy but the name, he was exceedingly pleased to discover what the diet and water treatments produced: "In ten days the hemorrhoids had nearly disappeared: the inflammation was gone; . . . a newly awakened appetite [had appeared] . . . and I have walked upon an average of five miles a day. . . . I find the whole habit of my system undergoing a rapid, most favorable change."[120]

While dyspepsia was particularly well suited to the entire arsenal of hygienic principles, other diseases, although indicating hygienic violations, necessitated immediate water-cure procedures. As the allopaths would commence bleeding and drugging and the homeopaths their infinitesimal dosages, the hydropaths began plunging, douching, and packing a patient who had an acute or chronic condition in an attempt to induce crisis, throw off the foreign matter, and foster a balance within the system, leading to a restoration of health.

Personal accounts of those treated by the water cure for acute and chronic diseases were next in popularity in the journal to articles on innovations in therapeutics. The ailments treated included surgery, burns, brain fever, paralytic disorders, fevers, bronchitis, eye diseases, hysteria, teething, flesh wounds, broken bones, dislocations, seasickness, ague, rattlesnake bite, sore throat, hernia, foot disease, worms, typhoid, yellow fever, spermatorrhea, sick headache, nervousness, psychosomatic illnesses, and hypochondria. In short, water-cure treatments existed for every ailment known to humanity.[121]

Hydropathic texts, like the *Water-Cure Journal*, focused on specific water-cure treatments. Gove Nichols's management of a case of scarlet fever, recorded in *Experience in Water-Cure* (1850), is a case in point:

> Miss —— was taken with a very malignant form of scarlet fever, which was then rife in the neighborhood. She was delirious, and the fever was of the worst type, and ran very high. She was first put under a pouring bath, then packed in the wet sheet. The wet sheet packs, and dripping sheet baths succeeded each other rapidly, for several days and nights, before the fever was subdued. The throat sloughed horridly, and large quantities of matter were thrown off. She took nothing but water for ten days, and four wet sheets in the twenty-four hours. She lay enveloped in wet linen when not in the wet sheet. The fever was then subdued, the appetite returned, the throat got well, and the patient fully recovered, with no drug poison in the system, and with health greatly better than she had ever before enjoyed.[122]

Self-Doctoring

By far the most common forum of education and cure through water therapy was the home. Texts, newly converted neighbors, and especially the *Water-Cure Journal* promulgated the desirability, ease, and efficacy of home self-doctoring. Domestic hydropathy succeeded because it followed the American tradition of self-care. For the segment of the population that "medicated without doctors" at home, numerous factors combined to validate hydropathy's near-extreme reliance on oneself. Allopathic therapeutic nihilism generated a sense of discouragement about the possibilities of curing the sick and preserving health. Hydropathy countered with its own systemic panacea. Further, the regular medical profession was not always accessible in certain geographic regions, especially rural areas. In addition, large numbers of the urban poor were unable to secure medical care through the insufficient and underfinanced institutions in the cities. Moreover, Americans' propensity for mobility (specifically westward expansion) and the problems associated with finding and affording medical care while traveling contributed to the need for self-help medicine. Medical self-reliance also found credibility and widespread appeal as a result of corollary developments that bolstered individualism: Americans' increased emphasis on social egalitarianism, glorification of the individual in literature and philosophy, a lessening of the hold of established religions, and a heightened emphasis on participation in the political process.[123] These themes in popular thought, the sects' increasing ability to print and distribute their tracts, and improved national literacy combined to produce a climate favorable to domestic medicine, as opposed to professional care.[124]

This self-care optimism reflected an attitude that people could influence and control what happened to their bodies and themselves. This belief mirrored popular religions that stressed self-help as an avenue to personal betterment.[125] The ideology of self-control emerging under expanding industrial capitalism, as well as the democratic ideology of managing one's own destiny, complemented the emphasis on self-care. Just as the "self-made man" in American popular thought reaps the accolades and rewards of personal advancement, so does he reap the blame and hardships of failure. The analogy to medical self-help is evident: The emphasis on patient self-care led to seeing ill health as one's own fault, perhaps even as a moral failing.[126] Adherence to the "systems" approach of the sects, and hydropathy in particular, served to allay these implicit accusations. *Some* responsibility for one's health was given over to the efficacy of the system itself, thus partially exonerating the individual.

Readers of the *Water-Cure Journal* were able to receive advice on home self-care for specific ailments in a question-and-answer column, "Professional Matters." A more complicated disease, such as bronchitis, found the editor referring the patient to a text, such as the *Hydropathic Encyclopedia*. But for simpler ailments, such as enlargement of the liver, the column told M.S. of Erie, Pennsylvania: "Your case is evidently an enlarged liver, and probably complicated with piles. Frequent hip baths, a wet sheet pack for an hour, two or three times a week, and a plain vegetable diet are the remedies."[127] J.P. of Auburn, Alabama, in the same 1853 column, received this advise on caring for a bothersome cutaneous eruption: "Your internal ailments are probably caused by the remedies you employed to repel the external one. You should take a wet-sheet pack daily, followed by a tepid half-bath, or dripping sheet, and live almost wholly on wheat-meal unfermented bread, with a little good fruit."[128]

The journal's editors also encouraged their readers with tales of successful home self-doctoring. An 1846 piece, "Facts in Domestic Practice of Water-Cure," tells of "Priscilla, a highly respected mulatto woman [who] has been for twenty years afflicted with many weaknesses."[129]

Depleted financially from physicians' fees, Priscilla was influenced by a benevolent lady sojourning at Fairfield, Connecticut. Suffering from piles, nervous trembling, severe headaches, distressing and excessive menstruation, and rheumatism, Priscilla used the water cure at home as follows: "Cold bathing twice a day, the sitting bath, drinking very freely of cold water, and strict attention to diet."[130] Applying these means, she was restored to perfect health within a month. Priscilla's daughter, taught in true hydropathic fashion by a converted believer, benefited from her mother's recovery. Her own discomforts from scrofula and rheumatism abated after she followed the same therapy as her mother (plus wearing a wet bandage), leaving her in *perfect health*, with an enormous appetite, and sleeping all night perfectly well."[131]

Throughout the decades of hydropathy's greatest popularity, the domestic use of the water cure was continuously promoted as the means by which all people, regardless of economic or social class, could participate in hygienic healing. (Live-in cures, however, were more class-determined, and they will be discussed in detail later.) As Shew reminded the journal's readers in "A Word to Water Patients on Household Treatment": "The writer has always maintained that the Water-Cure is eminently a DOMESTIC treatment. No method ever known by man can at all compare with it in this respect."[132] Shew went on to reassure readers that water therapy was simple and easily applicable. In fact, "It requires a great degree of awkwardness in its application for one to do any great harm."[133] Shew also highlighted the economic benefits of household treatment, prime among them that one saved on the fees of physicians and water establishments. Further, he reminded readers, expert physicians were available for cases demanding greater knowledge and for those who wished to consult a hydropath by letter (so that they could then treat themselves at home), Shew listed the particulars needed for a proper diagnosis.[134]

Numerous cases illustrated the efficacy of domestic use of the water cure, including "A Case of Home Treatment in Water-Cure" (1850). A husband refused to call a doctor for his fevered wife, preferring "with my wife's consent, [to] cure her myself."[135] Having attended L. N. Fowler's lectures and having read of the water cure, "he went to work on her according to rule: 'giving, all along, what cold water she desired to drink, keeping a circulation of pure air through the room, and the room and bed-room most scrupulously clean.'"[136] The husband–doctor reported his wife–patient up within a few days, well and hearty.

The prospectus for the *Water-Cure Journal* in 1851 listed among its year-long thematic headings "Water-Cure at Home."[137] Not surprisingly, therefore, a February letter from A.E.H. in Mississippi chronicled the writer's bouts with sick headache and hepatitis, which had been relieved through home self-doctoring. A.E.H., since recovery, had treated thirty cases without failure.[138] A month later, Jane V. Hull told of her use of the wet-sheet pack on her fevered child. Recalling her fear and trembling on using water therapies for the first time—alone at midnight with a delirious child—Hull joyfully reported:

> With what anxiety I watched the countenance, listened to the breathing, that I might note the smallest change! Gradually the little sufferer became calm . . . the breathing easy. The experiment was repeated, and with so happy a result, that I was able to take my little patient to bed, where we both slept comfortably until morning.[139]

Hull, interestingly, derived all her knowledge solely from reading, as she had "never seen any practice but my own."[140]

Later that same year, Solomon Freez, writing from an unidentified place in the West, urged readers to utilize domestic water cure instead of drugs and in cases where no hydropathic physician was available. Freez had treated and cured a bilious middle-aged man and a feverish four-year-old boy.[141]

A similar tale is "Domestic Practice of Hydropathy by an ex-Druggist." The druggist, on learning of his four-year-old son's depleted state from scarlet fever, applied a wet-sheet wrap and then a rubbing sheet to cure the child. He later applied similar techniques to his other three children, who had been comparably stricken, and cured them.[142] As a result of these episodes he gave up using drug medications. Other reports of home treatment included the successful management of wounds, hemorrhages, burns, and choking.[143]

"Home Voices: Extracts from Letters," a regular feature of the journal, also carefully chronicled the successes of the domestic use of the water cure.[144] Representative of these is a letter from a home user of water cure from Unionville Centre, Pennsylvania, who recalled his prolonged use of botanic medicine, which had failed to provide lasting relief for chronic indigestion. Having gradually become habituated to the exclusive use of water, and "my faith increasing in the efficacy of water to remove all curable diseases, I resolved to abandon the use of medicine, and rely wholly upon Nature's Physician, pure Water, for myself and family."[145] This Pennsylvania resident noted that in addition to water therapies, "we have also adopted the reform in diet, using neither tea, coffee, nor animal food. I now find myself much improved."[146] The editors, pleased that this correspondent had secured forty-four subscriptions for the journal from among neighbors, exclaimed: "This is the *true* missionary spirit. Think of it. Placing the WATER-CURE JOURNAL into the hands of *every* neighbor. May this noble co-worker in our glorious Reform, be rewarded for this manifestation of practical benevolence."[147]

In addition to testimonials offered by common folk, water-cure physicians continuously promoted the desirability of home doctoring.

Representative of these was Dr. James Caleb Jackson's "Sick-Headache," which appeared in the June 1862 issue of the *Water-Cure Journal*. Jackson recommended the following treatment, always emphasizing the necessity of hygienic living: (1) Cease to drink alcohol in any form; (2) "If the person be a female, to wear the American costume [a loose-fitting dress-reform outfit], and live largely in the open air"; (3) get abundant sleep; (4) avoid meat and spices; (5) bathe three times a week with water at a mild temperature and then have a rub by an attendant—lie down in bed, well-covered, for an hour afterward; (6) regulate the bowels either through diet or, if unsuccessful, tepid injections of water; and (7) arrange your life to be carefree. This, Jackson assured readers, would solve the sick headache.[148] Other physician-authored articles, such as "Nurses for the Sick" (1855), "Domestic Practice—No. 2" by Dr. W. T. Vail (1864), J. H. Hero's "Errors in Home Practice" (1855), Dr. Howard Johnson's review of "Domestic Practice of Hydropathy" (1849), and Dr. E. P. Miller's "Hygienic Home Treatment of Diseases" (1867), were similarly instructive and enthusiastic toward self-doctoring.[149]

Domestic use of the water cure, therefore, combined the most salient features of hydropathic philosophy. Water processes, rationally applied and coupled with hygienic living principles, produced patient responsibility leading to home self-doctoring and eventual autonomy, the adoption of corollary hygienic reforms, and an advocacy of the hydropathic system to others. The convergence of these factors (variations among practitioners and therapeutic management aside) formed the core of the hydropathic world view, a view particularly directed toward, and appealing to, nineteenth-century women.

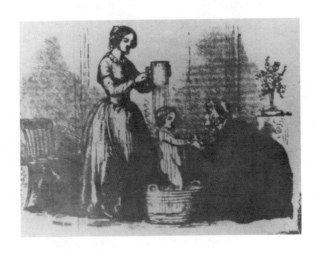

Chapter Two

Hydropathy, Woman's Physiology, and Her Role

The hydropathic management of female physiology encouraged self-doctoring, which gave women responsibility for and control over their bodies. In addition, the social ideology of the movement urged women to care for their families' health and to participate in social-reform activism to bring about healthier living conditions for all Americans. This was to be the special mission of female hydropathic followers and practitioners, a mission begun with one's own cure.

Cured and Converted

The newly cured often reacted with the enthusiasm of the religious convert. Jemima Pringle, in a letter to Trall in 1864 after a lengthy stay at his Hygeio-Therapeutic Cure, wrote:

> Permit me to submit my testimony of the saving efficacies of Hygeio-Therapy . . . in the hope that others may be induced to do likewise and have occasion to rejoice likewise.
>
> Two weeks previous to my arrival at your Cure . . . I had then experienced most miserable health for sixteen months, and had tried drugs and drug doctors unavailingly. . . . My ailments were various and complicated and among them were the horrors of dyspepsia, the depressions of nervous debility, the terrors of congestion of the brain &c.[1]

Pringle recalled that her life had "seemed to hang, as it were, by a thread, vibrating between life and death." In three weeks at Trall's Cure she "experienced a decided change for the better; and for five months [she] was a faithful observer of all [Trall's] directions and prescriptions." After recollecting that she had scarcely been able to walk on commencing treatment, she joyfully reported that she could by then walk three miles without resting. Shifting her narrative to praise Trall and hydropathy directly, Pringle used religious metaphors that were unmistakable and powerful:

> I feel as though I had been born again; your system has been my salvation; and I feel like bidding an eternal farewell to drugopathy and all of its abominations, while praying fervently that the system of truth which you are ably advocating, and so successfully practicing may soon extend to the uttermost parts of the earth.[2]

Pringle was not content to let her discoveries and revelations remain a private matter. "Spreading the word" seemed the ultimate validation of her cure and the metaphorical mission she had assumed: "Could I stand on the summit of some vast mountain and proclaim with the voice of a Stentor, that this is the way, the truth, and the life, for diseased mortals, methinks the millennium would soon dawn upon the earth."[3] Pringle concluded her testimony by wishing Trall every success in his good cause and signed her epistle, "I remain, gratefully yours."[4]

Pringle's narrative reveals the considerable consistency between the rhetoric of the hydropathic leadership and the reality (i.e., "felt" experience) of the hydropathic following. Because the water cure was a profoundly ideological system that demanded of its followers a solid working knowledge of the tenets, principles, and, one might argue, world view of hydropathic living, the narrated experiences of water-cure patients often closely reflect the words of hydropathic leaders. Many narratives contain the same elements as Priessnitz's conversion. Pringle's emphasis on the restoration and maintenance of her health, abhorrence for allopathic therapeutics, "born again" testimony, desire to proselytize, and heartfelt belief in the efficacy of hydropathic therapeutics all resound as familiar chants of the larger movement. Patients' narratives, were they not signed, could at times be taken for statements by the leaders themselves. There is no evidence, however, in this direction. They did follow a typical format: description of early ill health; unsuccessful encounters with allopaths; (for some) a life-and-death turning point; discovery of the water cure; utilization of hydropathic therapeutics and habit changes; improved health; conversion to hydropathy; desire to convince others of its efficacy; and, often, near-reverent praise for the hydropathic healer.

Consider the narrative of "I," who wrote a friend from a water-cure establishment:

> I myself was much weaker and more diseased every day, when I came here eight weeks ago. . . . I [had] employed an Allopathic

physician [before arriving at the cure]. . . . He gave me medicine that made me sicker and weaker. . . . Since I came here . . . I have gone daily, Sunday excepted, to the bath-room, and taken from one to four baths daily, and eat plain, simple food, twice per day, and slept nights without anybody sitting up all night to wait on me.[5]

"I" went on to report that she was by then walking two or three miles a day (something she could never do before), "Yes! in the snow." This walking was facilitated by her new, lighter garments and more sensible shoes. "I" concluded her letter with verbal testimony to the worthiness of the water cure and her hope that others would follow: "I have come to love Water-Cure, and I would wish that everyone knew more about it than I do, then they would love it too, and cease to poison themselves or their friends, in the erroneous hope of driving disease from their system."[6]

Mary Jenks of Springfield, Massachusetts, reported her "Astonishing Cure" in the May 1853 issue of the *Water-Cure Journal*. Jenks recited her legacy of sickness, including scrofula, which had produced huge swellings on her neck and side that, when treated with plastering, powders, and calomel by the allopaths, became open sores. For fifteen years Jenks had "continued to linger between life and death, sometimes in the most subject condition." Her disease imbedded itself in her colon and rectum, "till a place of discharge came near [her] right hip, from which the feces of the bowels passed at every discharge." Desperate, Jenks applied to Dr. Snell of the Easthampton Water Cure despite the warnings of her friends, who "said it would certainly kill me; but as a drowning person will catch at a straw, and having some independence of my own, I resolved to try, and accordingly was carried to the establishment."[7] Snell was more encouraging than she had anticipated, and began treatment after one week's consideration. Jenks noticed little improvement in the first four weeks of treatment. Then, "After this I began to gain in every respect, it seemed to me almost a miracle, I found myself gaining in flesh, and getting the use of my eye and arm."[8] Jenks chronicled the disappearance of swelling and abnormal bowel discharges and noted that, to her delight, she had gained thirty pounds in four months. Shortly thereafter, she was able to return to her responsibilities. Her disease came to crisis in the form of forty boils, which discharged profusely. "When these passed off, I found myself in the possession of health, which I had not known for more than fifteen years."[9] Jenks, noting the simultaneous relief she experienced from a variety of female complaints, described her new-found belief and reverence for the water cure, and promised to make herself useful in the healing art:

Thanks to a kind Providence for making me willing to try the Water-Cure before it was too late. And now, sisters, don't stay at home dreading it, . . . but esteem your baths a great luxury. . . . Do not wait for your friends to advise you to go; had I done so the grass would now have been growing upon my grave.[10]

Similarly, an anonymous correspondent wrote Shew in 1847, "I shall never forget nor regret the few days I spent in your institution, for they have been the means of bringing about a great change, not only in my diet and manner of living, but also in my general health."[11] This patient, "now able to labor on the farm and perform more hard work in a day, than at any time in years previously," clearly attributed her successful rejuvenation to her healer–physician, and to the system itself: "And this improvement I owe wholly to the instructions gained at your institution, and the thorough and constant application of the means recommended."[12] One need only be briefly reacquainted with the narrative of Fanny Johnson, who at the fiftieth anniversary celebration of the Dansville Water-Cure in 1907 recalled that decades earlier "Dr. James C. Jackson was then at the height of his power to lift and carry his patients along the often difficult road to health and to impress them with his fresh thought."[13]

It would be naive to argue that all adherents to the system were drawn by its ideological position (exceptions are discussed later), but the trend *was* marked. Further evidence for this consistency lies in the ready integration of newcomers such as Mary Jenks into the middle levels of authority and expertise in the movement. Her personal cure, revelation, and decision to pursue a hydropathic course of study represent a significant amount of agreement with the basic premises and goals of the system.

The Dual Appeal: "Physicians'" Hydropathy and Self-Doctoring

Another aspect of hydropathy complements the compatibility of leaders' and followers' perceptions of the system. The *rhetoric* of water-cure philosophy viewed the hydropathic physician as a guide, a hygienic teacher to patients; it urged patients, once supplied with the information, to assume responsibility for their own physical future. The success of the therapeutic encounter, however, was predicated on the spiritual as well as physical effects of the healer on the patient; whereas the rhetoric stressed self-sufficiency, the lived experience, for many who utilized hydropathic physicians, flourished because of a tight, albeit episodic, bonding. The philosophy of the water cure, therefore, stressed a moving away from the therapeutic power of the (often charismatic) healer–patient dyad.

So there is a fascinating paradox in the hydropathic physician–patient relationship: an articulated goal of separation with a simultaneous reliance on the healing dyad—the *bond* of trust, faith, and hope that in turn yields loyalty and reverence for the one who has "shown the way." This reliance on the power inherent in the healer's role actually *facilitated* the realization of self-care and an efficacious therapeutic encounter. The healer's role as mentor inspired trust, which, when coupled with ideological agreement, merged to form empowering self-care. Thus, while hydropaths were more *theoretically* supportive of patient self-care than were practitioners of other sects, they were also able to inspire more confidence in their patients through the bonds formed at live-in cures. Other sects, Thomsonians and homeopaths prime among them, succeeded similarly because they too followed in the tradition of American self-care. But if hydropaths were not alone in this regard, they were singularly successful in balancing the appeal of domestic therapeutics with "physicians'" hydropathy. This dual approach enabled the movement's leadership to appeal to (1) educated urban and rural reform-minded folks attracted by self-doctoring (laboring *and* middle-class people alike), and (2) to educated urban and rural reform-minded folks who sought physician care (largely middle- and upper-middle class, although not exclusively). Urban and rural followers were possible because the domestic mode could be—and was—practiced anywhere, and cures were located in both venues. Reform orientation and education seem likely prerequisites for hydropathic followers because of the movement's reliance on printed material and its emphasis on vegetarianism, dress reform, and all-encompassing temperance, ideals and views not shared by most mid-century Americans.

The source of hydropathic success, therefore, lies in its dual appeal as well as in the ability of hydropaths, unrestrained by the detachment and uncertainty of "scientific" medicine and its attendant therapeutics, to utilize curative aspects of the healer–patient dyad: presence, touch, communication, arousing hope and expectancy of cure, and the reinforcement of ties with the social group, thus minimizing the sense of isolation that so often accompanies sickness.

Echoing familiar strains in American popular thought, water-cure leaders argued that once patients began controlling their physical lives, the entire spectrum of self-determination and choice was within reach. Women patients were a prime case in point; after the hydropathic reconceptualization of disease management, a consideration of women's physiological abilities and sphere of influence inevitably followed.

Management of Women's Diseases

Hydropathy was particularly scornful of the allopathic handling of women's diseases. Hydropaths argued not only for the rejection of dramatic therapeutics in the management of women's diseases but also for a redefinition of women's physiological processes as nonpathological and natural, not as a series of repeated medical crises.

Hydropaths claimed that women's physiology was neither the cause nor the justification for women's social status. The hydropaths' approach to human physiology, and sexual physiology in particular, embodied their belief in human perfectibility through right living. As such, it embraced issues such as hereditary disease, regulation of offspring, spermatorrhea, and masturbation, all the while considering woman's physiology as a nonpathological series of occurrences. Adolescence, puberty, menstruation, childbearing, and menopause were seen as natural physiological processes. Yet hydropaths did believe that all aspects of women's health could benefit from the water-cure system and that difficult cases would be improved by therapeutic intervention (by physicians or others). Thus hydropaths were especially interested in female disorders because of women's critical role in nuturing the young and possible ensuing physiological complications. Female physiology per se was not seen as frail, but social conditions, habits of life, and nature's uncertainties made therapeutic *prevention* and intervention advisable.

In this spirit, masturbation and other sensitive topics found eager lecturers among the ranks of hydropaths. In 1846 Paulina S. Wright, a follower of Sylvester Graham, lectured to ladies in Pennsylvania, Maryland, New Jersey, and New England on anatomy, physiology, and health.[14] Similarly, Gove Nichols's "Lectures to Ladies, on Anatomy and Physiology" were nationally known for their frank discussion of such matters. The *Boston Quarterly Review* of April 1842, when speaking of her lectures, stated: "Sincerely do we thank Mrs. Gove for daring, in our falsely-delicate society, to raise her warning voice, which she has done, and in tones which can offend nobody."[15]

By publically addressing matters of sexuality with female lecturers, hydropaths were among the vanguard of health theorists. Many of their nineteenth-century counterparts either considered the topic taboo or considered women educators unfit or improper for the task. By affirming the need to speak of sexual subjects to help avoid "self-pollution," hydropaths, like their contemporaries, aligned themselves with the standard nineteenth-century denial of the acceptability of masturbation. One reason for this stance was the belief that loss of the "vital force" (which constituted the body's very life force) occurred through seminal emission. In fact, one medical theorist equated the loss of one ounce of seminal fluid with that of forty ounces of blood. For both men and women, masturbation disarranged the necessary balance of the life force and induced illness. Beyond this physiological rationale, however, lay a more culturally based reason for opposing masturbation. Unlike colonial Americans and their European counterparts, who had clearly developed positive ideas of the female sexual appetite, much nineteenth-century medical theory, while acknowledging it, worked hard to suppress it. Although hydropaths *did* articulate the necessity for a pleasurable expression of women's sexuality, their views reflected popular concerns and fears held by other healing sects, including the premise that the control of "problematic" (i.e., unnatural, unhealthy, and inappropriate) sexuality, which included masturbation, was a medical task. That their therapeutic approach, while interventionist, did not rival the virulence advocated elsewhere is attributable to the nature of hydropathic therapeutics, not to a sharp divergence in beliefs.

Among hydropathic practitioners, self-pollution, as Gove Nichols called it, was nearly always met with a rigorous regimen of hygienic practices. The hydropathic management of masturbation was exemplified at one water-cure establishment, where the "sweating process" was used to treat masturbators. This "consisted of encouraging perspiration and then altering it with cold air or baths; in another method, a wet sheet was wrapped around the person and as soon as he became warm, the sheet was replaced with another."[16] Trall, when discussing the "Solitary Vice," is cryptic, asserting that the infirmity and degradation that result can only be eliminated (as in the case of prostitution, which compares to masturbation) when people are educated about health. This education entails diet renovation to relieve congestion and constant irritation in the pelvic viscera, which, if unchecked, "result[s] in a precocious development and morbid intensity of amativeness."[17] Similarly, tea, coffee, meat, and sugar products contribute to the "sexual dissipation and debauchery" manifested by young children. Compared with straitjackets, genital cages, and Spanish fly blisters, this treatment demonstrates the hygienic reforms that hydropaths brought to their therapeutics amid a generally repressive approach to sexuality.

The nineteenth-century water-cure patient suffering from venereal disease would be met with similar hygienic therapeutics and would "undergo a course of purification, not of swallowing 'drugs and dye-stuffs,' but by means of a rigid dietary, fresh air, simple exercise, and abundant bathing."[18]

Similarly, spermatorrhea, that "preternatural, morbid discharge of the seminal secretion" was caused, according to Trall's *Pathology of the Reproductive Organs; Embracing All Forms of Sexual Disorders* (1863), by masturbation or some other form of sexual abuse, which in turn, he believed, was caused by "dietetic habits of children and youth." Other sources of inducement included "stimulating beverages, irritating condiments, gross food, and especially everything which induces constipation of the bowels . . . animal meat [and] *pestilent literature. The sensation* fictions of the 'great story papers' are doing immense mischief."[19] Treatment consisted of "a towel wash or dripping-sheet in the morning on rising, followed by thorough frictions with dry towels, or rubbing over the dry sheet [and] a hip or sitz bath twice a day—at 10 to 11 A.M., and again at 4 to 5 P.M."[20]

Trall concluded the seven-page section on spermatorrhea with more general hygienic rules: Drink a tumbler full of water each morning *after* ablution; eliminate all seasonings, stimulants, and grease from the diet; eat twice a day; avoid meat; exercise frequently; get solid sleep, although do not lie about in bed in the morning; and sleep on a hard bed only. Finally, successful cures necessitated being sensitive to the "passional and social influence" of the patient, specifically, the difficulty his friends and family will have in understanding his predicament.[21]

In other aspects of sexual physiology the hydropathic approach was similarly hygienic and interventionist. Simultaneously, it demonstrated a desire to conserve the "vital force" and to channel sexual expression appropriately. When discussing women's physiology, several hydropathic leaders stressed the *naturalness* (their own word) of these functions. For example, Gove Nichols wrote in 1850, "Gestation and parturition are as natural functions as those of digestion."[22]

Like Gove Nichols, Trall repeatedly emphasized that rational thinking would demystify woman's physiology. Trall, a primary philosophical and systemic shaper of American hydropathy, was also the author of *Sexual Physiology: A Scientific and Popular Exposition of the Fundamental Problems in Sociology* (1861). His explicit goal was "to instruct the masses of the people on those subjects which have heretofore been to them as a sealed book." Discounting the arguments of indelicacy, Trall offered his beliefs as "contain[ing] a truth which the whole world would be benefited by understanding and practising."[23]

The views expressed in Trall's book, extremely forward-thinking for his time, were received with great enthusiasm by his hydropathic colleagues. In fact, some of his ideas had been articulated by others before his volume appeared; its distinction lay in its consolidated form, his merging of social philosophy with medical care, and the prominence that his stature as a water-cure leader lent to the undertaking. Publication was eagerly anticipated by the public, significant numbers of whom had sent in advance payment for the book.[24]

It is difficult to determine if Trall represented the views of all hydropathic adherents, although his adamantly demystifying approach throughout the book, as well as his relentless emphasis on the necessity to consider physiology, personal choices surrounding reproduction, and women's social role as one and the same issue echoed themes agreed on in hydropathic circles. Criticism of his social views by his hydropathic contemporaries is not evident, although his credibility in the larger medical community was damaged by his disavowal of the field of organic chemistry. He seemingly articulated the vanguard position among hydropaths, although he by no means occupied a fringe position. His writings were bolstered by agreeing colleagues and complete congruence with the social agenda of the hydropathic world view.

When speaking of the "Physiology of Menstruation," he wrote: "A woman was regarded as 'unclean' during menstruation and among other absurd vagaries of those who adopted this view of the process, a woman was regarded as a *dangerous character* during her 'monthly periods.'"[25] Trall went on to explain that menstruation was ovulation, "nothing more nor less than a discharge of ordinary blood."[26]

When discussing the physiological process of "Impregnation," Trall chose to subtitle a section "The Sexual Orgasm," wherein he remarked: "It is true that the sexual orgasm on the part of the female is just as normal as on the part of the male."[27] When responding to the question "Pregnancy, Normal or Abnormal?" Trall retorted, "I should as soon think of arguing whether sleeping or growing was a pathological condition!"[28] And when writing of the "Pleasure of Sexual Intercourse," he remarked: "Whatever may be the object of sexual intercourse—whether intended as a love embrace merely, or as a generative act—it is clear that it should be as pleasurable as possible to both parties. Indeed, when it is otherwise to either party, unless generation be intended, it is mere lust."[29] Concluded Trall, "Surely if sexual intercourse is worth doing at all, it is worth doing well."[30]

Cognizant of and articulate about woman's sexual desires and responses, Trall denied her "passionlessness"—a trait attributed to mid- and late-nineteenth-century women by many medical theorists and adopted by many women themselves.[31] Individual hydropathic physicians might not agree with or implement this opinion (just as allopaths varied in their perceptions), but the prevalent ideology supported and perpetuated these views.

Aware that sexual relations, unchecked, produced tangible results, Trall addressed the issue of "Regulation of the Number of Offspring." He subtitled the section "Woman's Rights" and stated that pregnancy was absolutely an issue that women should control.[32] To regulate the number of offspring, according to Trall, women should participate in the sexual embrace only when they felt inclined toward it:

> Woman's equality in all the relations of life implies her absolute supremacy in the sexual relation [since women's health, mental well being, and happiness are directly imperiled if they bear children against their will]. . . . It is her absolute and indefeasible right to determine when she will, and when she will not, be exposed to pregnancy.[33]

Trall then went on to describe the infallibility of abstinence, but noted:

> If sexual intercourse is intended as a love act, independent of reproduction, then it becomes expedient and proper, in all cases where married women do not desire children, and in all cases where they are not fitted bodily and mentally to nourish and train them properly, and in all cases where extreme poverty deprives them of the means of either mental or physical culture, to prevent pregnancy without interdicting sexual intercourse.[34]

For preventing pregnancy, Trall described in great detail the "safe" days of the month for intercourse (i.e., couples should begin abstaining ten or twelve days after the menstrual flow ceased). He noted, however, that this method was not infallible and recounted cases where pregnancy had resulted. He then suggested that women pay close attention to their menstrual flow and, in so doing, chart their fertile periods. If this is an uncertain method for some, Trall suggested watching the menstrual cloth for a clot, signifying the decay of the egg and hence indicating that intercourse is safe. It is worth noting that, according to modern medicine, ovulation usually occurs fourteen days before the next menstrual cycle; the most fertile period for most women is forty-eight to seventy-two hours from the time of ovulation.

Should all these measures fail to prevent pregnancy, Trall discussed abortive techniques in great detail. First he noted that "very soon after impregnation, or even conception, any sudden and violent motions which agitate the pelvic viscera and cause the uterus to contract vigorously, will prevent pregnancy." Equally efficacious were drastic purgatives and violent coughing or sneezing. Running, jumping, lifting, and dancing could be successful if resorted to immediately after "connection." Vaginal injections of cold water, or warm water "employed within a minute or two after coition, prevent pregnancy in a majority of cases."[35] Similarly, drugs such as bicarbonate of soda and other alkaline preparations, when injected into the vagina, would induce abortion. Trall also described self-induced abdominal manipulations, which "by a voluntary bearing-down effort, so compress the abdominal muscles upon the pelvic viscera as to cause the uterus to contract with a degree of force that expels [or moves] the impregnated egg."[36] Trall attributed significant success to this method and noted that "such an abdominal kneading and squeezing as would result in abortion [can be done] without the benefit of physicians or the aid of physiologists." A final method for preventing pregnancy is "a piece of soft sponge introduced as high up the vaginal canal as possible," although he cautioned about the likelihood of the sponge becoming dislodged and impregnation occurring.[37]

These graphic descriptions of contraceptives and abortifacients complete, Trall articulated one sweeping disclaimer as to the desirability and wisdom of abortion: "Let it be distinctly understood that I do not approve any method for preventing pregnancy except that of abstinence, nor any means for producing abortion, on the ground that it is or can be in any sense physiological. It is only the least of two evils."[38]

The evil greater than birth control and abortion, according to Trall, was the enslavement of women through unwanted children. "When people will live physiologically . . . there will be no need of preventive measures, nor will there then be any need for works of this kind," he concluded. But since that day had not yet arrived and since women were "compelled" to bear children who could not possibly be reared and who would be a constant drain on their life force,

They have implored me for a remedy, and so long as the present ignorance prevails, or the present false habits of society exist, so long will there be a demand for relief in this direction. And if these sufferers cannot find the desired remedy in the knowledge imparted by this work, they will seek it in more desperate and more dangerous measures. Who can blame them?[39]

Trall's willingness to discuss birth-control techniques and abortion, despite his ambivalences, becomes further clarified and understandable when one considers his "Theory of Population." This theory posited that births should only replace deaths; therefore, each couple should have only two children. Trall's social goal that "the amount of life shall be the greatest possible, and the births and deaths the fewest possible" can be accomplished only by the vision of character and vitality proposed by "the Health Reformers, who are, therefore, the only ones who can hasten on the millennial period."[40] Here, he was critiquing the Malthusian doctrine, which views war, pestilence, famine, and intemperance as population "weeding-out factors." Dismayed, he noted that this doctrine made disorder the rule of the universe and order the exception. His vision entailed a "self-adjusting law," since progress "is the fundamental and all-pervading law of the universe." This self-adjusting law involved calculated manipulation of means to achieve desired ends (here, population control to arrive at health). Without this schema, "there can be no millennial period this side of 'the future state'; no rational basis on which to predicate any great reform among men, or advancement of the whole human family in knowledge, virtue and happiness."[41]

As Trall's views of birth control and abortion exemplify, hydropathy's goal was to perfect self-regulation, resulting in social virtue. His view of prostitution, the "Social Vice," demonstrates the interconnectedness of the two goals. Prostitution was more than a moral or sexual issue; it entailed economic, health, and societal factors as well. As Trall argued: "If young women were allowed equal opportunities with young men for education and occupation, one-half of the sum causes of prostitution would be removed at once."[42] Individual reform, therefore, would lead to social justice, and vice versa.

Care during Pregnancy and Childbirth: "The Curse Removed"

Therapeutically, the hydropathic management of women's physiology involved active interventionism, despite the belief in the "naturalness" of these processes. What was noteworthy was that the body was, essentially, left to heal itself. With water employed as the active agent, nothing interfered with that process. Hydropaths did believe that water was critical to the successful management of medical cases, as a tonic to the nerves, a cleansing agent, an enematic, a stimulant to the skin, a conduit for diseased fluids, a reliever of weaknesses, a toner for the system, and an aid in a variety of other specific medical situations.

Complaints during pregnancy, which allopaths treated by bleeding, cathartics, blister wraps, and mercury, met with wet sheets, packs, plunges, and sitz baths under hydropathic care. Gove Nichols wrote that

> the treatment I have adopted most generally, in pregnancy, has been daily wet sheet packing, which is a powerful tonic to the nerves. The patient has remained in this pack till a warm glow was established over the whole body. This is usually accomplished in an hour and a half, and sometimes in half that time. They have sometimes used the plunge bath, and sometimes the dripping sheet after the pack. The sitz bath once or twice a day, cold water enemas to keep the bowels open, if inclined to costiveness, and vaginal injections of cold water, particular attention to diet, pure air, and exercise, have also been carefully enjoined. Peculiar cases have needed peculiar treatment, but the above treatment has been used in a majority of cases.
>
> The consequence has been, that the duration of labors under my care has been from 20 minutes to 4½ hours. With one exception I have had no labor over 4½ hours. Ladies who have had long and severe labors before they came under water treatment, have had their time of suffering reduced from 48 hours to one hour, and in several instances the time of labor has been reduced to a few minutes.[43]

Reflecting similar procedures, Shew in 1846 recounted a case of pregnancy that he had handled in his private practice. "Pregnancy and Childbirth" explained the prenatal care for the mother:

> She performed two ablutions daily, and took sitz-baths; discontinued the use of tea and coffee, took very little animal food, living principally upon coarse bread, hominy, cracked wheat and fruits. She took frequent exercise in the open air, and by these means became sensibly invigorated in general health, and was kept perfectly free from unpleasant symptoms of every kind.[44]

Mrs. O.C.W. of Fairfield, New York, had a similarly positive childbirth experience. Her article in the journal was entitled "Childbirth—a Contrast." Her first child had been delivered by an allopathic physician, and she noted that "all the 'regular' results followed: A broken breast, sore nipples, O horror! and the like, kept me confined to my bed nearly two months; and it was not until about the middle of the following summer that I attained my former health and strength."[45] On May 17, 1850, Mrs.

O.C.W. was again confined. This time she had practiced daily bathing and also made use of the wet bandages. She had followed a hydropathic diet and been attended by

> intelligent females of the Water-Cure order. Of doctors we had no need. . . . At the commencement of labor, I took a sitz bath, and an enema of cold water; these soothed me into a quiet sleep, and seemed to prepare me for my coming trials. After the birth of the child, I was allowed to remain about an hour; I was then bathed in cool water, and linen towels wet in cold water were applied to the abdomen.[46]

Mrs. O.C.W. concluded her tale with descriptions of the diet she followed, daily ablutions, and her speedy recovery. Aware that her use of the water cure in pregnancy had stirred some local gossip, she remarked:

> In this vicinity . . . my practice in hydropathy, which has been variously termed rashness, presumption, and folly, furnished, for some time, a general topic for conversation among the neighboring pro allopathies. Well, let them talk, we can, we need not care, when the world is thereby to be benefited.[47]

The theme of self-doctoring raised by Mrs. O.C.W. was repeated in a brief "filler" in the August 1853 issue of the journal. A father from Petersburg, New York, wrote that because his wife had practiced hydropathy, no physician was needed during her labor.[48]

Ever mindful that the successful and undramatic treatment of pregnancy could do much to secure a loyal female following, Shew's two-part "Twelve Cases in Midwifery with Details of Treatment" used case studies from his private practice to illustrate the efficacy of water cure in parturition. Case 3, from July 31, 1850, details the delivery of a woman's tenth child:

> She ate no flesh-meat during pregnancy [and drank] pure water only. . . . Labor commenced in the evening, and soon after, at the recommendation of her husband, she was sponged over the whole surface with cold spring water, and soon after took a cold sitting bath. In about an hour after this she was delivered of a fine plump boy weighing ten pounds. After resting a little and being somewhat fatigued and suffering some pain, her husband proposed another ablution to which she readily consented. After this she slept well till sun-rise the next morning.[49]

T. L. Nichols maintained in "The Curse Removed" that water-cure treatment in pregnancy relieved women's weaknesses, radically altered women's mischievous clothing (under the cure, they did not wear tight clothes), restored the tone of the entire system, carried them safely through the period of gestation, shortened the duration and mitigated the pain of labor, allowed the immediate removal of the placenta and prevented hemorrhage and postbirth pains, removed all danger of puerperal fever and inflammation, secured a rapid recovery and freedom from *prolapsus uteri,* and promoted healthy and well-developed offspring.[50] The claims of Gove Nichols, Shew, and T. L. Nichols, and the testimonies of women who had used water-cure therapies in pregnancy, all asserted that hydropathy offered the best treatment for pregnancy. In specific instances, unsubstantiated claims are made by these proponents, such as that the water cure "removes all danger of puerperal fever and inflammation." Whether hydropathy offered the best treatment is debatable. What it did offer was an active role for the delivering woman that engaged her physically, emotionally, and mentally; much tactile stimulation; near-constant attendants (thus providing support and communication); noninterference with nature's ability to heal; and therapeutics that did not induce further feelings of suffering and distress (which drugs and purgatives were known to produce).

Menstruation and Other Female Conditions

Menstruation received significant attention. Once again, the emphasis was on understanding women's physiology, on hygiene, and on water processes. Treatment was delineated in "Bathing to Be Practiced during the Time of Menstruation—Treatment in Suppressed and Painful Menstruation"[51] and in Trall's *Pathology of the Reproductive Organs,* which described the cause, symptoms, and treatment for retained menstruation, suppressed menstruation, dysmenorrhea, excessive menstruation, vicarious menstruation, and irregular cessation of menstruation.[52] An example of hydropathic management of dysmenorrhea (painful menstruation) entailed

alleviat[ing] the suffering of the patient [during the attack]. The cure must be attempted by means of treatment during the intervals. Fomentations, vaginal injections of warm water, and warm or hot sitz-baths, as in *suppression* [of menstruation], are the leading measures. Should there be constipation, the bowels should be freed by enema of tepid water. The full warm-bath, for fifteen to twenty minutes, or, better still, the electro-chemical or hydro-chemical bath, when practicable, should be employed daily in severe cases.[53]

Water therapy for older women was also proclaimed for its the general promotion of good health. Mrs. Scott, a New Yorker, wrote in the journal in 1847:

I commenced bathing last spring, and it certainly appears to have done me much good. Although I am sixty-nine years of age, I went out every morning to the bath room and took my cold bath until after Christmas. I yet continue my ablutions and have not taken colds as I did before I commenced the baths. I feel better, and in every respect improved.[54]

At the end of this testimony the editor encouragingly asked, "Aged mothers, how many of you will follow the example of our worthy friend, Mrs. Scott?"[55]

In acute female diseases, hydropaths were ready with emergency therapeutics. A woman suffering from uterine hemorrhage had come to Gove Nichols greatly alarmed by her weakened condition and loss of blood due to hemorrhage. Treatment by allopathic physicians had failed. Gove Nichols, on seeing the patient, "ordered a deep sitz bath from a very cold well. She remained in this bath half an hour, and then was wrapped about the abdomen and limbs in a wet sheet. . . . There was at first but slight abatement of the hemorrhage, and I ordered the half bath for two hours."[56] On the fourth day of treatment the patient was able to resume her regular duties, while she employed diet modifications to stave off further hemorrhages, a seemingly successful regimen that occasioned only one relapse, several months later, which was also checked with water.

Like pregnancy, childbirth, problematic menstruation, and uterine hemorrhage, *prolapsus uteri* (displaced womb, a common problem caused by, among other factors, incorrect use of obstetrical instruments) was particularly conducive to home self-doctoring. As Mercy P. Howes wrote in 1847, she had been severely debilitated with a fallen womb (and much attendant inflammation) since 1840. After unsuccessful treatment by two allopaths, during which time she suffered from dyspepsia, dysentery, diarrhea, and cholic, Howes visited the Massachusetts General Hospital but found no relief. According to her narrative, Dr. Bigelow, the head physician at the hospital, advised her to try the water cure. So instructed,

I returned home and immediately commenced the treatment. I used the sitting bath daily, except when too much fatigued. [Then, if too tired to bathe] I would . . . apply ice to my bowels, letting it remain on the parts for an hour. This I found to be very soothing, and always refreshed me. I took a sponge bath occasionally, but kept the head cool.[57]

This done for two years, Howes improved markedly. She then utilized the wet sheet and shower bath, which "had a better effect than my former applications." The combined therapeutics enabled her to walk again and abandon the use of her "chair with wheels."

P. H. Hayes, several years later, corroborated Howes's experience in a two-part article in the journal. Hayes reported that "we believe the baths, exercises and diet of the Water-Cure thoroughly and philosophically adapted to the cure of this disorder, and if combined with a more physiological treatment than supporters and pessaries for overcoming displacement, are almost infallibly successful."[58] Hayes wrote of a young woman who had been brought to the Wyoming, New York, Water-Cure on a bed. She had been an invalid for nine years, and her nervous system was exhausted from uterine and other displacements, misdirected medication, and poor digestion. Under the water-cure treatment for eight months, she was eventually able to walk four to eight miles daily. "She was restored to good health."[59]

Hydropaths also devoted attention to barrenness, long thought to have been helped at Europe's spas.[60] Shew and Pierson, writing as the editors in an 1847 *Water-Cure Journal* article, attributed fertile properties to water on *hygienic,* not *mystical* (or mineral), grounds:

> I have known and heard of numbers of cases, in which by a prudent course of bathing, exercise, &c., the use of a plain and unstimulating diet, and the observing of proper temperance in the marital privileges, persons have borne children when most earnestly, and by a great variety of means, that object had been sought in vain.[61]

Treatment of Nonorganic Complaints

Hydropaths also offered insights, and remedies, for women with nonorganic complaints. Observing hysterics—those who manifested nervousness and frustration—they noted that such patients usually "select a comfortable place for this fit." As appropriate treatment they counseled:

> Place the head over a basin, and pour water from a jug over the head and chest till the patient becomes chilly and relieves. Never use anything but cold water for the hysterical fit, unless the party turns very cold, when you should discontinue it, and apply warmth to the feet. I once saw the cold applied for three hours, but the patient was quite well the next day.[62]

This treatment, used for nervousness and insanity, while brusque—even severe—sought to quieten the patient.[63]

Dr. L. Reuben, in an 1850 essay, "Imaginary Diseases," lamented the ridiculing by supposedly learned people of patients with nervous ailments as "'*hypos*' or NOTHING BUT HYSTERICS!" Reuben contended that these diseases were the most debilitating: "When will such persons learn that there is not such a thing as an imaginary disease under heaven;

and that those diseases which they call imaginary, are positively *the most real and tormenting* that poor human flesh ever writhed and groaned under, this side of paradise?"[64] All such ailments, he concluded, have a "*bodily something* grating upon the nerves, and thus producing those unhappy sensations, no matter whether we can or cannot see it—can or cannot name it!"[65]

While validating the real discomfort brought by nervous ailments, Reuben, like his colleagues, urged the sufferers to adjust their life habits via dietary changes, frequent exercise, bathing, and dress reform. By so doing, he turned the focus away from the symptoms and toward the cause. The patient's passive expression of malaise, discontent, and frustration was transformed into an active participation in recovery and self-determination: Preventive measures were stressed over symptomatic interventionism. In nervous ailments, perhaps more clearly than in organic medical problems, the potency of the healing dyad was evident. Here, the water treatment itself did not yield a demonstrable and replicable link between treatment and effect, just as in heroic medicine. Sedation or patient weariness were probably the most likely somatic outcomes of the hydropathic therapeutics. In both hydropathy and allopathy, therefore, the presence of the healer and the attention given to the condition were the strongest assets. In this instance, it is likely that "being cared for" could be measured in terms of not producing further suffering and discomfort.

In fact, all of the hydropathic movement's writings on the subject of women's diseases and their treatment stressed the cessation of suffering, often through a virulent antiallopathic sentiment. Texts and the journal alike directed a veritable rage at the allopaths. Trall described the regular therapeutics for ovaritis in *Pathology of the Reproductive Organs:*

> The "drug and destructive" medication prescribed for ovaritis in the "regular" medical books on the Diseases of Women, is if possible, a little more deadly than anything we have yet seen. It is summed up by Churchill [an allopathic physician] in a single bloody and *murderous* sentence: "Venesection, leeches to the iliac region, to the groin, anus or labia, poultice and fomentations to the lower belly, calomel and opium."[66]

In articles such as "Allopathic Midwifery" and "Bleeding during Pregnancy" the water-curers unleashed their scorn on allopathic theory and therapeutics.[67]

In addition to the cessation of suffering, a consistent theme was the urging of female readers to adopt not only hygienic living principles but other reforms as well. Caring for one's own health was but the first step in an ever-broadening sphere of female influence. Trall, in *Pathology of the Reproductive Organs,* implored a woman suffering from leukorrhea ("whites") to adopt the bloomer costume. Dr. Ellen H. Goodell, in describing "The Cause of Female Diseases," cited numerous "physical transgressions" including unventilated rooms; restrictive clothing assigned to female children; requiring young girls to play indoors only; unwholesome food; excessive drugging of girls at puberty; tight dressing as an adult; and a lack of reproductive information, leading to unwanted pregnancies, unhealthy maternity, and a premature grave.[68] For each of these "violations of hygienic law," a corollary reform was offered as a solution. The alternatives inherent in vegetarianism, dress reform, physical education, temperance, and birth-control information were all explicitly stated in the theory and therapeutics behind the hydropathic management of women's diseases and promised painless pregnancies and healthy later years. Encouraged to be active shapers of their own physiological futures, women in the water-cure movement found other, wider, issues of female autonomy and reform awaiting their attention.

New Horizons for Women

Consciously citing the cultural connection between "woman's character" and her nurturant roles and responsibilities, the *Water-Cure Journal* authors continuously addressed articles to the interests of women (as mothers and nurturers and, later, as prospective brides and unmarried women). The editors of the journal, not unlike most of their contemporaries, believed that the future of the nation lay in woman's protective power and moral influence over hearth and family. By addressing women on issues not directly related to health and by expanding the definition of health to include nearly every aspect of human activity, the water-cure movement additionally sought to encourage women's interest and activism not only in the traditional female spheres of influence but also in the social and political realms. This expanded definition of health served a second purpose: It led to increased medical claims and broadened the possibilities for intervention.[69] In short, hydropaths encouraged female participation in the public as well as the private domain, thus widening their sphere of influence.

Indicative of the writings that promoted women's expanded spheres of influence is Gove Nichols's article, "Education. A Letter from Mrs. Gove Nichols." She urged women to take primary responsibility for the health of themselves and their families.[70] In the same 1852 issue Mrs. C.M.S. from Waukesha County, Wisconsin, wrote an impassioned letter proclaiming the benefits of water treatment and speaking adamantly against the use of tobacco. The editors, pleased with her letter, titled it "Our Mothers Are the Best Reformers."[71] A third article in the issue, "Physical Development the Duty of Mothers," by R. Roxana, spoke strongly about a mother's duty to raise her daughters to be strong. Of the daughters, she wrote: "Moored and kept in the soft and downy nest of physical ease and inactivity; reared and nurtured in the hot-house of parental indulgence; or made the pampered weaklings of air tight nurseries how poorly will they be fitted for the competent discharge of the duties of the maternal office!"[72] A fourth and final article in the issue, "Advice to Weakly Females," by Theodosia, confirms that hydropathy was as much a woman's health movement as it was a larger health reform.[73] In fact, many a yearly prospectus for the journal featured a subheading "To Women and Mothers," thus emphasizing the natural applicability of the water cure for women's purposes.[74]

Numerous articles appealed to women, as mothers and as nurturers, by way of their children's health. For example, "To Mothers" by "A Mother" testified that the water cure had saved her baby boy. Shew's "For Mothers. A Short Case" discussed jaundice, nursing, sore mouth, indigestion, wind, colic, and constipation in a young child; and the poem "Thank God for Water" was written by a mother whose fevered daughter had been saved.[75] Other reform journals of the day often published similar accounts on the efficacy of the water cure, for example, "Daisy Has Left Us" in *The Sibyl—For Reforms* in 1860.[76] In this article, bereaved parents lamented having strayed from strict water-cure processes, which had saved their daughter once before.

In addition to advice on child care, articles in the *Water-Cure Journal* on home management were aimed at capturing the general female readership. In December 1848 "A Good Mother" argued that all young women should learn to cook.[77] Still affirming women's domestic role, Rachel Brooks Gleason (cofounder of the Elmira, New York, Water-Cure and spouse of Silas O. Gleason, a hydropath) in "Letters to Ladies" (July 1867) discussed how to make culinary chores easier.[78] Similarly, "Women at Home," a lead article by the Reverend O. B. Frothingham, discussed the problems that ensue when women's work in the home is done largely by machines. In an oft-repeated cross-class emphasis, Frothingham also depicted the difficulties of women wage earners.[79] Other issues pertinent to women's familial and social responsibilities received attention, such as "Letters to Ladies' Society," which detailed how to bear the demands of visiting, and Mollie Bryant's "Visiting the Sick," which described the courtesies and etiquette surrounding that task.[80]

Husband–wife relations were a popular journal topic, with authors aiming for stabilization and equalization in the marriage relationship. A June 1861 article, "Scissoring. How to Heal a Longing for Divorce," was followed in August by "Married Life," which spoke of the importance of the wife's influence.[81] Two months later, Louisa Bell's "The Paternal Headship" conducted a frank discussion of the necessary limits of a father's authority.[82] A six-year pause found these issues still popular in 1867, when F.G.'s "How to Keep a Husband," in a more conservative tone, urged women to continue to woo their mate. To this end they must keep the house neat and in order, adjust the household to suit the husband, and continue to grow "in knowledge and graces of the mind and heart."[83] "Wooing" in this sense entailed keeping the initial attraction and stimulation ever present.

Occasionally, columns of this nature were addressed to men, who had similar gender-specific obligations, such as Dr. Ellen H. Goodell's "Responsibilities of Fathers." Arguing first for male sexual restraint and then for masculine support of the wife's daily role, Goodell wrote: "Never, oh, never! impose upon her the duties of maternity until she is prepared to meet them; never cease your devotion to that wife who is part of yourself. . . . Aid her in every possible way, let her pleasure be yours also . . . and you will be amply repaid."[84] Two years later, the Reverend Henry Ward Beecher's "How to Choose a Wife" again addressed a male readership. Health, he argued, was the main physical criterion.[85]

By urging their female readers to act as guardians of their family's health, overseers of their children's physical future, home managers, and equal partners in the marriage relationship, hydropathic leaders addressed issues of primary concern within the female sphere of home and family. Yet while all these writers stressed health as the common thread of women's participation in the movement, they did not encourage women to participate solely as home practitioners and as patients. Once the foundation was laid for communication and rapport through these domestic issues, hydropathic philosophy consciously urged women to expand their participation in the movement *beyond* the domestic sphere. Since health was women's province and since health touched every aspect of human activity, they argued, women needed to use their reformist zeal in the public realm.

Women as Physicians: "Never has woman had such an opening for usefulness and influence as this"

One of the first areas in which the hydropathic leaders sought to implement this public participation was in the movement's need for women physicians. As numerous historians have noted, much nineteenth-century medical practice was not open to women.[86] Opponents of female physicians employed the familiar arguments of mental inferiority, erratic physiological processes that rendered women unfit, inability to travel in the wilderness, and the unsettling prospect that if women were admitted, Negroes would surely be next.[87] The 1840s, 1850s, and 1860s were peppered with the names of women who sought admission to allopathic medical facilities: Harriet Hunt applied to the Harvard Medical School in 1847 and 1850; in 1852 Dr. Nancy Talbot Clark was the first woman to seek certification from a state medical society; and by 1850 the Boston City Directory listed six female doctors, which was 2 percent of the physician population.[88]

Perhaps the saga (for indeed it was that) of Elizabeth Blackwell best symbolizes women's reception in allopathic institutions. Incorrectly known as the first woman physician (she was, in fact, the first woman to graduate from an allopathic college), Blackwell received her degree from the Geneva Medical College in western New York, where the all-male student body had voted her in as a prank. Blackwell experienced severe difficulty (and often humiliation) in her professional training and on graduation could not find placement at any hospital in New York. (It will be remembered that she sought refuge as a patient at the Grafenberg Water-Cure in the 1850s after having graduated.) Blackwell finally started a private practice, and she eventually opened the Woman's Medical College of the New York Infirmary for Women and Children in 1868.[89] Blackwell, with similar-minded women who sought admission to and credibility within allopathy, did succeed in attaining, by 1900, "approximately five thousand trained women doctors in the land, fifteen hundred female medical students and seven medical schools exclusively for women."[90]

In the early years of the nineteenth century, many women committed to the practice of medicine followed neither Blackwell's path nor her reasoning.[91] As the "conversion narratives" suggest, many women chose to doctor through the water cure deliberately, not because they were excluded from allopathic schools; unlike Blackwell, they decided to practice healing through the hygienic, reformist sects. Adhering to beliefs of nature's ability to heal, the notion that the milder therapeutics of these sects were more in keeping with women's nature, and the conviction that women's modesty might best be preserved through the use of physicians of their own sex (a belief often shared by allopathic women practitioners), these self-conscious sectarian reformers turned, instead, to hygienic medicine that emphasized domestic self-doctoring. It is possible, of course, that some women joined reform sects because they were barred from regular medicine. Evidence suggests, however, that women did not become hydropathic practitioners because they were barred from regular medical schools or because of a general public abhorrence of women in a "male" profession. Instead, bad experiences as patients, a reformist nature, dichotomous cultural perceptions of allopathy and hydropathy as they "courted" women's participation, and the positive gender consciousness of the water-cure movement make *choice* and a compatible belief system a far more likely explanation than rejection.[92]

It is possible that hydropathy was not alone on this score, since, as one historian noted, "Most of the women who obtained medical training or degrees before 1851 went to . . . Eclectic or other irregular institutions."[93] Botanics, homeopaths, mesmerists, Thomsonians, and eclectics all welcomed women in their ranks. But no sect was quite so eager, so totally committed, to the full participation of female physicians as was hydropathy.

Leaders in the water-cure movement argued for women's *right* to

practice medicine, and from the inception of the American Hydropathic
Institute (the New York City Water-Cure college founded by Gove Nichols
and T. L. Nichols in 1851), the total involvement of women was solicited.
A passage from T. L. Nichols's article on the principles of hydropathic
medical education presents the argument in favor of women physicians:

> Never has woman had such an opening for usefulness and influence,
> as this. No Water-Cure establishment is complete without a qualified
> female physician. No community will be long content without one.
> Dealing out drugs, bleeding, blistering and torturing, are not woman's
> work; but the gentle ministrations of the Water-Cure, especially as
> applied to her own sex and to children, belong peculiarly to
> her. . . . So few are the avenues of useful and honorable labor open
> to women, that when a new one offers there should be no lack of
> candidates.[94]

The inaugural address delivered at the opening of the American
Hydropathic Institute in September 1851 was reprinted as the lead article
in the next month's *Water-Cure Journal.* "Woman the Physician" was
delivered by Gove Nichols, who was herself the embodiment of the kind
of woman hydropathic leaders hoped to attract to the movement. She
reviewed the "fortunate" exclusion of women from allopathy and their
noticeable presence in homeopathy. As medicine became more humane,
she predicted, women's participation would increase, and that was as it
should be, since "women are peculiarly fitted to practice the art of healing [because of their] tenderer love, the sublimer devotion, the never to
be wearied patience and kindness of woman."[95]

Relying on a fascinating combination of arguments that ranged from
traditional perceptions of "woman's nature" to a classic egalitarian rationale,
Gove Nichols believed that all of humanity would benefit from the use
of women physicians. She stressed a clear-cut feminist and emancipationist
rationale:

> We want truer and more elevated ideas of womanhood. We must
> have free, noble, healthy mothers, before we can have men. The
> cramped waist, the crushed vitals, the loaded spine, the trailing
> skirts, the fettered limbs, the feeble, fearful being, who has no
> rights but to be maintained, protected, and doctored, can train us
> no Washingtons, Franklins, or Jeffersons, no wise or great men, and
> no women worthier the name than their mothers. We want women
> who can break the bonds of custom, who are great enough to be
> emancipated from all that weakens, degrades, and destroys, and
> who will teach others the holy lessons of a true freedom, not to be
> independent of man, but that man and woman should be mutually
> dependent.[96]

The *Water-Cure Journal* reported on every aspect of women in medicine. It covered such issues and events as the formation of the Ladies Medical Missionary Society, whose secretary, Mrs. S. J. Hale, supported female physicians and missionaries; the contemporary debate surrounding the use of male midwives (Trall and four readers were against male midwifery); and the decision, derisively entitled "A Step Backward," by the Cincinnati Eclectic Medical College to exclude women from its 1858 winter term to protect their health.[97] Interestingly, in the college controversy the editors of the journal quoted the feminist paper *The Lily,* which reminded the excluded women students that they had women-only schools to turn to. To this, the editors responded: "We would beg leave to remind *The Lily* that special schools for the education of female physicians exclusively, are as unnatural and unphysiological as are schools for males exclusively. A medical school should educate doctors, not sex."[98] This disapproval of women-only schools was based on the recurring premise that the natures of men and women combine to produce the most effective, and socially beneficial, result. This emphasis on the complementary nature of men and women did not, however, prohibit hydropathic support for gender-specific issues and goals. The *Water-Cure Journal* traced the progress of the all-women schools, even though it disagreed with their premise. "Female Physicians" discussed the attack the Female Medical College of Pennsylvania had undergone at the hands of male allopathic colleagues, and while the journal was in favor of neither single-sex schools nor allopathic therapeutics, it called the allopaths' accusations against the women's school unfair and unfounded.[99]

The hydropathic leadership also sought to legitimize and popularize hygienic nursing. Dr. Huldah Allen urged that "hundreds of young women, middle-aged women and old women, should qualify themselves, especially, for Hygienic Nurses."[100]

Articles discussing the propriety, wisdom, and necessity of female practitioners seemed never-ending. An 1867 piece, "Shall Women Be Doctors?" sounds very similar to Gove Nichols's 1851 "Woman the Physician." Sixteen years had passed, but the arguments remained similar:

> Give woman a profession of honor, of trust, of usefulness, and of dignity, and you give her motives for cultivating womanliness, higher graces, a more devoted life. . . . Our advice, therefore, to women is to become physicians wherever they have the taste, the necessary qualification, the head and the heart.[101]

Hydropathic theorists—and followers—believed that medical practice would provide the wedge for women's further instrumentality in health—and beyond—as Dr. M. L. Holbrook concluded in his oratory: "It is in this field that we hope to see woman labor; and here we bid her a hearty welcome, and will say and do all in our power to help her to achieve a useful destiny."[102]

While theoretical arguments may have remained virtually unchanged, the number and force of female water-cure physicians had not. Although only Gove Nichols, Harriet N. Austin, and Rachel Brooks Gleason (of the Elmira Water-Cure) are even slightly remembered as trained female hydropathic practitioners, numerous women underwent the course of study at the American Hydropathic Institute (later, the Hygeio-Therapeutic College) in New York City or elsewhere. Commencement notices from the institute, as published in the *Water-Cure Journal*, carefully noted the size and gender composition of each class. In addition, the marital status of the graduating women (only) was noted; perhaps to encourage husband–wife teams such as the Shews, Tralls, Nicholses, Gleasons, and Jacksons; to emphasize the possibility of linking medical work and married life; or to advertise the feasibility, for unmarried women, of becoming a physician. This meticulous recording of a class's gender breakdown reflected a self-conscious attempt to encourage and highlight female enrollment. From May 1852 through May 1862 the data available reveal gender percentages as follows: May 1852—9 graduates, 4 women; July 1854—15 graduates, 3 Mrs., 3 Misses; May 1856—20 graduates, 4 Mrs., 3 Misses; August 1858—"A large enrollment with 50 percent women is expected"; May 1859—25 graduates, 7 Mrs., 5 Misses; May 1861—20 graduates, 3 Mrs., 4 Misses; May 1862—16 graduates, 8 women.[103]

Women graduates went on to be affiliated with private practices or water-cure establishments; those connected with specific cures in western Massachusetts and upstate New York are discussed in Chapter Three. Some women water-cure practitioners went on to found or manage their own establishments to serve women only. These included Dr. Amelia W. Lines (in the Williamsburg section of Brooklyn) and Dr. Mary Ann Case (Norwich, New York).[104]

Other women practitioners, who did not go the route of the American Hydropathic Institute, the Hygeio-Therapeutic College, or a similar school,[105] and therefore had no formal training, also had their activities charted in the journal. It is likely that many of these practitioners learned hydropathic techniques within a loosely organized "apprenticeship" relationship with a practicing hydropath. Indicative of the hydropathic practitioners whose educational backgrounds, institutional affiliations, and professional activities were charted despite their lack of hard credentials is a "Letter from Miss Coggswell, M.D.," which tells of her travels, her observations of water-cure establishments, and her upcoming summer in Hudson, Ohio, to care for a sick sister.[106] A similar piece by Dr. Adaline M. W. Weed tells of her "Water-Cure Travel on the Pacific Coast."[107]

Women water-cure physicians, then, were the clearest manifestation of hydropathy's consciously articulated goal of expanding woman's opportunities for moral influence and her just rewards from the domestic sphere into the larger social realm. The philosophy reflected in hydropathic writings and by the hydropathic leadership evinced an emancipationist feminism that, although based on the ideology of domesticity, sanctioned—even impelled—an extension of women's abilities and activities into the *in*formally political world.[108]

Solicited for their womanly qualities and strong minds, women physicians were utilized to their fullest and implored not to abandon their moble mission. As Mrs. McAndrew, a graduate of the American Hydropathic Institute, wrote to her female co-graduates in 1859 through the *Water-Cure Journal:*

> My Dear Sisters—I often think of you. . . . As a general thing, we are far apart from each other and our chances for sweet communion and fellowship are but few. . . . Some few years ago, in many instances, we were objects of scorn and suspicion. We were looked upon as singular beings, as "strong-minded women," who were out of their spheres. . . . But, my dear sisters, nothing can harm us, if we be followers of that which is good. . . . Let us continue to do our duty unflinchingly. Let us teach the principles of our hygienic system with unremitting diligence. Let us hold forth by the bedside, by the fireside, and by the wayside, and let us fearlessly tell our patients the reason why they or their children are sick, whether they will hear or whether they will forebear: and in due time blessings shall descend upon our heads. At all events, we must "learn to labor, and to wait."[109]

The reformist zeal and self-sacrifice so evident in this communication illustrate the life commitment that often accompanied the practice of hydropathy. And as the testimony of Mrs. McAndrew embodies that commitment, her training represents the hydropathic belief in woman's *right*, natural affinity, and inclination (via her gender propensity to nurture and to act as moral educator) to practice medicine. This inducement for women to practice medicine, preceded by the hydropathic renovation of medical practice itself, reflected the reform ideology that characterized the hydropathic movement.

Conclusions

The female audience for and the practitioners of hydropathy were attracted to the theoretical and therapeutic empowerment inherent in the system. The therapeutically moderate, interventionist, and hygienic approach to disease management, the deemphasis of physician omnipotence, and the self-doctoring that hydropathy emphasized naturally carried over into the management of women's diseases. Not now seen as sickness, women's physiology and reproductive processes were hygienically treated with water and alterations in personal living habits.

In addition to their approach to women's diseases, and because they did not view women's intellectual abilities as inextricably linked to their sexual physiology, hydropaths were able to reconceptualize both women's capacity for intellectual work and their sphere of social influence. Thus the hydropathic movement actively solicited female physicians and urged women to utilize water-cure philosophy as a positive alternative to the passive social role available to them elsewhere.

Through this combination of therapeutics, the redefining of women's physiology, the solicitation of women's activism, and the advocacy of corollary reforms, the hydropathic movement advocated an expansion of women's sphere. For these reasons, the ideology and opportunities provided through hydropathy became a retreat for the nineteenth-century woman searching for an alternative philosophy that stressed her capabilities, strengths, and potentialities. Ideally, this vision could be realized communally and unequivocally at a live-in cure.

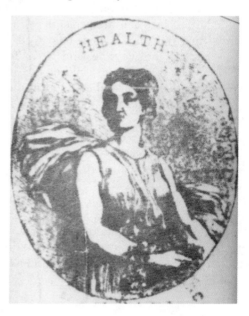

Chapter Three

Ideology in Practice
Water-Cure Establishments

Yet, just as physically the institution towered above the valley, so in its mental and spiritual outlook it seemed to rise above earthly turmoil. Owned and managed by human beings, the Jackson Health Resort never claimed perfection. Evidence is ample, however, that patients and guests found there not only help for their bodies but an atmosphere of serenity, unobtrusive hospitality, genuine friendliness, and goodwill. To many, this place became Utopia.—William D. Conklin, The Jackson Health Resort

If the reader indulges the idea that life at a water cure in the city or in the country is a stupid, frigid, formal, unsocial affair, I beg leave most respectfully to undeceive him. . . . Walk or ride with me to the famous establishment located at 15 Laight Street [Trall's water cure in New York City]. . . . Are you ill, the doctor will give a diagnosis of your case, and put you at once on the road to health. If you are well, and desire to find a first-class boarding-house, he will strike a bargain with you, and you can have hotel fare, or vegetable fare, or both, as you please. . . . [The dining] tables are lined with men, women, and children. Some of them are celebrities. . . . There are doctors, lawyers, clergymen, editors, merchants, mechanics, farmers, manufacturers, clerks, students, and others. . . . [A male attendant will] introduce us to Miss Higgins, the female physician, a lady of rare attainments and unquestionable skill. . . . [I] promise to write better next time.—G. W. Bungay, "Life at a City Water-Cure"

Life at a cure seemingly reinforced all the positive elements of hydropathic living. Well over two hundred water-cure centers of healing existed from San Francisco to Maine, reflecting the immense popularity of the hydropathic movement. Their survival ranged from a few months to over a hundred years, and they were especially numerous in the East, particularly in New York, New Jersey, and Pennsylvania. The particular appeal of New York for water-cure establishments may have stemmed in part from the rich tradition of evangelical religious reform that flourished there in the first half of the nineteenth century. But as the enthusiasm for revivals waned, people's attention was turned toward phrenology, mesmerism, land reform, living experiments, and faith sects—in short, other panaceas.[1] Although the geographical overlap between the religious belt and the center of hydropathy's popularity is not always exact (in Dansville, the site of the cure *is* in the midst of the "Burned-Over District," so dubbed for the religious revivalism that flourished in the region), it seems reasonable to hypothesize that the ebbing of the religious revivals left thousands of people with energies to devote anew to the social redemption of American society. For some, the water cure was just such a calling, hence the testimonials read like conversion narratives.

In this chapter, six establishments, three in western New York and three in western Massachusetts, demonstrate the typical characteristics of a cure. These were located in Binghamton, Dansville, and Elmira, New York, and in Athol, Northampton, and Springfield, Massachusetts. All these cures promoted their facilities in the pages of the *Water-Cure Journal;* several distributed pamphlets and brochures that are still intact at local historical societies; and still others had their doings diligently charted by local newspapers. The Dansville Cure published a newsletter (the "Letter Box") detailing daily life at the cure. Letters published in the journal from patients who had frequented the cures lend insight into their life situations, surroundings, therapeutics, and communal experience. And references in autobiographical memoirs and biographical texts of cure patrons address the question of life at a cure. All these sources illuminate the composition of the clientele; exact information as to gender, place of origin, length of stay, type of ailment, and so on, can be verified either where the chronicler specifically noted them or, as to gender, where lists or estimates appeared in the journal advertisements or the cures' records and self-descriptions. A justification exists in these sources for inferences about gender consciousness and the significance of the cures for women. The sources clearly reveal a significant female clientele—which, given the impediments to women's mobility, is notable—and a positive gender-conscious sensibility pervading the larger cures.

These six establishments had diverse histories and by no means demonstrated equal longevity or stability of proprietorship. But they did have several common features: the reform activity that emanated from them, their commitment to water-cure principles that gradually expanded to include other healing methods, conflicts between the movement's philosophy and the practitioners' methods, and their use by women as a retreat. (Although these cures were not "women-only" communities, and often housed more men than women,[2] they conveyed a positive gender consciousness that appealed to and attracted women.)

Advertisements and Endorsements

Convinced that natural surroundings were the first step in determining a new outlook for patients, many hydropathic establishments stressed their country settings. Although urban establishments (e.g., Trall's Laight Street Cure) existed and flourished, patients were encouraged to stay at a rural establishment. In fact, physicians and family members who recommended a sojourn at a cure cited the curative element of travel and a change of scenery as part of the healing process. For example, Dr. Silas O. Gleason, of the Elmira Water Cure, found that

> there was a large class of patients for whom physicians could do little in their home environment. They needed change of scene, systematic and constant oversight and the most healthful of mental, moral and physical aid, free from the cares and despondency that came of routine that had grown depressing.[3]

The cure establishments advertised in the *Water-Cure Journal* and published their own literature, which heralded their facilities, staff, and successes. From the journal and the literature, a colorful and enticing picture of life at a water-cure establishment emerges.[4]

The publications of cure establishments competed to portray the beauty and serenity of their settings. Since potential patients probably governed their choice of establishment through advertisements and word-of-mouth, these broadsides and graphics, along with advertisements in the journal, were extremely important in determining an establishment's success. The Mount Prospect Water-Cure in Binghamton, New York, in a broadside distributed by Dr. J. H. North and Dr. Martha French, painted a scene of unrivaled beauty:

> The Water Cure House is situated one mile from the centre of the town, on the side of MOUNT PROSPECT, commanding a beautiful view. The hill rises four hundred feet above the House to the northward, completely sheltering it from the cold winds of winter. In summer the trees shade it, and make it cool and pleasant. The groves upon the hill afford beautiful walks, and charming views of the town, the valleys through which the Chenango and Susquehanna rivers flow to their confluence, of the surrounding mountains, and the numerous trains of the Railroads. It is believed that no similar Establishment has a finer natural location.[5]

Less than a hundred miles away, the Elmira Water Cure, under the leadership of Rachel Brooks Gleason and S. O. Gleason, overlooked a panoramic view of sweeping hills and lush woods. Even now, the unspoiled countryside and the street that has been named in more recent years "Water-Cure Hill Road" make envisioning a nineteenth-century cure an easy and pleasurable task.[6] An 1869 leaflet described the site:

> The establishment is just out of the city, on the hillside, overlooking the entire city, the river and valley of the Chemung, and the hills around, giving miles of the most varied and beautiful scenery. Our elevation gives us a dry and bracing air, so necessary in the cure of Catarrah, Throat and Lung diseases, Rheumatism, Neuralgia, and Scrofula.[7]

Massachusetts cures were no less exacting in their selection of their environs, as shown in this quote from the *Daily Hampshire Gazette* (1847) in Northampton depicting the glorious setting of Round Hill House:

> The situation of the establishment is well known to be not only *unsurpassed* but *unequalled* in beauty by any in the country. . . . From the windows . . . are spread the beautiful meadows, at one time clad in verdure redolent in Spring at another, radiant with the golden wealth of Autumn; in the distance is the pretty town of Amherst, with its college crowning the summit of a gentle acclivity, and backed by a finely undulating line of eastern horizon. . . . There is one more charming feature, which we should not omit to mention. In front of the building is the finest terrace imaginable, commanding the unrivaled prospect we have faintly described, on which the patients may promenade, and in the rear, is a beautiful wood intersected with walks, and fitted with seats, to which they can retire at pleasure, and enjoy the soothing influence of shade and cool breezes in the more heated state of the Summer atmosphere.[8]

The article goes on to note the surroundings, which included Mount Holyoke, Mount Tom, the Connecticut River, the Connecticut River Railroad, and the Farmington Canal.

Offering scenes of "unrivaled beauty" and removal from stressful situations, these cures were pastoral lures for many urban women and men suffering from organic or nonspecific ailments. The cures aimed to provide not only the most congenial setting but sex-segregated modern hydropathic conveniences and comforts as well. The buildings ranged in size from a modest one-family dwelling that housed twenty patients to mammoth structures that served as home for hundreds. The Springfield Water Cure, for example, under the proprietorship of Jasper Severance and Dr. E. Snell, was 200 feet long by 50 feet wide, three stories high, with nearly fifty rooms, separate bathing facilities for women and men, and large dressing rooms connected by an abundant supply of pure soft water.[9] Nearby, also in the Connecticut River Valley, the facilities of the Round Hill Water Cure (also called the Round Hill House) exemplified the success enjoyed by one of the larger, more prosperous cures. Reporters of the *Northampton Herald* reported in 1847:

> In the first place, we remark, that they contain over one hundred rooms. On the first floor is the great Dining Hall, which is indeed a magnificent room. It is 14 feet high, and measures 50 by 36 feet on the floor; the Saloon, which measures 38 by 35 feet; several Reception rooms; the Office; the Kitchen, &c. On the second and third floors, are numerous handsome, and most conveniently furnished chambers, with beds peculiarly adapted to the wants of invalids. From the chambers we descended to the basement, where were shown us the various conveniences for bathing, &c. . . . In addition to these, are bathing conveniences for the exclusive use of ladies.[10]

A study of Round Hill affords the rare chance to follow the growth of a cure, since it passed through several proprietors, all of whom added facilities. An 1855 article in the local newspaper reiterated some of the points of the earlier account, but several noteworthy changes had occurred, including a basement "devoted to bathing, dressing and packing rooms, including all varieties and baths, accommodated with ample heating apparatus for the winter months." Further, the cure now claims "about 150 sleeping rooms—many of them with each a handsome bathroom connected, and furnished with both hot and cold water. . . . Among the out-of-door beauties, are the piazzas, the shady walks, and various accommodations for bodily exercise and amusement combined."[11]

Other cures offered similar facilities, which invariably included sleeping quarters, a dining hall, a bathing area and, often, "an exercising hall," which at the Binghamton Water Cure was "65 feet long and 20 wide, which is provided with all the requisite appliances for the most approved gymnastic exercises."[12] Advertisements often mentioned their "ladies' bathing facilities" separately, since they were aware that these accommodations would largely determine their appeal to a female clientele. Genteel women would hesitate to entrust themselves to a practitioner or system that might offend their modesty. The reassurances that there were separate facilities and practitioners specifically trained in women's diseases fostered trust, consciously solicited women's patronage, and appealed to women's gender consciousness. Advertisements stressing that modesty would be preserved also served to allay the fears of the women's husbands (often the financiers of the stay) about the suitability of the environment. In fact, women would write home on arrival at a cure reassuring their mate or family members on just these issues.

In keeping with this solicitation of a female clientele, the Northampton Water Cure (to be distinguished from the Round Hill Water
Cure, or House, also in Northampton) specifically advertised that "the
ladies' plunge is 6 by 10 feet," and quite deep.[13] At this cure, interestingly,
the proprietor, David Ruggles, insisted that he would admit only those
patients who applied to him beforehand in writing so that he might
ascertain their suitability for water therapies. This was prompted by his
less-than-total faith in hydropathy (discussed below).[14]

The cures' advertisements either described or included sketches of
their grounds and indoor lounging rooms. The Elmira Water Cure's office for example, had a stained-glass window refracting light on the
carpeted floor and numerous wicker rockers and inviting bookshelves. A
wood stove in the corner promised winter warmth, while newspapers
and magazines scattered on the reading table implied that readers had
just left or were about to arrive. Two large pairs of antlers and a few
taxidermied fowl reminded the visitors of their rural surroundings. The
solarium was a study in comfort and hominess. In a large, glass-walled
room, rockers sat on scatter rugs interspersed among huge, healthy pot-
ted plants. The late-nineteenth-century photographs conveyed the serene
atmosphere that characterized a stay at the cure.[15]

Clients of the Cures

Cures often appealed to a specific clientele (e.g., women, sufferers
from certain ailments, physicians, weary clergy, or exhausted teachers),
yet they serviced a variety of patients, who made their choices by the
setting and accoutrements offered, the reputation of the physician in
charge, the therapies employed, and the proximity of the establishment
to the patient's home. Both male and female patients noted a discernible
"emancipationist" ideology as well as a "feminized sensibility" (particularly
at the larger cures), which affected many who frequented the cures.[16]

Isabella Waite of Savannah, Georgia, in a letter to her husband
shortly after her arrival at the cure in June 1846, recounts the range of
backgrounds and ills that her co-patients brought to "the cold water
fountains":

> No one could for a moment conceive what astounding results I
> have learned of the water-cure since I came to this place. Here may
> be seen the pious and zealous devine, his nervous system a perfect
> wreck, . . . the youthful and accomplished lady emaciated and wan
> with your hectic glow, which tells too plainly of the devouring
> disease [tuberculosis, most likely], . . . the talented physician of the
> old school, his constitution ruined with the too great a quantity of
> drugs [and] the accomplished gentleman, with his constitution ruined
> by the abuse of mercury. One man . . . had been afflicted for 25

years with paralysis of the extremities. . . . Suffice it to say, that all the patients who are here . . . are of the most decided opinion that cold water is the only universal elixir for disease. . . . Oh! you can never know the pleasure I experience at finding all my anticipations of the water-cure more than realized. When—when shall we learn that God accomplishes his mightiest works through his simplest agencies?[17]

An 1873 article on the Elmira Water Cure displayed a client population not unlike that described by Waite twenty-seven years earlier:

Within its walls have been harbored some of the foremost men and women of the age. Men of leisure and literature have here sought health and recreation. Pastors and their wives, worn with their parish work, have found rest. Physicians, ceasing for a time from their weary round, have waited themselves to be healed.

Reformers, turning for a time from their reformation, have found here fresh strength to renew their struggle. The woman of fashion, the peaceful Friend, the child and the old man, are all gathered within its walls to seek the lost boon and to find again the new fountain of youth.[18]

Because many of the staff members at Elmira had a traditional medical background before becoming "believers," they attracted a significant number of allopathic physicians seeking medical help from the water cure. The Gleasons' varied reform interests also appealed to nineteenth-century activists, to Quakers, and to clergy. Some of the illustrious patients they treated were the Beechers (Thomas, James, and Catharine), the Samuel Clemenses (who lived in Elmira), and the Langdons.[19] Of the cure, Thomas Beecher wrote:

Twenty-three years ago come June, as I strolled one Monday . . . I spied on the hillside a huge, chalky, sun-smitten building which was called the Water Cure. I went for it, I found it new, cheap, clean, honest. For three years it was my home as a single man; for three more years it was home as a married man; and for 17 years it has been our neighbor toward which the board-walk leads.[20]

The cure also treated Schuyler Colfax, vice-president of the United States under President Ulysses S. Grant; Congressman Samuel Cox, scholar and writer; the son of Brigham Young, who brought other family members; May Riley Smith, a popular literary figure of the day; Virginia Townsend, an author; and Susan B. Anthony, the women's rights activist (who also visited the Worcester, Massachusetts, Water-Cure).[21] It is unclear whether Elizabeth Cady Stanton, lifelong coworker in the cause of woman's suffrage with Anthony, ever stayed at one of the water cures, but she was clearly aware of the powerful reform influence they had. When speaking on the adoption of reform dress, she pointed out it was "worn by skaters, gymnasts, tourists, and in sanitariums. . . . Among those who wore it were Paulina Wright Davis, . . . Dr. Harriet N. Austin, and many patients in sanitariums, whose names I cannot recall."[22]

On occasion, married couples would frequent a cure together, as did the Howes in the summer of 1846. Seeking rest and recuperation, Dr. Samuel Gridley Howe, a renowned reformer, who was subject to agonizing headaches after his service in the Greek revolution, resolved in the summer of 1846 "to try the water-cure, then considered by many a sovereign remedy for all human ailments."[23] Julia Ward Howe (playwright, author, suffrage leader, Women's Club activist, and author of the "Battle Hymn of the Republic") accompanied the doctor on this trip, and they spent some delightful weeks at the cure in Brattleboro, Vermont.[24]

Since the water cures tended to publicize visits of well-known patrons, this could reflect some uneasiness on the part of hydropaths about the legitimacy or status of the establishments. Equally plausible would be the use of "celebrity" names to lure prospective patients with a certain cultured ambiance as well as with therapeutic validity. Most patients, however, were ordinary people seeking rest and recuperation. One among them, Maria Waterbury, had been serving as a teacher among the freed slaves in Mobile, Alabama, when she was taken ill with a throat affliction. She traveled to the Elmira Water Cure, where, according to her journal, the physician who greeted her was not surprised to find a sickly teacher.

> "We have the most trouble with teachers of any class of patients. They are worn out. They wear out faster than any other class of people. Orders: Hot baths; high diet—beefsteak, eggs, milk, fruit, oysters, everything the health cure has on the table; ride for exercise; sleep late in the morning; never mind the breakfast bell. . . . We'll see if you can be toned up, for some more teaching."[25]

Waterbury was greatly impressed with her accommodations and her roommates:

> A lovely room, with all needful modern improvements—couches, that are so tasteful they look like resting; lovely views of the Allegheny mountains from the windows; three room-mates—all of them high-toned southern ladies, from West Virginia; stiff silk dresses, but very plain, one of them a young woman, but wears a white cap. Can it be? Yes; they are Quakers.[26]

Apparently the cure rejuvenated her sufficiently so that she could return to teaching, as Waterbury was one of the "long list of every day folk who went forth strengthened for usefulness and comfort."[27] Elmira was, in short, a haven for simple folk as well as "a rendezvous for leaders of thought in questions of social and political import, hospitable alike in intellectual understanding and sympathy and practical helpfulness."[28] As for "everyday folks" using the cures, the rhetoric of an establishment's owners reflected an ideological commitment to economic accessibility, but in reality that vision was difficult to achieve; people still had to have money and leisure to stay there.

The physically debilitated were joined by clients less interested in medical care than the recreational facilities. Round Hill consciously recruited healthy people, and "invites to its enchanting retreats the pleasure-seeking, and those who wish for a season of recreation from the cares of business, where pure air, pure water, lovely walks and rides, and captivating scenery, may be enjoyed, without 'stint or measure.'"[29] The director, Captain Brewster, former manager of the Mansion House in Northampton and a hotel at Nahant, also reassured the guests that "those of healthy stomachs, need have no apprehension of being brought down to the scanty diet of the invalid."[30] Round Hill, eager to point out its versatility, courted invalids, pleasure seekers, weakly children, and "those who have induced Chronic Affections of the Throat, by exposure, by public speaking, or by over exertion in business or study."[31]

The cure met with considerable success, as a list of seventy former patients available as references attests. Among them were people from Rhode Island, Massachusetts, Connecticut, New York, Ohio, Michigan, Illinois, Indiana, Missouri, Kentucky, Virginia, Pennsylvania, Georgia, Washington, D.C., South Carolina, and New Jersey. They included numerous women, a judge, professors, ministers, doctors, and a sea captain.[32] The crowning compliment came from Jenny Lind, the renowned soprano, who, after a three-month stay, called Round Hill "the Paradise of America."[33]

Affordable Hydropathic Care

A look at practitioners' views on fees is indicated before examining the costs at individual cures, the wages of different occupational groups, and the cures' consequent affordability—or lack of it. In addition to attracting the well-off, the hydropathic movement's leadership and the individual cures emphasized the necessity of remaining economically accessible to large numbers of people. From the beginning, the leaders were committed to remaining affordable so that their work could reach the hundreds of thousands they hoped it would. Early writers in the *Water-Cure Journal* noted that the cost of a subscription ($1 per year) would save a family much in the way of doctor bills, and for those who could not afford it, the information was sent free.[34] Shew reminded readers in an 1854 article, "To Cheapen Water-Cure," that the system was accessible to all through home use. Further, to cut the cost at the cures, he suggested that patients help one another with the processes that required attendants, thus removing the fees of bath attendants from the overall cost.[35] Other writers argued that charitable benevolence could make hydropathy accessible to poor patients, as could treating the needy at a nominal fee or promoting free physician advice.[36] Even with the lowered costs of the journal and treatments at the cures, there was an identifiable strain of genteel noblesse oblige operating when the way of poorer people was paid by patrons. It is here that the greatest difference between the two kinds of water cure—domestic and physicians'—is evidenced: The former was truly available to the masses, but the latter was essentially possible only for the middle and upper classes and certain laborers, charitable exceptions notwithstanding.

Hydropaths, undaunted by these difficulties, encouraged charitable benevolence for those unable to afford their fees. Ann Turner, age fifteen, "owed her Hydropathic treatment to the liberality and benevolence of Asheton Smith, Esq., of No. 13 Hyde Park Gardens (well known as one of the most zealous and active patrons of Hydropathy), and who sent her, at his own expense, to the *Experimental Baths* at Harrow."[37] Turner remained three months, during which time she recovered totally from scrofula. In a piece written four years later, Shew stressed another kind of charitable benevolence when he counseled (regarding write-in advice from hydropathic physicians): "If you are in reality poor, and not able to buy or beg money for tea, coffee, tobacco, spirits, &c., let some responsible friend, the minister, the postmaster, magistrate, or doctor write for you, and be assured no true hydropathist will send you away empty."[38]

One 1858 article, "Salaries of Professional Men," went so far as to declare that physicians should be salaried, not paid on a fee-for-service basis. Arguing that this would encourage *both* the doctor and the patient to emphasize keeping the patient well (versus curing sickness), the author stressed:

> It is a great mistake on the part of the people to suppose that the private interests and professional reputation of the physician are best subserved by curing his patient as soon as possible. It is precisely the other way. If the patient has a long and severe sickness, the doctor gets correspondingly well paid. . . . In any event, the *worse* he does for the patient, the *better* it seems to be for himself.[39]

Noting that a salaried arrangement between doctor and patient would encourage health, the author continued: "When we pay our physicians salaries, they will have a motive—a selfish motive—for preserving our health. They will then study first above all things else, the laws of health. Their main skill will be directed to keeping us well."[40] In addition, an article by Trall in the February 1864 issue of the *Herald of Health* urged the adoption of "The Contract System vs. Fees," which proposed

> to pay the doctor a stipulated salary for ordinary professional services, and fees only for extraordinary work. Ordinary work was defined to mean periodical visits, attending to the health of the patient, etc; and extraordinary work was held to be such exceptional services as calls to attend on patients immediately, accidents and so on.[41]

This arrangement, he concluded, would make prevention and cure equal priorities and assimilate the interests of physician and patient. One month later, the editor encouraged patients not to abandon the subject of medical rates if doctors do, because it is of critical concern to the health and well-being of so many.[42]

The thinly veiled strain of hostility that these writings reflect toward the allopaths' economic relationship with medical practice has a complementary theme in what can best be categorized as a belligerently pro-laboring-class sentiment. The scorn and ridicule heaped on allopaths was spread to the allopathic clientele, who were branded too lazy—and elitist—to adopt hydropathic principles. As James Caleb Jackson wrote in "Considerations for Commonfolks—No. 2": "This earth of ours is peopled with two classes of human beings—the *common*, working, toiling, plodding, back-bent class [and] the *un*common class, made up of those who look on labor as a *curse*, divinely inflicted, but to be avoided by all means, if possible."[43] This latter group Jackson derided for their powers of deception, exploitation of others' labor, emphasis on capital gain versus muscle, and belief in land rights over human rights. Aware that his followers did not come from this class, Jackson angrily wrote: "For this *latter* class I am *not* writing—I can do them no good. My name lacks prestige, I am not adequately heralded, I lack titles, place, position, power."[44] His prescriptions, he concluded, would not reach this wealthy class, since "its vital essence would consist in demanding an abandonment of habits which they would rather die than give up."[45]

In a real sense, these writings reveal a class enmity and struggle being waged through a debate on medical systems and beliefs. The ire and disgust expressed by hydropathic practitioners and followers transcended a medical or philosophical disagreement. It reflected, in instances such as this, a demand for personal freedom and self-determination in all areas of one's life—from wage labor to medical care—a demand asserted by the ordinary people who used hydropathy against their "social opposites" (the nontoiling classes), who benefited from human passivity, personal irresponsibility, and the unfair distribution of wealth at the expense of others' labors.

This active commitment to economic accessibility can be seen in a comparison of water-cure costs with the average wages of workers, the cost of living, and the costs of allopathic medical care. The water-cure rates, it must be remembered, included not only medical care but also accommodations, meals, and entertainment.

From 1840 to 1870, the rates at the seven cures examined held steady at roughly $5 to $15 per week. The Mount Prospect Water Cure in Binghamton, for example, charged "from $5 to $10 per week, according to room and attention required."[46] Additional fees were incurred for ordinary washing (60 cents per dozen items), for meals sent to rooms when the patient was not confined by sickness, and for fuel in winter. One advertisement noted that a deduction was made on large bills to those who remained over six months or who paid in advance.[47] The nearby Elmira Water Cure, in an advertisement from the early 1860s, described their terms as "$7, $7.50, $8, $9, $10, pr. Week, according to size and location of the room required. Each patient expected to furnish, for Bath purposes, 2 Comforters, 1 Blanket, 2 Sheets—linen preferred—and 6 bath Towels. But these may be rented at the Cure."[48] By encouraging patients to bring their own linens, the managements of the cures kept the costs lower and freed the establishment from the herculean task of providing laundry. Using these strategies, the Elmira Water Cure was able to maintain reasonable rates during its century of activity. In the late 1890s and early 1900s the same establishment (by then called the Gleason Health Resort) increased its rates to $14 to $18 per week for a single room and $21 to $28 per week for double and corner rooms. This included board, baths, and medical attention.[49] In 1955 the rates were $29 and up for single occupancy per week, including all the necessary staples.[50]

The Dansville Water Cure, which also enjoyed a long life, later became the Jackson Sanitarium. In 1887 "the San" charged $10 to $30 per week, with an average of $15 to $18, and established a "clergyman's price" of $2.50 a week, which the management extended to all interested men of the cloth. The sliding scale was flexible and was applied at the discretion of the Jackson family. For example, when the Seventh-Day Adventists wrote in 1863 that they and their families wanted to come but had little money, the clergyman's price was extended to them all.[51]

Massachusetts cures also reflected and maintained this rate scale. The Easthampton Water Cure charged, in the 1850s, $6 per week with an examination fee of $2, while patients could board a private nurse for an additional $2 per week.[52] Close by, the Springfield Water Cure charged $5 to $10 per week and reminded prospective patients to bring two linen sheets, two cotton sheets, two woolen blankets, two comforters, and some towels and linen for bandages.[53] For in-home treatment, patients could either consult a physician in his office for a "reasonable charge," or the physician could do in-home visits.[54] The Northampton Water Cure, under the auspices of Dr. Ruggles in 1847, charged $5.50 per week.[55] The Springfield Water Cure in the late 1840s and early 1850s charged markedly higher rates, averaging $5 to $10 per week.

The nearest year with available statistics on wages and cost of living is 1850, during which the average farm laborer earned $12.98 per month in New England and $11.17 in the mid-Atlantic region.[56] The costs of common foods at this time included wheat at $1.27 a bushel and sugar at 7 cents a pound; raw cotton sold for 12 cents a pound.[57] Further, in 1850 the average family (calculated nationally) spent $84 of its income on all commodities (calculated to include a "food basket" base of numerous staple items).[58] In short, a farm laborer earned roughly $134 to $156 in 1850, out of which $84 went to purchasing "all commodities." This left a disposable annual surplus of $50 to $72, some of which was doubtlessly available for medical care.

The daily wage rates on the Erie Canal for five decades beginning in the 1850s reveal that in 1860, when a common laborer earned $6 per week (or $312 per year), the nearby Elmira Water Cure charged $7 to $10 per week, a fee that was not likely to be affordable to a laborer's family. For more skilled workers (masons among them, whose yearly salary in 1860 was $624 per year), an away-from-home water cure *was* within their economic reach.[59] In regions that did not experience the building bonanza and high wages the Erie Canal region did, the economic picture was less optimistic.[60]

In the 1870s when the Jacksons' Dansville "San" (Sanitarium) averaged $15 to $18 per week, a carpenter (in 1870) earned $21 per week in the Erie Canal region. By this time, the "all-commodities" (wholesale) index of goods had climbed to $135,[61] meaning that of a carpenter's $1,092 annual wage a significant portion remained as disposable income. For skilled workers, therefore, medical care within the cures' price range was feasible. In 1860 the average painter, for example, earned $1.62 per day ($9.72 per week, or $505.44 per year). This increased to $833.04 annually in 1870, but dropped to $689.52 in 1880.[62]

Physicians, military personnel, and those who worked in finance and commerce fared even better.[63] All military personnel, for example, averaged $231 for 1865 ($510 including allowances). For officers, the annual pay was $717 basic, yielding $1,912 when allowances are included.[64] Clearly then, certain income groups had more choices when seeking fee-for-service health care; this further illuminates the hydropathic leadership's advocacy of the abandonment of fee-for-service care. The ability of a given family or individual to afford a stay at a water cure depended ultimately on a variety of factors that included regional economic opportunities, earned wage, the region's cost of living, and fluctuations in pay and costs of consumed commodities.

For women who were self-supporting, the economic and social limitations of their lives (large number of hours worked per week, and lack of mobility and autonomy) made them unlikely, although not impossible, patients at cure establishments. In nearly all instances, women's wages did not approximate those of skilled male workers. Before the 1850s, when women figured most prominently in textile employment, the reasons that caused women to seek paid labor—a ne'er-do-well husband, economic distress of the natal family, or a belief that factory work was a road to self-betterment—often precluded their considering an away-from-home cure. Women were also employed in domestic work, agricultural labor, and the sewing trades, and as teachers, laundresses, bookkeepers, nurses, and employees of hotels and restaurants. From 1870 to 1940, "servant" was the most prevalent occupation of women.[65] Irish domestic servants in the mid-1850s made from $4 to $10 per month and averaged $6. This wage was less than a third of the $21.12 a male common laborer—the lowest-paid of four work categories—earned in the same decade. In the same era chambermaids and women doing housework received $5 to $6 monthly and slopwomen $4 monthly. Cooks, ladies' maids, nurses, and waiters earned more, lived more comfortably, and were paid additionally if they cared for children.[66] Dressmakers who did piecework in their homes received $1 to $3 for each dress in the 1850s, and privately employed seamstresses earned from 62 cents to $1 per day. Seamstresses in the ready-made clothing industry saw their wages kept low by the competition of country women coming to New York seeking employment, and found themselves in dire straits: "In 1845 the journeymen dressmakers toiled fourteen to sixteen hours a day for the weekly pittance of $1.25 to $1.50. Apprentices worked for six months without wages and frequently paid their employers $10 to $15 for the privilege of learning the trade."[67] By 1870, the economic prospects for wage-earning women were still bleak; they still earned below the national average for all nonfarm employees.[68]

Limited by sex-specific work, low wages, social strictures surrounding their social mobility, and, often, the demands of childrearing, wage-earning women had numerous difficulties to overcome before frequenting a cure. These obstacles account, in part, for the tremendous emphasis put on sliding fee scales at the cures, and the establishments' recurring appeal to the charitable benevolence of the friends of hydropathy, but particularly for the solicitation of support from male relatives, who often paid for a woman's cure. Aware that many of their female clientele could afford these fees only with their husband's sanction, hydropaths stressed the comparatively affordable rates of the water-cure system and, simultaneously, acknowledged a husband's financial concerns. Recalling the words of Fanny B. Johnson, who first frequented the Dansville Cure in 1857: "This [sending her to the cure] was at a considerable sacrifice on my husband's part, both as concerned the feelings and the purse, for it was a year of panic in the financial world, but I often heard him say afterward that he never made another investment that paid him so well."[69] There were frequent casual references in the *Water-Cure Journal* that a healthy wife and mother could do much to aid her family's physical and economic well-being.

While the cures were profit making, their managers consciously sought to keep them accessible to everyone, realizing that their rates would determine not only their popular appeal and economic "health" but also their ability to spread hygienic teachings. People's health, not the accumulation of wealth, was the priority of the idealistic managements. Despite this goal of accessibility, it was difficult if not impossible for the lower economic classes to afford a cure from their own earnings. Yet, rates of water-cure establishments seem relatively low when compared with allopathic medical care and, interestingly, even with hydropathic rates for outpatient services.

In 1848, for example, a Philadelphia allopath charged $5 to $10 for a single visit and advice in a case where no further visits were required.[70] This in a decade when a *week* at the Northampton Water-Cure cost $5.50. In the 1860s in Cincinnati an allopathic physician charged $1 to $2 for "ordinary office advice," $5 for a "letter of advice," $3 to $6 for a "visit, in haste," a fee of 50 cents to $1 per mile for all distances over one and a half miles from the physician's residence, plus the cost of any specific service.[71] Simultaneously, the Elmira Cure charged $7 to $10 per week throughout the 1860s. Rural allopathic fees were considerably lower. For example, in the 1880s an allopath's first visit in North Parma, New York, cost $1.50, subsequent visits 75 cents, and each hour detained, $1; there was a doubled fee for consultations outside the village, the service fees themselves, and pharmaceutical charges.[72]

In comparison with live-in cures, the rates of outpatient establishments seem disproportionately high. Thus, in an 1864 article, Trall responded to charges that the water cure was more expensive than allopathy. He argued that when this was so, the reasons were (1) a hydropath's services were worth more (a delightfully unembarrassed self-justifying retort); (2) hydropaths could not make business (by keeping their patients dependent and unhealthy) as allopaths did; (3) hydropaths usually saw their patients once, whereas drug doctors saw them several times (charging anew each time); (4) allopaths charged for nurses and medicines; (5) hydropaths spent more time with their patients; and (6) hygienic physicians taught their patients to be independent of them, thus running their business down.[73] Except where fees were reduced or waived, recommended fees for outpatient water-cure visits were as follows (depending on the region and its density): $5 for the first office examination; $1 for each subsequent prescription, the same charge for consultations by letter, and $10 to $20 for obstetric cases. (Allopaths in rural North Parma charged $8 to $20 for attendance during natural labor, $15 to $25 for delivery by instruments or turning, $5 for removing the placenta, and other costs).[74] Hydropathic country patients who necessitated great traveling by the practitioner and required prolonged stays were charged $25 per day plus expenses, and surgical cases ranged from $25 to $200,[75] which seems roughly comparable to allopathic rates.

A stay at a water-cure establishment, therefore, was financially feasible for family members of skilled workers, professionals, and those who qualified under the loosely defined "clergyman's price," which may have included an occasional farm laborer, unskilled worker, or self-supporting woman. The inability to leave responsibilities (specifically work) behind, however, limited the cures largely to the middle and upper classes or, possibly, recipients of charity, and seasonal workers such as farmers or teachers.

It is significant, too, that a stay at a water-cure establishment was economically feasible for people who were able to afford other kinds of health care. That is, hydropaths competed for clientele with allopaths; both sets of practitioners sought to attract patients with at least minimal purchasing power. But hydropathy's philosophical emphasis on economic accessibility and home self-doctoring appealed consciously to a more diverse patient population than did allopathy's strictly fee-for-service emphasis.[76]

At the live-in cures, fees were kept low by employing several innovative methods. These included a centralized medical staff, which reduced per visit charges; modest dietary regimens; sliding fee scales, which included "clergyman's prices" extended generously to reformers; and a fee reduction for long stays. Patients were also asked to supply their own linens and to serve as one another's attendants. Through these procedures, numerous patients could receive constant supervision at reasonable rates.

Physicians at the Cures

In a setting that fostered daily proximity between physician and patients and sought a bonding in that relationship, physicians at the cures did not function only as medical advisers. The supervising physician was also overseer of all medical attendants, consultant to the kitchen staff, and the role model demonstrating habit alterations for patients. The individual physician was closely connected to the success of the establishment; some cures actually failed after the departure of a particularly charismatic or hard-working physician.

The personal competency and training of these physicians, coupled with the frequency with which they moved from cure to cure, were primary determinants in the success or failure of an establishment. Further, each individual physician brought unique additions to water-cure philosophy; these, in turn, influenced their patients to explore wider medical innovations and reform activities.

No description would cover all water-cure physicians, whose backgrounds varied considerably. At one time, for example, the medical staff at the Glen Haven Water Cure consisted of three physicians. Dr. J. P. Wallace "was educated in the old school of Allopathy, but, after dealing out poisons four years, a reformation came over him. . . . He now gives no drugs. He stands very high in his profession as a Hydropathist, Surgeon, and Obstetrician."[77] (Often, the "conversion" of an allopath served as grist for the hydropaths' contention that every individual possessed the potential for change and rejuvenation.) Wallace's colleagues were Dr. Jansen (background not specified) and Dr. Ellen Beard, a graduate of the New York Hydropathic College.[78]

At the Mount Prospect Water Cure, the founder, Dr. Orson V. Thayer, was an eclectic.[79] He was followed by Dr. J. H. North, who had himself been cured by water therapies after being pronounced incurable. He then studied medicine and obtained a knowledge of regular practice, which was followed by five years as an assistant in one of the country's largest water cures. North's associate, Dr. Martha French, according to the broadside,

> has enjoyed the best advantage for a medical education, and has had an experience of several years in the treatment of diseases peculiar to her own sex. For three years past she has been constantly in attendance at a large Water Cure. Ladies will find her fully competent to treat their diseases, and may consult her with confidence.[80]

Water-cure establishments found it to their advantage to employ female physicians to assuage any doubts female patients might have had about the intimacies of the physician–patient relationship. While it is difficult to estimate the percentage of water-cure physicians who were women, the larger establishments made an attempt to employ *at least* one woman physician. At the water-cure colleges the gender ratio of students was roughly 1:1, and the larger (often family-owned) cures recruited and trained women physicians. A few cures had staffs and clientele who were exclusively female. More specifically, advertisements in the journal reveal that the establishments most likely *not* to have a woman physician in attendance were the smaller cures, often operated out of a single-family dwelling unit. These cures focused more on an outpatient, fee-for-service population and were more often operated by a single proprietor who could not reasonably afford a partner.

One can conjecture that cures without a female physician in attendance might have had problems of credibility in a movement whose followers so articulately supported gender-matched physician–patient health care. The prevalence of female physicians at the cures seemingly increased after the middle of the nineteenth century. This stemmed from hydropathy's corollary social-reform activism, which took on an increasingly gender-conscious component through the influence of the political woman's rights movement, whose participants argued for the legitimacy of women physicians (although much of that support was aimed at women pursuing traditional medical careers). Other factors were the training of women physicians at the cures and the large "homosocial" (i.e., gender-identified women who sought same-sex bonding, companionship, and intimacy) clientele that preferred female physicians for modest and gentle medical care and rest and recuperation in a female environment. Finally, despite (or, possibly, spurred by) the founding of female-only regular hospitals, numerous reform-minded women pursued hydropathic practice in the second half of the nineteenth century in the belief that their services were critical to refuting this threat to hygienic healing.

The Elmira Water Cure thrived for over a century because of the skill, reputation, and gender consciousness of its attending physicians, Drs. Silas O. and Rachel Brooks Gleason.[81] Silas Gleason was born in Massachusetts in 1818 and spent most of his childhood and youth in Vermont. He attended Oberlin College in Ohio and graduated in 1844 from Castleton Medical College in Vermont. Later he served as attending physician at the water cure in Cuba, New York (the first cure west of the Hudson River and the third in the United States), cofounded (with James C. Jackson) the Glen Haven Water Cure on Skeneatelas Lake, lectured on hygiene at the Eclectic College, and took charge of the Forest City Water Cure on Cayuga Lake.[82]

Silas Gleason's reputation was founded on a traditional medical background, but it was Rachel Gleason through whom reform activity and gender consciousness found expression. She was a long-time sympathizer with the antislavery movement and an active friend of freedmen's schools. She earned her medical degree through private lessons with her husband, since no eastern medical school would accept women. Before founding Elmira with Gleason, she had five years of sanitarium work in Cuba, New York, and at the Forest City Water Cure.[83]

As in so many male–female or husband–wife physician teams, Rachel Gleason made a specialty of the diseases of women, and her reputation attracted many women to Elmira. She was known for her "origination of methods in treatment and operation, since adopted by the most successful and distinguished practitioners."[84]

The Gleasons opened the Elmira Water Cure (later called the Gleason Sanitarium and, later yet, the Gleason Health Resort) in 1852. They stood at the helm of the cure until 1868, sixteen years after its inception, until Silas's ill health forced them to seek the warmer climate of Florida.[85] The competence, commitment, and consistency of their leadership helped the establishment to overcome economic and cultural lulls and, ultimately, survive until 1959. In addition, under their leadership physicians were trained to carry on their work.

In the training of physicians a few select water-cure establishments were similar to another well-developed nineteenth-century institution, the dispensary.[86] A largely urban phenomenon, the dispensary arose to meet the needs of the urban poor who could not afford private-physician health care. Before the inclusion of clinical training in medical education, dispensaries provided a career step for aspiring physicians.[87] Thus the role of dispensaries in medical education can be likened to the water-cure physician-trainee's "apprenticeship" at a cure, in that both provided experience and case materials. Two more similarities exist between the two institutions. Both operated from a notion that medicine must reflect an awareness of the patient's environment and the patient's moral decisions. In this sense, the emphasis on integrative health care was a common value, although hydropaths strove for life-habit renovations, whereas dispensary physicians, convinced that such fundamental changes were unlikely, if not impossible, responded with drug therapy.[88] Finally, both flourished as long as the parameters of medical science provided them with a contribution to make, a clientele to serve, and a rationale for their existence. The decline of the dispensary in the last third of the nineteenth century coincides with both the decline of the cures and the rise of hospital innovations such as the germ theory of disease, antisepsis, modern surgery, the X ray, and clinical laboratory methods.[89] For a few decades in mid-nineteenth-century America, however, the cures and the dispensaries were ideologically similar institutions that played vital roles in training young physicians, albeit of different persuasions.

Among nineteenth-century water cures that served as training grounds for physicians, none was more effective than the Elmira Water Cure. Under the leadership of Rachel Gleason, whose parlor talks on the physiology of women and *Talks with My Patients* argued for female health and personal responsibility, the cure trained female and male doctors. The original medical staff, for instance, was composed of the two Gleasons, Dr. Theron Augustus Wales from the University of Pennsylvania, his wife, Zippie Brooks Wales, and Miss Eddy from the Woman's Medical College of Pennsylvania.[90] Theron and Zippie Wales later served as assistant physicians at the establishment from 1873 to 1897. After the retirement of the Gleasons, Dr. Edith Flower Wheeler, Dr. Clarabell M. Hutchinson, and Dr. Fanny Brown followed. In 1927, when Brown moved to Washington, Dr. John C. Doyle and his wife, Dr. Gertrude Davies Doyle, staffed the sanitarium.[91]

Not only was the attending staff predominantly female, but the Gleasons trained, by one count, eighteen women who went on to practice medicine. Among them were the Gleasons' daughter, Adele, who attended Elmira College and received her M.D. from the University of Michigan (she returned to work at the cure and served with the Red Cross during World War I); Dr. Anna Stuart, in 1895 the first woman graduate of the University of Buffalo's School of Dentistry (she went on to found the still-flourishing Arnot–Ogden Hospital); and Dr. Jessie Herrick, the first Elmira physician to use radium in the treatment of skin cancer.[92] As these later examples demonstrate, some women originally trained in hydropathy, particularly in the late nineteenth century, went on to adopt and participate in the methods and advances of scientific medicine.

Stable Cures: Elmira and Dansville

Chroniclers of the Elmira Water Cure (Gleason Health Resort) attribute the establishment's longevity to the Gleasons' unswerving commitment and influence, commenting that "it became and remained an intellectual and social center by reason of the brilliant man and perceiving woman at its head."[93]

The Dansville Water Cure offers a similar history; under James Caleb Jackson it also enjoyed a tenure of over one hundred years. Before Jackson's management, the cure had suffered from instability. In the four years preceding his arrival it passed through the hands of four owners and three physicians-in-charge. Originally founded in 1854 by Nathaniel Bingham, a lifelong invalid, and Lyman Granger, both of Rochester, it was soon sold because of Bingham's failing health and their inability to meet the demands of the business. It failed twice more until taken over by T. S. Ripley, who also could not run a successful operation. "Once more it was turned over to the birds and the bats, and it thus remained until September of 1858 when it was purchased of Mr. Pennell and F. Wilson Hurd and Company, at a very low figure."[94] Hurd, who had been Gleason's patient at Glen Haven, recruited Jackson to fill the position of physician-in-charge. Thus began a hundred-year family commitment to the operation of the Dansville Water Cure.

Jackson brought several years of experience as a physician to Dansville. While his wife, "Mother Jackson," as she was affectionately called, did not possess a medical degree, she was overseer of the establishment's management. His adopted daughter, Dr. Harriet N. Austin, a trained medical practitioner, catered to the interests of female patients and gained national recognition for her advocacy of the American costume.[95]

Like Elmira, Dansville reflected the reform interests of its leaders and served as a training ground for women physicians. The reform activity at Dansville included dress reform, Jackson's involvement with the Seventh-Day Adventist health empire, and the invention of Granula (1863), in keeping with his desire to make a vegetarian diet more appealing. Granula was a breadcrumb mixture made of graham flour and water, the first cold cereal breakfast food, and precursor to John Harvey Kellogg's Grape Nuts.[96] In addition, Jackson's interest in abolition, temperance, women's rights, the cooperative union of labor and capital, and mental therapeutics placed Dansville at the center of national reform politics.[97] The numerous luminaries who traveled there reflected the prominence he and the cure had gained. Among those who spoke at "Our Home," as

Dansville was called, were prominent activists in nearly every nineteenth-century reform, exceptional women particularly prominent among them. The speakers included Sojourner Truth, Frederick Douglass, Elizabeth Cady Stanton, Susan B. Anthony, Frances E. Willard, Bronson Alcott, Clara Barton, Jerry McCauley (slum mission founder), Mrs. Ballington Booth and Edith Marshall (Salvation Army leaders), Mary Low Dickinson and Margaret Bottome (leaders in the Order of the King's Daughters), and the authors Kate Douglas Wiggin, William Dean Howells, and Ruth McEnery Stuart.[98]

Several women physicians trained at the cure later played central roles in the management of the institution. Among them were Dr. Kate J. Jackson, Dr. Fanny Hurd Brown (daughter of F. Wilson Hurd, the owner), Dr. Agnes L. Brown (daughter of Hugh and Fanny Hurd Brown), and Dr. Elizabeth Fear (second wife of Albert J. Leffingwell, the nephew of James Caleb Jackson). In addition, ten male members of the Jackson family later earned an M.D.[99] As at Elmira, later generations of the Jackson "family" were not necessarily opposed to pursuing regular medical degrees, and many, in fact, did so. The Jackson Health Resort, as it was later called, also produced a number of nurses. Seven women from the sanitarium's class of 1907 and one from the class of 1905 successfully passed the Regents exam.[100]

The effect of "Our Home" on its women physicians was recorded at the fiftieth anniversary celebration in Dansville in 1908. In brief messages sent to Dansville, Dr. Sarah J. McNutt of New York City, Dr. Susanna W. Dodds of Saint Louis, and Dr. Mary Emma Dickinson of Rochester, New York, paused to honor both the founder of the institution and the establishment's success. As Dodds wrote:

> It was from your founder's lips that I first heard the a-b-c of the true healing art. He taught that disease is remedial action—not a thing to be destroyed. He also taught his patients that drug poisons do not "act" on the living system, but are acted upon it. He taught us that good health is secured by strict obedience to physiological law, and that the same agents which maintain health—pure air, pure water, good food, etc.—are the one [sic] to be employed in restoring it when lost.[101]

Unstable Cures

The Elmira and Dansville water cures, with their consistent leadership and genuine family commitments, flourished for decades, but they were more the exception than the rule. Four cures in western Massachusetts—at Athol, Westboro, Easthampton, and Northampton—demonstrated less continuity in leadership. These cures experienced physician mobility, frequent periods of decreased use, and earlier closings. The

Athol Water Cure, for example, was run by Dr. George Hoyt. Hoyt was born in Deerfield, Massachusetts, in 1801, attended Deerfield Academy and the reputable Pittsfield Medical School, practiced in a Boston hospital for two years, specializing in surgery, and started a practice in Hubbardston, Massachusetts, before arriving in Athol in 1832. Hoyt succeeded Dr. Jacob Holmes "and was one of the first to introduce the use of water medicinally in baths, etc., establishing a Water Cure, which became quite extensively known."[102]

The Southard House, where Hoyt established his cure, is remembered not only as a water cure but also as a station on the Underground Railroad, since Hoyt was one of the state's most active abolitionists. He played a major role in the liberation of a young slave and later enrolled him in the Athol public schools. This case, the first of its kind in Massachusetts, provoked Hoyt's antagonists to violent acts, so much so that he did not dare ride around town in his gig without carrying stones as weapons. Hoyt's friendship with William Lloyd Garrison and other prominent abolitionists protected his person and reputation from harm.[103]

Hoyt operated the Athol Water Cure and won a respected position in the town and state through his water-cure and antislavery efforts. In addition, he was one of the earliest match manufacturers in the country.[104] When Hoyt left Athol in 1851 to move to Boston, he sold the cure to Dr. J. H. Hero, who "is said to have been a man of unusual natural ability, endowed by nature with a commanding physique and a pleasing manner."[105] Years earlier, Hero had been Hoyt's patient at the cure. Hero studied medicine in a New York medical college and later practiced in Milford, Massachusetts, before buying the Athol Cure.

Hero conducted the cure for nearly two years and had an extensive outpatient practice. Following that, "In 1853 in company with his preceptor, Dr. Wilmarth, he bought the old Wesson Hotel property in Westborough and established the 'Willow Park Water Cure.'"[106] Wilmarth died two months later in a railroad accident, and Hero was left to manage Willow Park. Hero, always interested in innovative modes of treatment, introduced the Turkish bath in 1866, the first in New England outside of Boston.

Hero apparently owned another cure in Westboro, the New Malvern Water-Cure (circa 1855), from which he wrote an article for the *Water-Cure Journal* entitled "Errors in Home Practice." In this piece he derided water-cure "fanatics" whose in-home treatment was too severe, whose water temperature was too cold (40°F. to 50°F.), and whose lack of knowledge of the true tenets of the system caused them to debilitate those they were trying to help.[107]

In 1867 Hero established the Willow Park Seminary. The school combined mental and physical culture in its curriculum and had many illustrious alumni. In 1876 Hero moved to Worcester, Massachusetts, where he conducted a Turkish bath establishment for three years at No. 58

Summer Street.[108] It was in Worcester that he began to manufacture a cough syrup that he had used successfully in private practice. Never one to become sedentary, Hero returned to Westboro, while the manufacture of the syrup met with large-scale success. Other remedies were added, and later the Hero Cough Syrup Company was formed, and its agents covered a large area of New England. Hero also dabbled in the raising of fancy stock and peach culture, but his belief in, and commitment to, water cure lived on in his work and in his two sons, Butler Wilmarth and George Hoyt, who were named after his two medical mentors.[109] In the midst of his varied career Hero sold the Athol Water Cure to Dr. Field, who "was a physician of education and refinement, but he lacked the push and enthusiasm necessary to successfully run a Water Cure."[110] The cure faded out, and the building became a dwelling house.

The Athol Water Cure is interesting, since it survived roughly twenty-two years despite physician mobility and transiency. Hero is typical of a certain kind of water-cure physician whose energy and charm rendered his ventures successful but who seemed incapable of settling in one place. The result was a series of short-lived yet temporarily successful water-cure establishments that arose in the same vicinity but faded when the physician's interest waned.

Evidence suggests that Hero's cures did not close because of declining public interest, economic troubles, or internal strife. In fact, many patients apparently flourished under the care of charmers such as Hero. The physician-as-placebo factor, which has been observed in twentieth-century studies, would account for the near-reverence in which some water-cure physicians were held and the vital role that charismatic personalities played in the success of the cures and the movement as a whole. At successful water cures, personal charm, therapeutic efficacy, and faith and trust in the physician coalesced to produce smooth operation and strong popularity.

It seems as if a certain personality type was attracted to hydropathy, contributing to the instability of some of the cures, since the repeated startings and stoppings of these ventures cannot be attributed solely to commonly held idiosyncrasies. Somewhat too zealously idealistic, inspired by a series of moral and social revelations, creative, energetic, and not afraid to incorporate and experiment with complementary or conflicting methods and ideologies, these practitioners willingly sacrificed career stability in pursuit of the next horizon. The same enthusiasm, idealism, and eclectic vision that had brought them to hydropathy drew them away from the movement toward a new challenge. The nature of the next calling varied from the spiritual to the commercial, but it offered the lure of innovation, self-expression, and limitless potential.

This pattern of physician mobility was played out twice more in western Massachusetts cures. In Easthampton, "Dr. E. Snell, having removed his residence from Springfield Water-Cure on account of its bad location and great unfitness for the business, has located himself in the beautiful village of Easthampton, near the Williston Seminary, and has purchased and fitted the building known as Snow's Hotel for a Water-Cure."[111] It is reasonable to assume that Snell's new project in Easthampton lasted a year or so. It operated during 1853 under Snell's ownership. He was the sole physician and employed electrical cures in a great many cases. The brief tenure of his cure is difficult to explain, as it left little written evidence. Whether there was a more attractive prospect elsewhere or economic difficulties or a personal change of heart and mind is not known.

In the nearby town of Northampton, the Round Hill Water Cure was unique for its survival in the face of constant turmoil. From its purchase in 1846 until its sale in 1870, the cure passed through the hands of seven owners and six physicians. Samuel Whitmarsh purchased the Round Hill estate (formerly a school) in 1846 to open a water cure. His associate and the medical superintendent was to be Dr. E. E. Dennison, a European-educated regular physician.[112] Dennison barely had the chance to apply his expertise, since Round Hill was bought after only one year by Dr. J. A. Cummings and Albert Clark (of the firm of Holman and Clark, U.S. Hotel) of Boston. Cummings and Clark promised to make extensive additions and introduced as their physicians, in addition to Cummings, Dr. C. A. Hall and Dr. Samuel B. Woodward, "so distinguished as the late Superintendent of the State Lunatic Hospital at Worcester."[113] Six months later, in May 1848, a newspaper article revealed that the medical superintendence had changed again.[114] Dennison, meanwhile, had struck out on his own and opened "Dr. E. E. Denniston's [sic] Water Cure, At Springdale, Northampton, Mass." Dennison's cure was run out of a small house that could accommodate twenty to forty patients. This cure, too, had a dubious tenure, although it did gain the support of eight regular physicians.[115]

Dr. Dexter, who was put in charge of the Round Hill Hydropathic Department under the new ownership, was no neophyte in water-cure circles. He had been an early advocate of water treatment and had studied European water practices.[116] Dexter conducted a water cure in Morristown, New Jersey, for several years before his arrival in Northampton; his hydropathic skills were complemented by Woodward and Hall's attention to "those invalids who object to the water treatment, or to whose cases that practice does not seem to be adapted."[117] Round Hill, more so than other prominent cures, exhibited early on a willingness to integrate varied therapeutics and to let its facilities be used as a physiological retreat.

This seemingly smooth mesh of physicians and owners lasted seven years before the entire staff underwent another upheaval. An 1855 article in the *Daily Hampshire Gazette* discussed the qualifications of the new owner and physicians, and the establishment's growth:

The establishment is managed with much tact and skill by its energetic proprietor, Dr. Halsted, assisted by his son-in-law, Dr. Strong, who, by his scientific learning and gentlemanly address, is admirably qualified for his position. The number of persons now residing there, we learn, is about 250. The number will soon be greatly increased.[118]

Halsted's management lent consistency to the establishment. After his arrival in 1855, he built an excellent reputation that followed him throughout his fifteen years as owner and physician. It was said of him that "the many, whom he has almost raised from the dead, have gone away holding him in everlasting rememberance [sic] and gratitude, and to be living monuments of his great skill."[119]

Halsted, weary from his labors, finally sold Round Hill in 1870 to fifteen Northampton businessmen. Despite all the turnover, Round Hill continued to be one of the most popular cures in the country.

Hydropathy and Professionalism

As we have seen, the histories of individual cures were extremely diverse, as were the backgrounds of the physicians who managed them. In the cures examined, all the attending physicians had medical training, and several had practiced or studied regular medicine before coming to hydropathy. It is likely that their varied backgrounds account for the wide spectrum of ideas and goals they held regarding hydropathic professionalism.

Professionalization, including medical education, training, and the forming of a medical society, was never significantly embraced by hydropathy. In the fall of 1851 Mary Gove and Thomas Nichols opened their American Hydropathic Institute in New York City. They operated the school for three terms and then abandoned it as they drifted toward other interests. Shortly thereafter, Trall opened the New York Hydropathic School (1853) and four years later changed its name to the New York Hygeio-Therapeutic College (1857), which became the water-cure center of the United States with Trall as mentor. Orson Squire Fowler was on the original faculty as lecturer on phrenology and mental science. The Hygeio-Therapeutic College seems to have suffered from a decided informality, resulting in a questionable degree. As one chronicler noted:

Standards and staff alike were woefully inadequate. On opening day, when Trall found his faculty short two teachers (he had three on hand, including himself), he improvised by pressing Merritt (Kellogg, a new graduate of the College who went on to become a full-time health lecturer for the Seventh-Day Adventists) into service as instructor in anatomy and John (Kellogg) as lecturer in chemistry. The arrangement worked reasonably well until John innocently wandered onto the forbidden field of *organic* chemistry—a science Trall insisted did not exist—and was subsequently relieved of his duties. . . . Despite the fact that he never examined his students, and that some were not old enough to practice medicine, Trall awarded them each a handsome diploma and sent them out to ply their trade on an unsuspecting world.[120]

Other, less-well-known hydropathic schools included the New Jersey Hydropathic Collegiate Institute at South Orange, founded in 1853, but short lived; the Hydropathic College and Institute of Loretta, Pennsylvania, 1859; Franklin Water-Cure and Physiological School, near Winchester, Tennessee; Dansville's Water-Cure College, circa 1861; and the Minnesota Hygeio-Therapeutic College, circa 1865.[121]

Although important questions have been raised about the value of Trall's degree, it was not dissimilar from numerous other medical diplomas of the time.[122] Moreover, rigorous standards of professionalism and training were contrary to many of the tenets of hydropathy. Unlike regular medicine, hydropathy considered experiential expertise to be a satisfactory credential for practicing. Thus the formation of the American Hydropathic Society in June 1849 is instructive. Of the fifteen practitioners listed, eleven held an M.D.[123] The society was open to all men and women (it seems unlikely that women served on the governing board) of good moral character who signed the constitution or wrote their assent to it and paid $5. It was formed "for the general purposes of collecting and disseminating information concerning the doctrines and practice of the Water-Cure among the people." It sought to provide "theoretical and practical instruction to proper persons in the principles and details of hydropathy, for the purpose of supplying the country with competent practitioners."[124]

A second society, seemingly displeased with the first, met in June 1850. The group's name was changed to the American Hygienic and Hydropathic Association of Physicians and Surgeons.[125] At this meeting a tumultuous debate arose over whether members *must* have an M.D. or a license to practice the healing art before they could be voted in by the membership. As reported by T. L. Nichols, the secretary:

> While a majority of the Convention insisted that all future members should have received the degree of M.D., or a legal license, several members were for placing the test of membership upon qualifications alone. It was urged upon one side, that a conformity to medical usages would give the society the stamp of respectability—on the other, it was urged that a Hydropathic Society, composed of those who profess to be the vanguard of medical reformers, ought not to stand upon the musty precedents of the past, or practice the ex-

clusiveism of older schools, by the adoption of a rule which would exclude from the society the Founder of Hydropathy, and many of his most eminent disciples; much less that a body of water-cure physicians should make the diplomas of Allopathic faculties, or the licenses of Allopathic board of examiners, the test of membership.[126]

Nichols could not resist interjecting his own view of licensure, which he deemed "far behind the spirit of the age, truckling to the low forms of the schools of medicine we are exterminating, and utterly opposed to the liberal and enlightened public sentiment upon which all the success of our system of practice depends."[127]

The delegates did vote to require regular licensing to practice hydropathy, but before adjournment Dr. B. Wilmarth, one of the vice-presidents, gave notice that at the next meeting he would make a motion to make qualification the sole test of membership. At the next meeting, in May 1851, four hydropaths were denied membership because they lacked proper training. At Shew's suggestion, however, the four were voted in as honorary members.[128] While the attempt to change the criteria for membership failed at this meeting, it appears that all those not accepted for membership were given honorary memberships, although Dr. Broadbent declined the offer. Thus the intent of educational standards was intentionally downplayed and virtually circumscribed.

The association had a short life. At the 1851 meeting, only eight members and approximately six visitors attended. Membership fees totaled $32, and after convention expenses of $20, $12 was left. Small membership, negligible finances, and a deep-seated ambivalence over the licensing issue dissipated the association. The *Water-Cure Journal* assumed many of the tasks the group had attempted and handled them much more ably than a convention format was able to do. Thus the issue of licensing was, essentially, abandoned.[129]

Because hydropathy was *not* based on a traditional definition of professionalism entailing exclusionary tactics and special knowledge and precisely because it was a self-conscious reform movement, professional criteria were largely shunned, and experience was an acceptable measure of skill. Further, as the conversion narratives demonstrate, since some had been "called" to practice hydropathy as a result of a personal revelation, there was certainly no way to evaluate their training objectively or their claim to being practitioners. That many of these people ventured forth to treat kin and neighbors was precisely what the rhetoric of the system advocated. To circumscribe these informal healers' influence would have undercut hydropathy's own premises. For a system that prospered, by and large, on self-doctoring and eventual patient self-determination, licensing and professional standards were antithetical.

The attending physicians at the New York and Massachusetts cures reflect this acceptability of diverse backgrounds. Three or four had complemented American study with study abroad, and one brought expertise from a lunatic asylum to his hydropathic labors. These physicians' lengths of employment at a cure also differed considerably. Elmira and Dansville, for example, were under virtually the same familial leadership for over a century, while the Athol and Northampton cures devoured physicians and proprietors alike. Although the rate of physician and management turnover affected the stability of a cure, it was not the sole cause of longevity, as the lengthy survival of the erratically governed Round Hill Water Cure demonstrates. Similarly, the reform interests of individual physicians, such as Austin's dress reform, Jackson's cereal invention and temperance beliefs, and Hoyt's antislavery efforts, determined which reform activities were sponsored by a specific cure. In addition, the varied interests of energetic physicians led many successful hydropaths to start and stop their water-cure efforts in the pursuit of other reform or money-making ventures.

It seems clear that only the two establishments with the greatest longevity and gender-conscious leadership, Elmira and Dansville, provided an environment in which large numbers of women physicians were fostered and trained. Other, more erratic cures were too embroiled in their internal machinations to pursue any long-term projects, although individual female practitioners and "apprentices" did find employment at the smaller cures.

Textual Teachings versus Physicians

With standardized criteria often lacking and cure managements in flux, conflicts between water-cure philosophy and an individual physician's practices were inevitable. Ruggles, for example, in his Northampton Water Cure (1847), earned himself an ambivalent rebuke from Shew as the editor of the journal:

> The peculiar doctrines of Mr. Ruggles concerning electricity, &c., we do not wish to be understood as advocating. We may notice them hereafter. Mr. Ruggles has proved himself to be a judicious and efficient practitioner of the new system, and this is sufficient for our present purpose. He has our best wishes for his success.[130]

Had the national leadership not been this flexible, it is doubtful they would have had much of a following.

While nearly all practitioners agreed on the ABCs of water-cure philosophy, dogmatic adherence to the exclusive use of water was not enforced, and this trend escalated in the later decades of the century. The Binghamton Mount Prospect Cure, for example, while it did not stipulate specific alternatives, asserted that "in a majority of cases water and the hygienic remedies are all sufficient. If, however, it is desirable to use other means to relieve pain, or facilitate a cure, the Physicians will use such remedies as their experience has approved."[131] Other cures were even more explicit about their willingness to integrate nonhydropathic therapies. The advertisement for the Elmira Water Cure, which appeared in Brigham's *Elmira Directory, 1863–1864*, stated:

> We do not pursue the extremes of Hydropathy or of Vegetarianism. We intend the condition of the patient shall indicate the diet and regimen necessary to promote health in each case. We seek, first of all, TO CURE OUR PATIENTS. Water is our Chief Remedy. But we do not hesitate to use Homeopathic remedies, Electricity, or any other means within our knowledge to facilitate the recovery of the Sick. We are Eclectic in our practice—using all the means that in our judgment shall do any good to any patient. Those who come to us shall have the benefit of our best skill and care.[132]

This statement is particularly surprising because it legitimizes the use of homeopathic medicine, which, while entailing minute doses, nonetheless constitutes drug therapy. Here the Gleasons were contradicting one of the basic principles of water-cure philosophy, yet this deviation did not prevent their cure from being one of the most popular and respected in the country.

In fact, as hydropathy gained in national prominence, the "ideological purity" of the movement's institutional practitioners steadily decreased. The journal continued to promote a doctrine of unadultered cold-water therapy and no drug use while carrying articles and advertisements for electrochemical treatments and various pieces of exercise equipment (the former transgressed systemic teaching, whereas the latter simply reflected an eclectic awareness of complementary devices). Individual establishments, meanwhile, varied greatly in their adherence to the original philosophy. This variety both reinforced the movement and sapped its strength. On the one hand, it helped recruit business from segments of the population that had followed other established systems (allopathy, homeopathy, and so on), as well as prospective patients infatuated with an experimental therapy. On the other hand, these smorgasbord therapeutics in the long run minimized the uniqueness of the water-cure system and diluted the movement's special properties. What is important is that hydropaths, although eager to embrace other sectarians' therapeutics, looked askance at allopathic innovations or therapeutics. This refusal cost hydropathy credibility as vaccination, vivisection, and other scientific procedures came into public acceptance.

Indicative of hydropaths' fleeting use of various therapeutic models (reflective of both the practitioners' changing beliefs and the consuming public's changing demands) was an 1873 article in the Elmira press. The

Gleasons once again explained their eclectic approach, but this time there was no mention of homeopathic therapies.

> While this is ostensibly a "water-cure" and has not taken refuge under any title of Sanitorium or "Institute," as of late has been the fashion, it is by no means bigoted or sectarian in its practice. Water, in its various applications, is used as a means—and a valuable means—for the relief of chronic or acute affections, but not the only means. The faculty are regularly educated physicians, and are graduates of the best medical colleges of our land; but they have thrown off the trammels of "school" and "party," and rejoice in the freedom of true physicians choosing their means from the best proved remedies of all sects.[133]

The article described the cure's use of electricity, Swedish movements, light gymnastics, and hygienic principles. Again in conflict with the strictest hydropathic principles, Gleason wrote, "We live like other folks, allow tea and coffee in moderation, the best of meats, and all other good, plain, wholesome food in abundance."[134] An 1889 pamphlet reveals another form of nonhydropathic treatment administered at Elmira. Mentioned only once in all the available literature, "the 'Weir Mitchell Rest Cure' is carried out scientifically in cases requiring it—time, six weeks."[135] The inclusion of this particular therapy, which by definition employed bed rest, frequent feeding, and inactivity, seems paradoxical and incompatible with the Gleasons' beliefs. Their use of the rest cure reflects the credibility it had gained as a therapeutic treatment among soldiers and nervous sufferers in the general populace, who sought to restore their lost "nerve force," and also their willingness to integrate nonhydropathic regimens.[136] While hydropathy and the rest cure both relied heavily on a charismatic physician, the physician's ability to convince patients they can be helped, and patient instruction and suggestion, it is likely that the (rhetorically) egalitarian model fostered between hydropathic physicians and their patients would modify some of the more power-laden dynamics of the Mitchell Rest Cure. Further speculation will reveal little, for Mrs. Gleason mentioned this therapy only once, with no attendant explanation.

The exceptionally long life of the Elmira Cure affords the opportunity to observe the repeated adoption of innovative and, at times, contradictory therapeutics. A pamphlet describing the resort at the turn of the century notes its ability to offer all kinds of baths (some mineral), including "Turkish, Russian, Roman, Sulphur, Cabinet, Electro-Thermal, Electro-Chemical, Foments, Douches, Hot and Cold Tub Baths, Sprays, and *Brine Baths*, both plain and *Carbonated*."[137] By 1912, the Gleasons' therapeutic offerings had expanded to include "static machines, high frequency and sinusoidal apparatus and electric light baths. For mechanical stimulation there are also vibrators, a vibrating chair and oscillator and for the administration of ozones in respiratory troubles and depletion there is an ozonizing machine."[138] In emphasizing the use of hot water, mineral baths, and machinery (which greatly minimized the "hands on" efficacy of the wrapping and rubbing of earlier treatments), the Gleasons had strayed considerably from the tenets of Priessnitz's cold-water cure. Sixty to seventy years had elapsed, however, and adherence to the original principles was far less zealous and, apparently, was even viewed as antiquated.

The Jacksons in Dansville also gradually moved away from the strictest hydropathic principles. In a letter in the *Dansville Advertiser* in 1876 James C. Jackson wrote, "Our Home is not a water cure, nor a diet cure; it is a great institution come to be widely known all over the land as a place where the sick can come, and having right condition of life created, get well."[139]

This trend toward integrating varied therapeutics was noticeable in Massachusetts as well, where Dr. E. Snell adopted at the Easthampton Water Cure "Coad's Patent Graduated Battery, which he has obtained at great expense [and found] very useful in many cases of Paralysis, Rheumatism, &c."[140] On moving to Springfield, Snell teamed with Dr. H. H. Sherwood of New York, a magnetic practitioner who dispensed medicines. These medicines, one of their advertisements states, could be given without water cure if the patient wished, "no questions asked," at a reasonable charge.[141]

Competition among the various cures, even the highly successful ones, seems to have required some variation from hydropathic practices. Round Hill's practitioners, aware that water-cure therapies might be a deterrent to some,

> have also made extensive arrangements, and have spared no pains in fitting up a part of the Retreat for the use and convenience of the friends of patients, for persons traveling for health or for pleasure, who will find this a rare location, combining a great variety of amusements and accommodations not inferior to any Hotel in the country.[142]

Provisions were even made for "those invalids who object to the water treatment."[143]

Several years later, under Halsted's auspices, the name of the cure was changed to Round Hill Water-Cure and Motorpathic Institute, which reflected his personal belief in motorpathy. Although he did not expect people unfamiliar with it to accept it readily, he advocated its adoption and praised its efficacy in glowing prose.[144] The movement cure, according to Halsted, promised relief to patients with spinal disease, paralysis, disease of the lungs and air passages, disease of the joints, and loss of the use of limbs. At the same time that Halsted introduced the movement cure to Round Hill, he purchased "one of Professor M. Vergnes' Electro Chemical Baths, for extracting from the human system all metallic substances, whether taken as medicine or otherwise absorbed."[145]

It has been shown that individual physicians had a significant impact on the therapeutics offered at their cures. Embracing therapies as diverse or contradictory as homeopathy, electromagnetism, drug medications, and movement cures and including culinary modifications that allowed meat eating and coffee drinking, these physicians consciously contradicted water-cure philosophy. The cures were nevertheless hydropathic as defined by individual practitioners, the movement's leadership, and patrons. These modifications sharply undermined the dogmatism of the purist water-cure philosophy. Such alterations, significantly, seemed to elicit little or no criticism from other hydropaths. Instead they were viewed as nonimpediments to the efficacy of water therapies, necessary adaptations to therapeutic innovations, and responses to the changing nature of health-care consumers, some of whom were attracted by the promises of new "isms" and mechanical gadgetry. It would be simplifying a complex set of expectations and goals, however, to attribute these therapeutic alterations solely to the public's demand for modifications in hydropathic practices—or to the reliefs promised in old and new panaceas.

Individual physicians undeniably had a significant impact on the therapeutics offered at their cures, but a more general trend of "therapeutic revisionism" emerged in nearly all the cures. This move away from doctrinaire hygienic principles created a fascinating contradiction between the teachings of the leadership (in the journal—still essentially purist) and the increasing adoption of fringe methods by individual practitioners. One can conjecture that hydropathic home self-doctorers, meanwhile, operating out of personal conversions, older literature, and minimal access to electronic devices, brine and sulfur baths, and vibrating machines, retained a longer hold on the unadulterated (textual) ideology than the practitioners, whose energies and interests could easily be swayed by a new intellectual lure or therapeutic addition. This would partially explain the laments of hydropathic authors over the excesses practiced by home self-doctorers. For many of the latter, the curative element still lay in the water; perhaps they reasoned that more and colder water applications facilitated healing. Those patients able to attend an away-from-home cure were exposed to diverse therapeutics, but it was still most likely that they could doctor at home with only "water, pure and simple." That a straying from vegetarianism and the resumption of coffee and tea *did* filter down to these followers is possible; the consensual system allowed for individuation at home as well as at the cures.

Since the adoption of hydropathic principles complemented the ideology of self-determination so popular in American cultural thought, self-regulating behaviors, such as strict diet and water therapies, appealed to hydropathic followers and were congruent with their world view—they were not imposed upon them. It is possible, and even likely, then, that "loyalty to the system" remained more intact among the following than among the practitioners. The sense of control and ordering experienced by self-doctorers might have been experienced as a sense of limitation or narrowness by the more eccentric practitioners, whose interests, life experiences, and opportunities for mobility were far more diverse. For a certain type of hydropathic practitioner, self-determination presented itself in the next panacea or in the next moneymaking venture. Their choices were greater than those of the following, and as a result they were attracted to an ideology of self-betterment through risk and innovation rather than self-betterment through control and moderation.

Thus the ideology of hydropathy would appeal to different constituencies within the movement on diverse grounds; it was modified to suit its various believers and practitioners. There was, in short, much individuation within the consensual system. The longevity and intensity of one's ideological adherence to hydropathy would be determined by factors well beyond the direct influence of the movement: to the extent that the hydropathic system *served* its constituencies and validated or reflected their world view, they would be loyal to it.

Conclusions

Widely varying water-cure "paradises," whether utilized by infirm married or single women, clergy, Quakers, weary professionals, or reformers, provided physiological and psychological sanctuary to their clientele. Placed most often in rural settings that strove for beauty and serenity, the cures combined removal from stressful and routine environments with the latest in hygienic therapies and water-cure methods.

The cures operated from a common basis of water-cure philosophy, but there were considerable fluctuations among them in longevity, physician mobility, reform activity, and patient population. Their success was largely determined by the energies and interests of individual physicians. The cures studied in detail had varied histories; some survived only a few months, while two flourished for over a hundred years. They also employed a great variety of nonhydropathic therapeutics and supported a cross-section of reform activities.

The individual cures' clientele also reflected the recruitment practices of the ownership. Reformers, clergy, and intellectuals found the Dansville and Elmira cures particularly inviting; reformers and vacationers were drawn to Round Hill in Northampton. Ideologically committed to being economically affordable, the cures were possible, realistically, largely for the middle and upper classes. Thus the hydropathic leadership, through charity, sliding fees, and, most important, home self-doctoring, sought to expand their accessibility. Perhaps the most important elements shared by the cures were the ambience, philosophy, and regimen that made them a temporary oasis from life's constant battles. Patients found a nurturant and genuinely caring community that reflected and perpetuated a world view congruent with their own. Finally, the variations implemented at individual cures speak to both the reform backgrounds of the individual practitioners and the role hygiene played in hydropathic living. Practitioners were of necessity concerned with corollary reforms, such as vegetarianism, temperance, discouraging the use of tobacco, and dress reform. This combination of reform activities rendered the water-cure movement not only a woman's retreat but a reformer's haven as well. Such corollary reforms complemented hydropathic principles and reflected the leadership's belief in the ever-widening capabilities of, and choices for, American women.

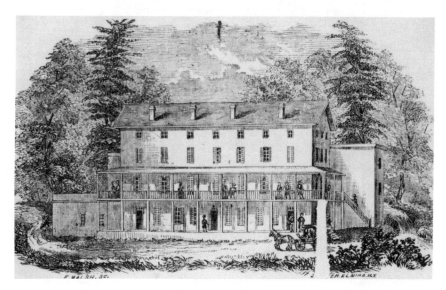

Chapter Four

Hydropathy and the Reform Movements

The Water Cure is most intimately connected with the Temperance cause. There is a strong affinity between drugs, medicines, and tobacco and liquors. They all belong to the same class of substances—foreign, exciting stimulants; and when the system becomes habituated to the use of one, it craves for all. The Water Cure is one of the greatest levers in the Temperance movement because its processes purify the system of all foreign substances and clogged excretions, and leave nature to act free, in harmony with herself.—Water-Cure Journal, 1853

As H.C.F. of Huron, Ohio, wrote in this article, the alliances between hydropathy and other nineteenth-century reforms were extensive: These various movements shared a belief in the desirability of reforming personal living habits as a means of uplifting humanity. Point the way to personal physiological and mental salvation, they believed, and the human will to improve will intercede and follow the calling. Hydropaths realized that the likelihood of actually achieving this "perfection of humankind" was remote, although continual striving was valued and encouraged. Realistically appraising their work, an editor of the journal remarked, "We shall never look for 'perfection' either in man or woman, yet we may hope for a high state of physical and mental cultures."[1] To accomplish this, the editor counseled, people must observe the laws of nature in order to ascertain the rights and duties of both sexes. As the frontispiece of the *Water-Cure Journal* argued:

> We labor for the Physical Regeneration of the Race, well knowing
> that only through this can we successfully promote the Intellectual
> and Moral Elevation of our fellow-men. . . . It is the appointed and
> glorious mission of the WATER-CURE JOURNAL to proclaim and has-
> ten the advent of UNIVERSAL HEALTH, VIRTUE, AND HAPPINESS. We
> ask all who have brothers and sisters of the Human Family, to aid in
> this work, by becoming Co-Workers with us in the great cause of
> HUMAN HEALTH.[2]

To achieve its goal, the hydropathic movement, operating in the
social context of other nineteenth-century reforms, did not view its labors
as an isolated pursuit. Since numerous hydropathic leaders had discovered
the water cure through other reform activities, they adopted and integrated corollary reforms, thus strengthening hydropathy's credibility in
a national reform network. It is important to note, however, that while
hydropathy embraced the breadth of reform sentiment and popular interest in health, it advocated a reform of personal life, but eschewed
more *formal* political involvement.

Hydropaths' Reform Activities

A study of the earlier reform activities of influential and eclectically
representative hydropathic leaders clarifies the leaders' adoption of
hydropathy as well as their activity in corollary concerns. The reform
network that radiated to and from the hydropathic movement illuminates
how adherence to water-cure principles naturally intersected with other
revisionist concerns. As a result, the hydropathic movement embraced
not only those reforms articulated by its stated philosophy but also others
that reflected individuals' backgrounds and priorities. The network was
described in the pages of the *Water-Cure Journal* and encompassed
vegetarianism, temperance, physical education, and, most important, dress
reform and an expanding domestic and social realm of influence for
women.

One of the earliest examples of a hydropathic advocate arriving at
the movement through corollary reforms was Sylvester Graham. Graham
first brought his tireless efforts to reform as a temperance lecturer in
Pennsylvania in the 1830s. Originally inspired by religion, he expanded
his concerns to include vegetarianism, bathing, fresh air, sunlight, dress
reform, and sex hygiene.[3] His notion of sex hygiene was based on his
belief that any sensual stimulation, including marital intercourse, depleted
the body. To prevent such depletion one employed moderate diet, simple
clothing, unarousing reading, and controlled contact between the sexes.[4]
These multifaceted beliefs found expression and support in numerous
issues of the *Water-Cure Journal.*[5]

A contemporary of Graham's, Orson Squire Fowler, brought to the movement his advocacy of the wonders of the Combe's *Elements of Phrenology*. Fowler's interest prompted him to synthesize phrenological principles with hydropathic ones. Originally prepared for a life in the ministry, he found his ultimate summons in phrenology. A prolific lecturer, writer, and publisher, he expanded his concept of reform until phrenology included nearly all other reforms: education, penology, diet, treatment of the insane, dress reform, women's rights, octagonal houses (to let in more light and air) and the water cure. Demonstrative of his growing commitment to hydropathy, he and his brother Lorenzo N. Fowler, who taught phrenology and mental science at Trall's New York Hydropathic School (1853), became the publishers of the *Water-Cure Journal* (1848) and maintained their support of the movement throughout their lifetime.[6]

Two other contemporaries (and disciples) of Graham's, Mary Gove Nichols and Paulina Wright Davis, began their activism in health reform by lecturing to audiences on hygiene, dress reform, and the water cure.[7] Gove Nichols, in particular, led a life that reflected a commitment to numerous reforms. At age fifteen she converted to Quakerism, and in 1831, at age twenty-two, she married Hiram Gove. Although her first-born (1832) lived, four subsequent pregnancies ended in miscarriages or stillbirths. Her own early sufferings convinced her of the necessity to focus on women's health, and to this end she utilized cold-water therapeutics on other women, beginning in 1832.[8] In 1837 she opened a girls' school in Lynn, Massachusetts, and shortly thereafter she began lecturing women on anatomy, physiology, and hygiene—"apparently the first of her sex to undertake this bold enterprise."[9]

Gove Nichols embraced Graham's brand of vegetarianism, considering him "one of the greatest benefactors the world ever had."[10] Since she believed that women's suffering originated from ignorance, especially in matters of sex, she cautioned repeatedly against masturbation, the "solitary vice," which, she believed, caused insanity but could be prevented by hygienic living and moral instruction. To achieve health she recommended a Grahamite regimen and plain diet, plus cold bathing and reform dress.[11]

Concurrent with her work on behalf of physiological reform, Gove Nichols struggled with a difficult and problematic marriage that demonstrated for her the need for women's full equality in that bond. In the early 1840s she left her husband, after years of emotional disquietude and monetary woes, and lectured on property rights for married women, general education, and freedom of thought and action. In this same period she was denounced by, and left, the Society of Friends, edited the *Health Journal and Advocate of Physiological Reform* (Worcester, Massachusetts), wrote *Lectures to Ladies on Anatomy and Physiology* (1842) and anonymous articles for the *Boston Medical and Surgical Journal* (anonymous because she was a woman), and established the *Health Journal and Independent Magazine* (1843), which lasted for only one issue.[12]

After an exhausting year in 1845 battling with her husband over their child, Gove Nichols, recently acquainted with Priessnitz's works, went to stay at the water cures in Brattleboro, Vermont, and Lebanon Springs, New York; at the latter, she lectured to women. Gove Nichols opened her own water cure on Tenth Street in New York City in May 1846,[13] and, aided by a mannequin, she gave instruction in anatomy and physiology. Later, she wrote, "My mission has been to instruct and help Woman, and for the furtherance of this end, I wish to use every means in my power."[14] Gove Nichols wrote frequently for the journal on water-cure therapeutics for mothers and infants, dress reform, and women's mission to be personally healthy and to serve as physicians.[15] She believed that controlling their physiological health was of extreme importance to women's ability to control their future. She addressed nearly all her "open letters" to journal readers as "My Dear Sisters," demonstrating the bonds she felt toward other women. Her prolific writing continued and included *Experience in Water-Cure* (1849) and numerous pieces of fiction. Active in a network of writers, reformers, musicians, and artists, Gove Nichols was a friend of Edgar Allan Poe and Albert Brisbane.[16]

Seeking a like-minded mate, she married Thomas Low Nichols shortly after her divorce. (She had met Nichols in 1847.) He was "a writer and editor with advanced views on the rights of women"[17] and one of the three most influential hydropathic leaders (along with Shew and Trall). He, too, had been greatly influenced by Graham and advocated dietary reform. They were married by a Swedenborgian clergyman in July 1848.[18]

Nichols received his M.D. in 1850 from New York University, and wrote his first book, *A Journal in Jail,* while serving a four-month prison term resulting from a libel suit. Together he and Mary turned their tireless energies to hydropathy, the reform that had become their first priority.

In the spring of 1850 the Nicholses opened a cure on West 22nd Street in New York City, and Thomas became a steady writer for the *Water-Cure Journal.* His contributions ranged from chatty essays that enumerated his reasons for becoming a water-cure physician to scientific articles on human physiology.[19] In a candid essay published in 1850, he credited his conversion to hydropathy to his meeting Mary Gove: "I found in her a thorough understanding of the principles and practice of Water-Cure in its purest and highest sense. A thorough anatomist, a profound physician, and a woman of remarkable philosophic powers, she had penetrated more deeply the mysteries of life than any one I had ever seen."[20] Also active in vegetarian reform efforts, he was elected secretary of the American Hygienic and Hydropathic Association of Physicians and Surgeons (1850) and was one of nine vice-presidents of the American Vegetarian Society.[21]

Utilizing their combined skills, the couple opened the American Hydropathic Institute, a water-cure college, in September 1851.[22] The institute succeeded for two terms, and the Nicholses turned their zeal toward a new water-cure establishment in Port Chester, New York.[23] During this time Thomas published *Women, in All Ages and Nations* (1849), a chronicle of women's history, and *Esoteric Anthropology* (1853), noteworthy for its forthright handling of sexual intercourse.

Committed as he was to furthering water-cure philosophy, but experiencing difficulties with the editor of the *Water-Cure Journal*, who saw his teachings as "free love" that blackened the reputation of hydropathy,[24] Thomas began his own publication, *Journal of Health, Water-Cure and Human Progress*, in April 1853. This journal's masthead demonstrates his commitment to reorganizing social priorities. It was "opposed to all existing forms of governments and all religious sects; to the prevailing systems of Finance, Commerce, Law, and Industry; to the institutions of Marriage, Slavery, and all forms of oppression and plunder."[25] Attracted as they both were to the complete reform of society, Thomas and Mary planned to join, in 1853, the community of Modern Times (founded by Josiah Warren in 1851) on Long Island, New York. Based on the principles of "individual sovereignty," complete self-expression, and noncompetitiveness, the community counted one hundred families in eighty dwellings. The Nicholses' connection to the community, while tenuous, served to reinforce their desire to open a "School of Life."[26] Their simultaneous founding of the first water-cure college and planned participation in a utopian community speaks to the breadth and diversity, if not the implementation, of their concerns.

The Nicholses' growing fascination with larger and more complex social innovations led them to devote two years to lecturing on socialism, spiritualism, and the harmonic life. On completion of their tours, their desire to link personal and professional ideals led them once again to an experimental community, the Memnonia Institute in Yellow Spring, Ohio. At Memnonia they joined hydropathic practices to the institute's facilities when they took over the water-cure establishment (from the Hoyts, later of the Athol Water Cure) amid much controversy. Apparently, Horace Mann, president of Antioch College, did not want what he perceived to be a colony of free-lovers near his campus. Friction in the community abated when the renowned spiritualist J. B. Conklin visited and calmed the rising tensions between the Nicholses and the community, while spawning much interest in his beliefs.[27]

The Memnonia Institute apparently did not reflect fully enough the Nicholses' concerns, because their interest in spiritualism led them to the Roman Catholic Church. Devoid of their former zeal, their experimental community failed. After opening one more water cure (the Central Park Water-Cure in New York City), the Nicholses left for England, where they continued to "write extensively on sanitation, health, human physiology, food reform, and related subjects."[28] The broad and erratic careers of Mary Gove and Thomas Low Nichols demonstrated their undying commitment to the principles and philosophy of hydropathy, their corollary efforts on behalf of numerous other reforms, and the often short-lived projects that they abandoned in the search for a fuller "vision."

Joel Shew, one of the triumvirate with Nichols and Trall and the original editor of the *Water-Cure Journal*, began lecturing on similar issues as Mary Gove Nichols at approximately the same time. Shew seems to have come to the hydropathic movement rather directly. Having learned of Priessnitz's successful water treatments during at least two visits to Grafenberg during the 1840s, Shew returned to New York and adopted significant portions of the Silesian's ideology and treatment. He added friction and massage treatments, as well as rest, exercise and dietary reform. Shew founded and edited the *Water-Cure Journal* in New York in 1844. A second series, also under his editorship, began in 1845. He remained in this capacity (with the brief assistance of F. D. Pierson) until the Fowlers and Wells took it over (circa 1848, until 1864). Then the editorship was briefly taken over by Trall.[29] Shew, like his colleagues, contributed frequently to the journal on the philosophy of the water cure and specific water-cure processes, and he kept readers informed about the doings at his own cures in New York City and Syosset (Oyster Bay), New York.[30] He also wrote the *The Water-Cure and Health Almanac* (1847), which was quite popular.

Trall, already described in some detail, entered health reform by way of temperance and combined hydropathy with advocacy of proper diet, fresh air, exercise, and rest. He took over the editing of the *Water-Cure Journal* in 1849, and as editor published numerous pieces about his professional travels that expounded on water processes and their efficacy.[31] In one 1864 article, revealing the breadth of his reform concerns, he derided the practices of hunting and fishing for sport.[32] He also filled the journal's pages with treatments for specific diseases and expounded on the natural bonds between hydropathy and kindred reforms.[33] A tireless educator, lecturer, and writer, Trall was the principal and founder of the New York and Minnesota Hygeio-Therapeutic colleges. He transformed the *Water-Cure Journal* into the *Herald of Health* in 1863, and was described by a contemporary as having "comparatively little deference for old theories and opinions, and is thoroughly progressive in all things." He continued to contribute to other health journals while writing reform-oriented books.[34]

One other New York hydropath qualifies as both an exceptional leader and a multifaceted reformer. A friend and coworker of Gerritt Smith in the antislavery and temperance causes, James Caleb Jackson turned his attention to health reform after an illness and stay at Dr. Silas O. Gleason's Greenwood Spring Water Cure at Cuba, New York, in 1847. After his recovery, Jackson, Gleason, and Theodosia Gilbert started a hygienic institute near Scott, New York, called Glen Haven Water Cure. Gleason left the institute three years later, and after Gilbert's death and a fire in the main building, Jackson rented a shabby structure in Dansville

(1858) and named it "Our Home on the Hillside" (later called the Jackson Sanatorium). Dr. Harriet N. Austin, his adopted daughter and a graduate of the Nicholses' college, joined him in this venture.[35] Austin, a prolific writer and lecturer, contributed to the journal on dress reform, women's rights, dancing, water-cure philosophy, and exercise, often addressing her readership, as Gove Nichols did, as "My Dear Sisters."[36]

Austin, like her father, viewed water cure as a vital link in an all-encompassing reform movement. Committed as she was to expanding and redefining the physical and social roles available to women, she designed a bloomerlike costume that she called the "American costume." Although patients at Our Home were not required to wear it, its adoption, like vegetarianism, was definitely applauded.

In addition to supporting Austin's work in dress reform, Jackson invented Granula and Somo, "a health coffee," and founded Our Home Granula Company to manufacture the products. The combination of dietary innovation and the charms of Jackson and Austin seem to have been successful, as the list of illustrious patients grew: Clara Barton stayed at Our Home after the Franco-Prussian War; Horace Greeley, Robert Dale Owens, and Baynard Taylor (a lecturer on Moscow) were also patients.[37]

Jackson's and Austin's hydropathic methods and reform activities, especially dress reform and dietary innovations, had an immense impact on the Seventh-Day Adventist movement and, consequently, on hydropathy and hygiene globally, as influential Adventists sought and found relief at Our Home in the 1860s. This inspired Ellen G. White, spiritual mentor of the Adventists, to go to Dansville, where she received "heavenly instructions" to set up a Dansville-type water cure in Battle Creek, Michigan, the headquarters of her church. In 1866 one of the earlier-cured Adventists left the staff of Our Home and went to Battle Creek to open the first Seventh-Day Adventist water cure, the Western Health Reform Institute (WHRI). Jackson, whose cure was being emulated, was a significant influence and lectured at the institute, but Ellen G. White and Dr. John Harvey Kellogg are most often remembered as the forces that built the Seventh-Day Adventist health "empire."[38]

Trall, invited by White and her husband, James, an elder in the church, went west to lecture with Jackson. Shortly after these visits, Ellen White's visions returned. In these she was directed to pursue hygienic living. A great point of controversy among Adventists, the "visions," in fact, closely resembled the written works of her health-reform contemporaries, which she claimed not to have read before her own visionary writings.[39]

Regardless of the origin of her information or her claims, White's impact on hydropathy was profound. For the publication of a series of six pamphlets that would advance her vision, *Health, or How to Live* (1865), White employed the services of Kellogg, son of Seventh-Day Adventist parents who had raised all thirteen of their children according to the principles expounded in the *Water-Cure Journal*. Kellogg then left Michigan to earn medical degrees from Trall's Hygeio-Therapeutic College, the University of Michigan (1873–1875), and Bellevue Hospital Medical School (1874–1875). On his return to Battle Creek he was appointed superintendent of the Western Health Reform Institute, "a water cure modeled after Our Home and the first link in what was to become a worldwide chain of Seventh-Day Adventist medical institutions."[40] Before Kellogg assumed his post, Horatio S. Lay, an Adventist whose wife had been cured in Dansville, was the chief physician with Phoebe Lamson, who graduated from Trall's Hygeio-Therapeutic College. In addition to overseeing the patients, Lay edited the monthly *Health Reformer*, a journal that began publication in August 1866.[41] Trall, a supporter and visitor to the institute, became a regular contributor to the *Reformer*, turned over the subscription list of his *Gospel of Health*, merging the two journals and giving Battle Creek a nationally influential role in the water-cure and health-reform movements.[42]

White also embraced complementary reforms. She devoted her attention, and encouraged her parishioners to do likewise, to the temperance cause via the Woman's Christian Temperance Union (in the form of the Battle Creek Reform Club). Further, the church's temperance pledge led to the American Health and Temperance Association, founded in 1879 and presided over by Kellogg. White also modified the American costume, which she had seen at Dansville, and sold the pattern for 25 cents through the *Health Reformer*. She advocated dress reform until a 1875 vision instructed her to abandon its use, a relief for her since there had been much infighting over the best design to wear. She advocated instead a simple, no-frills long dress that did not sweep the street.

A central figure alongside White in building the church's prominence, Kellogg, an orthodox-trained physician and eclectic health-reform activist, combined his adherence to hydropathic principles with other medical innovations. These included the student of surgery, the effects of electrical treatment when combined with hydropathy, and the invention of numerous exercise appliances. Also an avid advocate of dress reform and vegetarianism, Kellogg converted three dogs to vegetarianism and tried his luck on a wolf; he also corseted Mrs. Kellogg's collie to observe its reactions. After women gave up tightly laced garments, Kellogg turned his attention to male dress and urged daily changes of undergarments, use of porous fabrics, wearing white, and sensible shoes.[43]

Kellogg is best remembered for his attention to dietary reform. His manufactured cereal was originally used in the diet of water-cure patients; it eventually achieved international usage and success. He used the bakery in Battle Creek to produce his gluten water, Avenola, and granola, with Granose flakes following.[44]

The success and influence of Kellogg in the church led to tension among him, the Whites, and the Adventist leadership. This peaked in

1907 when the church expelled W. K. Kellogg, John's brother, heir, and the advertising innovator behind the eventual "cornflake empire." Shortly thereafter, John was expelled on the ground that he was "leading a movement to undermine the tenets of the church to disrespect toward Mrs. White." Kellogg, who for years had been embarrassed by White's "visions," one of his biographers has noted, was probably relieved to be disassociated from the church.[45]

As a result of the expulsion of Kellogg from the Seventh-Day Adventist church, his role has been downplayed in church history. But his legacy remains intact: The combined efforts of Ellen G. White and John Harvey Kellogg influenced the dress, health, and eating habits of 2.5 million Seventh-Day Adventists and promoted water-cure principles in thirty-three sanitariums and smaller treatment facilities globally.[46]

As these brief examinations of the backgrounds of hydropathic leaders demonstrate, they viewed themselves and the water cure as the central link in a national reform network. They felt it their duty to include complementary physical and social reforms as an extension of hydropathy's concerns. It is worth noting that the national leadership was predominantly male, the female side of husband–wife or father–daughter "teams" being the exception. So, even among the reformist leadership, there was not parity between women and men. In this, the water-cure movement mimicked other gender-mixed groups of that era; it further speaks to the limits of the movement's ability to reconceptualize gender relationships fundamentally. At the individual cures, as has been shown, there was greater opportunity for women to share positions of authority with men.

Physical Education

Among related reforms that received hydropathic acceptance and adoption was physical education. Physical training was furthered by Dio Lewis in later works such as *Our Girls* (1871), which advocated it particularly for young girls as future mothers and for women's development as thinking adults.[47] The *Water-Cure Journal* repeatedly stressed physical education's desirability in articles such as Dr. Antiseli's serialized "Physical Education," Trall's "Family Gymnastics," and Dr. Vail's "Exercise as a Remedial Measure." All argued for the positive, strengthening, and invigorating effects of physical education as a complementary hygienic reform to hydropathy.[48]

This early interest in physical education expanded to embrace "Kinesipathy, or the Movement Cure," in which specific motions were developed to aid the recovery of affected areas. Movement cures were also heralded by hydropaths as aids to the smooth operation of the circulatory, nervous, secretory, and muscular systems, as well as for spinal disorders.[49] In the United States, the coupling of hydropathy with kinesipathy and related movement cures was not uncommon. The Round Hill Water Cure in Northampton, Massachusetts, was particularly renowned for their integration.

Vegetarianism

Like physical education, vegetarianism was an outgrowth of the hydropathic emphasis on hygienic living. Beginning with the teachings of Sylvester Graham and William Alcott, hydropathic reformers very early adopted and advocated radical dietary platforms. Still active contributors to the *Water-Cure Journal*, Graham and Alcott preached the interconnectedness of diet and the cold-water cure. Indicative of this are Alcott's "Cold Water Facts" (1845) and Graham's "Fruits and Vegetables" (1851).[50] Trall's obituary of Graham in 1851, eight months after Graham's last contribution to the *Water-Cure Journal*, clearly reflects the admiration held for a colleague and mentor: "His powerful reasoning faculties and active cautiousness rendered him extremely devoted, searching, and guarded, as a scholar and author; while his large ideality caused him to spare no toil or pains to give finish and perfection to whatever went out to the world from his hands."[51]

The bond between hydropathy and vegetarianism was demonstrated again and again. Graham and Alcott argued that since fleshless life was morally superior, it must also be physiologically superior, since God's wisdom decreed both. Meatless eating, they claimed, was a natural use of reason, one in accord with God-given instinct; a vegetarian diet was more digestible and more nutritious than eating meat. While their physiological views have been characterized as self-serving, they did reflect the reformers' desire to "use science to improve the human condition without alienating man from nature in the process."[52] The work of the early dietary reformers was carried on admirably in the pages of the journal. Specific articles addressed the efficacy of single food items such as apples, Indian pudding, loaf bread, fruits, and potatoes.[53] Recipes appeared regularly, encouraging readers to abandon the unhealthy staples of the American diet. Recipes taught the how-to's of cooking biscuits, pastry, cake, corn, cucumbers, bread, and numerous other items.[54] Trall's recipe for water biscuits exemplifies the simplicity and wholesomeness of the food. The only ingredients were graham flour and warm water, baked into small, thin crackers that were advisable for those with weak stomachs and dyspectics.[55]

Dietary reforms encompassed more than food items. The time allowed for the proper digestion of different foods, the necessity of thorough mastication, and the abandonment of a very familiar kitchen utensil, the frying pan, were all discussed.[56] Dr. Andrew W. Combe, writing in "The Physiology of Digestion" (1850), compiled a table listing numerous common (and desirable) foods and the ideal times allotted for their digestion.[57] Combe's recommended times, given in hours and minutes, varied according to the method by which the food was prepared (fried, boiled, raw, stewed, broiled, or roasted). Hydropaths emphasized the importance of preparing food properly and bemoaned the fact that so much cooking done in frying pans used grease, lard, or shortening, ingredients that fattened, slowed, and debilitated the American populace. They believed that a desirable solution was the "outlawing" of the frying pan because it was an unhygienic cooking implement. In a mock law printed in the journal they proposed: "Thus—Be it enacted, that on the first day of January, 1852, every fyring-pan in the United States be broken up and sold for iron, and that no more be ever manufactured henceforth forever."[58]

The real heart of dietary reform, however, was an abandonment of "flesh eating." Arguing that meat products impaired physical health, were difficult to digest, carried contagious diseases, and were not hygienic, hydropaths were quite persuasive when they portrayed them as the foodstuffs of a lesser calling.[59]

The reform network between the water curers and the vegetarians was highly developed and extensive. In nineteenth-century America, meatless life was a legitimate social and moral issue.[60] Vegetarian boardinghouses and restaurants carried ads in the *Water-Cure Journal*. Vegetarianism became institutionalized through a national network of organizations. The first of these was begun at the American Vegetarian Convention held in New York City in May 1850 and religiously reported on in the journal. The list of participants read much like that of a water-cure conference, and the officers included the familiar names Alcott, Graham, Shew, Trall, and Wells. Of the ten officers, six were known practitioners or followers of hydropathy.[61] As the proceedings of the meeting revealed: "Dr. Bedortha, water-cure physician, of Troy, gave an interesting account of his experiments and observations, and one of the delegates from Philadelphia, a hale and hearty man of sixty-two, gave the pleasant result of forty years' use of a fleshless diet."[62] The *Water-Cure Journal* went on in great detail to print the declarations of the founding Vegetarian Convention,[63] and in the years that followed the constitution, philosophy, and leaders of the American Vegetarian Society were regular topics of discussion in the journal.

Of particular note within the hydropathic and vegetarian movements is the overlap in leadership. The third annual meeting, for example, was reported to have heard a brief address by President Alcott. T. L. Nichols was, by 1851, the first vice-president, and Mary Gove Nichols spoke at the convention.[64] In 1852 the *Water-Cure Journal* began covering the activities of the New York Vegetarian Society, of which Trall was president and a member of the Executive Committee.[65] In 1862 Trall was discussed again, this time as president of the New York Dietetic Reform Association.[66]

The overlapping membership was nowhere better demonstrated than in the company assembled at a vegetarian feast in the 1850s in western New York:

> There was a great vegetarian feast, with Horace Greeley presiding, and among the honored guests on the dais were Mrs. Lucy Stone, T. L. Nichols, after he was sprung from the Buffalo calaboose, Mrs. Amelia Bloomer and Susan B. Anthony. Dr. James Caleb Jackson, of the Glen Haven Water Cure at the head of Skaneatles Lake in New York, proposed a toast in a bumper of well water, "Total Abstinence, Women's Rights, and Vegetarianism."[67]

The reform network that existed between the vegetarian and hydropathic movements included philosophy, leadership, and practice. As vegetarianism grew out of hygienic living principles and dietary reform, so did temperance.

Temperance

Temperance, while nearly always taken to mean abstention from alcohol, was also used by the hydropaths in reference to coffee, tea, and tobacco. They believed that once the taste was whetted by these milder stimulants, the hard-core intoxicants were sure to follow. Articles whose titles leave little doubt as to their content, such as "Coffee as Narcotic or Poison" and "Palpitation of the Heart—Tea, Coffee and Tobacco," dramatized the physical and moral degeneracy that resulted from their use.[68] Alcott was inspired to write in the journal on this issue, and his "Effects of Coffee and Tea on Human Health" similarly addressed the physiological results of these stimulants.[69] Ever mindful of the impact a first-person testimony could make, the editor printed the story of a woman patient at a water-cure establishment who had been ordered by her physician to abstain from coffee and tea.

> Dr. Water-Cure [as we will call him] . . . strictly forbade the use of tea and coffee; it was hard work for me to give them up. No one but a person who has been in a similar position can tell how I felt. But there was no hope for it; my physician was decided on the point, and I was obliged to make the attempt. At last, however, I succeeded in overcoming my desires for these stimulants. My health was gradually improving all the time . . . and after a residence there of some months, I returned home greatly renovated.[70]

Tobacco met an even more hostile response from hydropaths than did coffee and tea. Numerous articles testified to the horrors of the substance, such as "Effects of Tobacco upon the Nerves," "Tobacco: Its Action upon the Health, and Its Influence upon the Morals and Intelligence of Man," and "On the Diseases Resulting from the Immoderate Use of Tobacco."[71] The consequences of smoking, according to this last article, "are manifested in the buccal and pharyngeal mucous membrane, and on the brain and nervous system."[72]

The journal's editors sought out reform leaders in other movements who adhered to abstinent principles. This was the motivation behind the reprinting in the journal of a letter from William Lloyd Garrison that had been read at the founding of the American Anti-Tobacco Society.[73] The journal also furnished a model petition that could be sent to one's legislature deploring the sale of tobacco to minors:

> The undersigned inhabitants of ___ Co., believing the use of tobacco predisposes strongly to the use of intoxicating drinks, besides the destruction of health and morals . . . therefore would respectfully ask of your Honorable Body the passage of a law prohibiting the sale or giving away of tobacco to minors, and that provision be made therein for arresting and detaining minors.[74]

Minors, the petition concluded, should be arrested and detained until they divulged who had supplied them with tobacco. In the event that the serious approach did not appeal to someone, the following "filler" made the same point: "There is a dog in Roxbury, Massachusetts who has acquired the habit of chewing tobacco. He is shunned by all the decent dogs of the neighborhood."[75]

Like abstention from coffee, tea, and tobacco, avoidance of alcohol received total hydropathic support. Trall, calling temperance one plank in the hydropaths' hygienic platform, wrote in 1865: "The effects of intemperance may be summed up in a few words—vice, crime, pauperism, social corruption and national decline, and the root of the evil is alcoholic medication."[76] Thus, water-cure leaders saw themselves at the helm of the temperance struggle because of the distressingly high alcohol content of many popular patent medicines. It varied from 20 percent to 80 percent, and hydropaths believed that until the general public could be made to understand that this, too, constituted intemperance, their work was not complete. Anxious to echo agreeing opinions, the *Water-Cure Journal* reprinted—as a lead story—Henry Ward Beecher's statements against alcoholic medication, but it entitled the article "Beecher in a Muddle" because, the editors felt, he had been unclear and unsteady in his contentions.[77] Two years later, Horace Greeley received a similar reprimand in the journal for having said that alcohol in medication was acceptable.[78] This debate had reached such proportions that the November 1865 issue carried as its lead article "A Muddled Muddlement," which encouraged temperance supporters to stop debating the efficacy of alcohol in medications with the allopaths and return to the work at hand—education and changing the public's reliance on alcohol-based medications.[79] Notwithstanding its own admonitions to desist from the debate, the journal printed an article in 1867, "Drunkenness among Women," which argued that American women were particularly susceptible to alcoholism because of the acceptability of drug medications.[80]

By entering into this discourse, hydropaths fueled the great attention being paid to the seemingly indiscriminate and largely uncondemned use of alcohol in medication. The use of alcohol for the treatment of virtually every disease was historically common, and it was discontinued (largely) only within the twentieth century.[81] The debate in mid-nineteenth-century America centered on the apparent contradictions inherent in the use of patent medicines by advocates of temperance as well as by the general public.

A case in point is the Lydia Pinkham Vegetable Compound, which, at its introduction in 1875, contained 19 percent alcohol (40 proof), much more than table wine or sherry.[82] This did not seem a problem to the temperate Pinkham family, since "alcohol, as far as they were concerned, was a legitimate medicinal substance."[83]

For women who were denied, through social proscription, the possibility of drinking in public barrooms or private parlors, patent medicines provided a socially sanctioned means of consuming alcohol. When the editor of the *Ladies' Home Journal* polled fifty members of the Women's Christian Temperance Union in the 1890s, he found that thirty-seven of them self-doctored regularly with alcoholic nostrums.[84]

Allopathic physicians contributed to the notion that alcohol was an effective and desirable form of medication. After having rejected depletive heroic therapeutics, allopaths prescribed drugs that, they believed, would sustain "the vital energy." They turned away from bleeding and calomel and toward opium and alcohol. As one chronicler has noted:

> The new therapy shared with the old an emphasis on demonstrable symptomatic relief at the expense of sound treatment. . . . Alcohol constituted a therapeutic mainstay in the late nineteenth century. Prescribed first for its tonic effects and later for its supposed ability to kill germs internally, alcohol was usually administered as whiskey or brandy. Physicians recommended doses equivalent to five shots a day for adults and dosed children with amounts sufficient to cause drunkenness.[85]

Also, the widespread use of the hypodermic syringe, when used with morphine, both of which were available over the counter and through the Sears, Roebuck catalogue, produced a generation all too familiar with socially acceptable, unnamed, and unchecked addictions.[86] Into this milieu, hydropaths injected their inflexible stance: No alcohol in any form or in any amount was permissible for either medicinal or recreational purposes.

In addition to being leaders in the alcohol-in-medication debate, hydropaths, through the *Water-Cure Journal*, were eager to note other links between the cure and temperance. This was exemplified in the enthusiastic introduction of a new contributor to the journal: "[Mr. Spencer], editor of the Ithaca Chronicle, a gentleman well known as an able editor and a champion of the Temperance cause, has written a number of articles on water-cure, which are richly worth a place in our Journal."[87] An October 1853 article, "Water-Cure and the Temperance Reform versus Drugs, Tobacco, and Liquor," left no doubt as to their common cause:

> The Water-Cure is most intimately connected with the Temperance cause. There is a strong affinity between drugs, medicines, and tobacco and liquors. They all belong to the same class of substances—foreign, exciting stimulants; and when the system becomes habituated to the use of one, it craves for all.[88]

The water cure, the author, H.C.F., argued, was vital to temperance because

> its processes purify the system of all foreign substances and clogged excretions, and leave nature to act free, in harmony with herself. . . . The Water-Cure is the "open sesame" to Temperance, progression and human improvement; the forerunner to sound health and elevated morals. . . . It is the hope of the million . . . for all sick or well, rich or poor, high or low, bond or free, white or black.[89]

This affinity found support in the *Water-Cure Journal* in a number of ways: in the publication of an intricate engraving of the New York State Temperance Medal, which commemorated the passage of the Prohibitory Liquor Law; in Trall's *The Alcoholic Controversy;* in articles such as "Temperance—What Is It?" and "How to Live; or, Temperance in a Nutshell," by L. N. Fowler; and in reports on the National Temperance Convention and the local temperance convention in Saratoga Springs, New York.[90]

The hydropaths' insistence on total temperance harmonized with their goal of individual perfectibility—how could one purify the body and assume a new level of health and self-determination with the effects of alcohol surging through one's blood? There was no middle ground in an issue as critical as this. Once again, the principles of hydropathy had found expression in a complementary reform. Temperance, like vegetarianism, diet reform, physical education, women's right to practice medicine, and the overhaul of therapeutic procedures, was an aspect of hygienic living.

The Civil War

In the reform network surrounding the water-cure movement, the absence of one issue is revealing. The posture of neutrality that the leadership adopted (through the *Herald of Health,* formerly the *Water-Cure Journal*) toward the Civil War seems puzzling and was unusual among nineteenth-century reformers. Convinced that the war would be short lived, the journal maintained a neutral position throughout its duration. At first glance the motivation appears to be pacifist. A closer reading reveals a hesitancy to alienate the South—by claiming allegiance to the North—since this would jeopardize what the editors predicted would become the new locus of health-reform activity.[91] As the war drew to a close, an editorial in the January 1864 issue spoke in noncommittal terms of its results: "Battles may still be fought, and victories won on either side, but surely and gradually are all things tending to the speedy termination of this gigantic strife." The editor, continuing, commented on the pending availability of the South for health-reform efforts:

> The sunny South will hereafter be more accessible than ever before to northern habits, and northern industry. . . . The Southern States, we predict, will be the best field in which to propagate our principles of Health Reform, and to practice the Hygienic system of the Healing Art. There are hundreds of places where soft water, mountain scenery, balmy and cool breezes, can be found in connection with a genial climate all the year round, with a soil of marvelous fertility.[92]

The editorial concluded with the observation that some water-cure graduates were already planning to locate in the South and, finally, with the hopeful prediction that the system was nearly ensured of success in New Orleans.

The South never became the new center of health reform. But the earlier hesitancy, if not outright failure, of the movement's leadership to confront the complex and painful issues surrounding the Civil War rendered the *Water-Cure Journal* strangely disengaged from the racial and political implications of the war. For example, in a July 1861 article Trall likened the deaths at Fort Sumter to the "deaths" of allopathic medical journals, an analogy that, while potent, resounded with poor taste.[93] Several months later, in January 1862, the journal ran an article asserting that the war on human constitutions was worse than the Civil War. A third piece, in March 1862, lamented that the war had diverted attention from health and other reforms.[94] In addition, several months' issues did not mention the war on the front page, an omission likely to have been unsettling to those in the movement who saw a connection between health reform and freeing the slaves. And for those not within the fold of hydropathy, the minimal attention paid to the political and moral aspects of the war probably served as more proof of the movement's exclusive obsession with health issues. Since no written records report the public response to this neutrality, it is difficult to measure its impact on the popularity of the cures and the credibility of the movement. Although this relative detachment from larger political issues was unusual for nineteenth-century reformers, hydropathy promoted one strain of perfectionism: an effort to reform the self and control the body that ends at those boundaries. Certainly contemporary (1980s) health-reform and self-help groups have something of that tendency.

This is not to say that the journal was oblivious to the medical aspects of the war. The editors included a "Soldier's Department," which addressed issues such as "Gymnastics Training for the Soldiers," "Value of Sanitary Measures in Armies," "The Deadly Virtues of Army Rations," and "Drunkenness in the Army."[95] This column was not introduced until 1864, but earlier articles had addressed general health issues surrounding the war and cited an increased need for hygienic principles to combat the effects of military life and battle casualties.

Although the *Water-Cure Journal* as the national voice for the movement avoided the issue of slavery, individual articles within the journal did mention whether the home practitioner of hydropathy was Negro or mulatto, and included "Negroes and whites" among the list of those who would surely benefit from the water cure. A case in point is the 1850 salutation in the correspondent Noggs's "Gossip from Boston," which begins: "Old and young, wise and ignorant, black, white and all the intermediate shades are being 'born of the water,' and great is the rejoicing in Franklin street."[96] In more concrete instances, individual water-cure physicians and establishments grappled with the issues of race and slavery head-on. Specific examples include the Athol, Massachusetts, cure's complicity in the Underground Railroad and the Dansville cure's linkages to antislavery efforts (both of which were discussed in Chapter Three). Hydropathic texts, meanwhile, although they denied the intellectual inferiority of Negroes, did echo other identifiably stereotypical and not always flattering portrayals of the black race.

Dress Reform and Women's Influence

Two related reforms complete the network that so intimately involved hydropathy, and similar hesitancies to enter the clearly political realm are again evident. Dress reform and an expanded role for women, closely resembling a domestic feminism, were carried into the public arena, although not necessarily the formal (male) political sphere. Both were essential concerns in the water-cure movement. Already demonstrated in the hydropathic conception of woman's physiology and her right to practice medicine, the issue of women's influence within the movement expanded to include these interrelated reforms, which demanded new definitions for women's physical, social, and intellectual abilities.

Articles in the journal were often labeled "woman's rights" without encompassing formal political issues and strategies. If the definition of "rights" is expanded to include actions that greatly affected social policy and customs, however, the "woman's rights" expounded by hydropaths were profoundly political.[97] These rights included the right to practice medicine, the right to participate in a family's economic decisions, and the right to be respected by children and workingmen. The term *woman's rights* in the strictly political sense—that is, implying legal or constitutional activism—does not figure prominently in the hydropathic vocabulary. Instead, it was used to signify woman's position, opportunities, and just rewards within a domestic realm *as well as* within the larger social realm: This was often referred to as "emancipation" by the leadership and the following. The hydropaths echoed a domestic–feminist rationale that empowered women within their own sphere and valued women as women within the home. This notion echoed sentiments that emphasized women's higher moral nature and "not only implied women's moral superiority but also created proud solidarity among women."[98]

Beyond contributing to the empowerment of women within the domestic realm, hydropaths advocated an extension of women's role into such social and intellectual activities as influencing opinion, educating family and neighbors, petition writing, pursuing hydropathic training, innovative types of paid work, and marriage-partner selection. This, they argued, would improve woman's self-image and her cultural status.

The hydropathic support of women's expanded roles was often argued through the issue of dress reform, which involved a fundamental critique of cultural concepts of feminity through the ignoring of fashion's dictates. The advocacy of immediate and substantial dress reform was argued first in the name of health and second for the sake of female advancement. Tight-lacing corsets, stays, high heels, voluminous yardage, heavy materials that trapped moisture against the body, and certain hats and shawls all came under scrutiny and then attack. Before 1851, the journal had printed a few scattered articles on dress reform, but the real commitment began in February 1851 after Rachel Brooks Gleason (later of the Elmira Water Cure) wrote urging it to print practical and comfortable fashion plates for women readers to emulate.[99] From that date onward, it was a rare edition of the *Water-Cure Journal* that did not devote at least one column to the issue; in fact, a "Dress Reform" column became a regular feature. The articles took essentially three approaches: The first approach urged the use of reform dress on hygienic grounds; the second contained testimonials from women who had found the new dress liberating; and the third argued that reform dress would elevate women's self-image and cultural status because they would no longer be slaves to fashion.

Indicative of the pieces that urged adoption of reform dress on the basis of hygienic principles are Dr. W. E. Coale's "Woman's Dress, a Cause of Uterine Displacements"; "Dress Reform. A Short Piece on Long Skirts," which argued that long dresses were a health hazard because they were cumbersome, picked up dirt, and absorbed dampness; "Tight Lacing," by Dr. D. W. Ranney; Madame Demorest's "Dress and Its Relation to Health"; and "Reform in Woman's Dress," which likened women's dressing habits to alcoholic addiction and medicinal poisoning.[100]

While these articles appealed to the intellectual bent of the readers, the editors were not unaware of the fact that the new costumes were meeting with scornful responses on the street and were considered by some to be quite unattractive. To combat this opposition, the journal devoted numerous full- and half-page spreads to intricate engravings of the various reform dresses in an attempt to portray their aesthetic value as well as their healthy attributes. Drawings contrasted American clothing with French fashions, Hungarian bloomers, Rocky Mountain bloomers, Bloomer and Webber dresses, and Water-Cure bloomers.[101] While the costumes varied in detail, they consisted basically of a loose-fitting pair of pantaloons (which either ended a few inches short of the ground, gathered in, or touched the top of the ankle in a square cut) and a tailored, loose-fitting dress that fell to below the knee (one costume had a top that fell just below the waist). The sleeves could be long or short, but no severe gatherings were allowed. Necklines varied from a V to oval-shaped but always left plenty of room for breathing and free movement. The outfit was completed with a belt at the waist that helped give it more shape but that never approximated the hourglass form so fashionable at the time.

Certain visual techniques employed in these journal drawings warrant mention. Quite often, the woman in reform dress was pictured alongside the "Allopathic Lady Who Considers It Vulgar to Enjoy Good Health." In these instances, the contrast was striking. Encased from head to foot and wearing a tight bonnet with her hair pinned to her head, the allopathic lady was a study in confined fashion. She had a tiny waist, a voluminous skirt that trailed the ground, and a parasol held precariously in one hand. A pinched if not stern expression graced her lips. To her right, the women in reform costume stood with their arms around one another, gesturing, hair loose or wearing ample hats. They seemed a study in camaraderie and comfort.[102]

Poems served as further evidence of the growing importance hydropaths placed on dress reform. Further, they served as comic relief in pointing out both the absurdity of fashionable dress and the public scorn levied against reform attire. Representative of these poems was "The Fashionable Lady's Prayer," which epitomized traits scorned by the hydropaths. Class resentments also are evidenced in references to the decadence of leisured women and the rich and indulgent diets of the wealthy.

"Give us this day our daily bread,"
    And pies and cakes besides,
To load the stomach, pain the head,
    And choke the vital tides,
And if too soon a friend decays,
    Or dies in agony—
We'll talk of "God's mysterious ways,"
    And lay it all to thee.

Give us, to please a morbid taste,
    In spite of pain and death,
Consumption-strings around the waist,
    Almost to stop the breath;
Then, if infirmity attends
    Our stinted progeny,
In visitation for our sins—
    We'll lay it all to thee.

. . .

We do disdain to toil and sweat,
    Like girls of vulgar blood!
Of labor, give us not a bit,
    For physic not for food;
And if for lack of exercise,
    We lack the stamina
Of those we trample and despise—
    We'll lay it all to thee.

. . .

Yes, give us coffee, wine and tea,
    And hot things introduce
The stomach's warm bath twice a day,
    To weaken and reduce;
And if defying nature's laws,
    Dyspeptic we must be—
We scorn to search for human cause,
    But lay it all to thee.[103]

Written with a similar message, "The Victim," by A.S.A. of Morris, New York, also urged dress reform on hygienic grounds.[104] Not to be outdone in wit and innovation, Mattie's "A Parody" poses the familiar-sounding refrain:

> To breathe, or not to breathe; that's the question
> Whether 'tis nobler in the mind to suffer
> The slings and arrows of outrageous fashion,
> Or to bear the scoffs and ridicule of those
> Who despise the Bloomer dresses.
>   In agony,
> No more?—and, by a dress to say we end
> The side-ache, and the thousand self-made aches,
> Which those are heir to, who, for mere fashion,
> Will dress so waspish.[105]

The poems found a musical counterpart in "Success to the Bloomers," a song of several stanzas complete with musical score that hoped to welcome in the new style.[106] These poetic forays enlarged not only the appeal of the reform but also the range of participants, since poems and songs probably came from different readers than those who submitted medical articles.

These not-so-subtle messages on the merits of dress reform, when coupled with first-person testimonies, had a persuasive effect on the journal's women readers. Once again, considerable overlap is evidenced between the rhetoric of the leadership and the "lived experience" of the followers: Women, famous and unknown, wrote in describing the liberating sensations and results that had accompanied their adoption of reform dress. One such letter, from Theodosia Gilbert, a cofounder of the Glen Haven Water Cure, is a case in point. An illness of hers necessitated much walking, and so:

> I conceived the notion of getting up a suit expressly for walk-ing. . . . And what a deliverance was that! The suit consisted simply of a pair of cassimere [sic] pantaloons, a frock of woollen material, loose, plain waist, and sleeves, with a skirt reaching to the knees, of decent dimensions in width, thickly lined throughout, a light cap or hat upon the head, and thick-soled, high topped boots.
>
> In this rig, I could just about double the distance, in the same length of time, which had been the extent of my ability with the accustomed appendages, and what is more, with half the fatigue.[107]

Gilbert went on to describe the shocked reaction she had met with, which soon turned to approval, then emulation, by many of the women patients. Noting that the Glen Haven Cure was in an isolated area, "One is altogether eased of an intolerant public opinion, and soon feels perfectly at home in the very comfortable *newness* of her attire."[108]

Reflecting the experience of a woman wearing the reform dress in a densely populated area, Mary Gove Nichols did not experience the cushion of isolation available to Gilbert:

> Every week that I wear my improved dress, gives me new health and courage. When I first put on the short dress, I was almost afraid of my shadow—at least I was afraid of the boys and rude women in the street, and used to beg my husband to go with me whenever he could. He said he "did not like a dress that had to be protected." I reminded him that our Republic had to be fought for and protected at first, and that all transitions were painful. Now, I hardly know fear, and we have outlived insult to a great degree.[109]

It is indicative of the evangelistic fervor of converts that wearing reform dress could be so easily compared to a war for freedom and autonomy.

In fact, the reform ambience and isolated nature of water-cure establishments made them havens for dress reform. Jackson's Dansville Water Cure has already been noted in this capacity as the point of origin for the American costume, which the Seventh-Day Adventists adopted and modified. Add to this the efforts of Jackson himself and of his daughter, Austin. Jackson, the *Water-Cure Journal* reported, delivered a speech before the first National Dress Reform Convention in Homer, New York, in August 1856. Austin, a regular contributor to the journal on dress reform, was herself a conscientious wearer of the new style and a frequent lecturer on its value, as her 1859 speech at the National Health Convention attests.[110] Like Dansville, Glen Haven and, later, the Elmira Water Cure (the latter two under the direction of the Gleasons) were focal points of dress reform. In addition, the costume was adopted at Trall's cure in New York City.[111] While articles from everyday readers, like Clara, highlighted this affinity between "Dress Reform and Water Cure,"[112] an excerpt from a correspondent of the *Georgia Citizen*, writing from the Mount Prospect Water-Cure, in Binghamton, New York, illustrates the widespread adoption of reform dress at the cures:

> Among some peculiarities of a Water-Cure establishment, none struck me with more force than that of the dress of females. . . . I have been [accustomed] all my life to seeing women arrayed in *tight* dresses only. . . . Hence I noticed, on my first visit to one of these "Cures," the peculiarity of loose dressing. . . . [I] saw its advantages in a remedial point of view, especially while under a treatment that required much outdoor exercise, in which the lungs and other vital organs have to perform a very vital part.[113]

Authors in the journal urged women not to abandon the reform dress on leaving the water-cure establishments. Citing the rising popularity of the garments, demonstrated by their usage by Amelia Bloomer, Anthony, and Lucy Stone, the *Water-Cure Journal* reprinted a passage from the *Franklin Democrat* that had noted the use of bloomers by these famous women and had gone on to remark that at a recent dinner party, "where [there] were over a dozen of the fair sex . . . some eight or ten of them had on a style and fit of 'Bloomer' that did credit to their taste, and proved very convenient and agreeable for their motive powers."[114]

Despite the growing popularity and credibility of reform dress and the persuasive tactics employed to encourage its adoption, journal authors remained sensitive to the ridicule that awaited a dress reformer, in articles such as "Bloomers; or, Is It a Duty to Wear the New Costume?"[115] This article, by Julia Kellogg, legitimized abandonment of the outfit when ridicule became overbearing. Perhaps, then, ideological principles took a back seat to embarrassment once one left the cure. (But as the "Matrimonial Correspondence" column, where one wrote in seeking like-minded reform mates, demonstrates, many water-cure believers adopted *and* maintained reform dress.) Two months later, a respondent took exception to this proposal, and in "Dress Reform. Is It Duty?" Mrs. E. Potter argued that it most certainly *was* a woman's duty, regardless of personal inconvenience.[116] *The Sybil—For Reforms,* a New York publication actively supportive of hydropathy and its attendant reforms, echoed the journal's position with an 1860 reader's letter entitled "Dress Reform Difficulties." The author, Mary V. W. Radcliff of Prairie du Chien, Wisconsin, noted that like the water cure, dress reform would eventually be seen as a must. For, as she succinctly stated, "I expect to see the majority of sensible women sensibly clad."[117]

In fact, among proponents, commitment to dress reform took on zealous, sweeping overtones. Arguing that dress reform was the first step necessary in elevating and revolutionizing women's self-image and cultural status, the most ardent reformers, personified in Gove Nichols, proclaimed:

I rejoice in all new freedom for women. We can expect but small achievement from women so long as it is the labor of their lives to carry about their clothes. Our present style of dress is enthralling and expensive. It is not adapted to the form as God made it, not to any form of work.[118]

Convinced that public reaction to dress reform revealed the power imbalance between the sexes, Gove Nichols continued: "The new style is opposed by bad men and weak men—by those who wish women to be weak, sickly and dependent—the pretty slave of man."[119]

Fashion, dependency, and femininity as traditionally defined were all portrayed by ardent water-cure dress reformers as demeaning and destructive for women. As Gove Nichols argued:

> The tender and confiding woman who is willing to be put in a bag to secure dependence and uselessness, and prove that she is not masculine, may be very pretty in story books, or to pass an idle hour with, but when poverty or disease palsies the hand that has fed her, when death takes away her protector . . . too often this crushed being becomes more utterly lost, because she has no self-sustaining power.[120]

In a revealing anecdote that starkly embodies societal intolerance for women's nontraditional appearance, the journal in 1864 recounted in great detail the case of Sallie M. Monroe of New Berlin, New York, a practicing physician, whose complete cross-dressing in male attire had irked some conservative contemporaries, who lamented the influence of dress reform on femininity. The editor of the journal, however, was delighted to discover that *"The said 'Sallie' is no woman at all, but a veritable man!"*[121] To protect the reputation of reform dressers, the androgynous one was deemed male. There were boundaries, apparently, to acceptable dress reform, even among the vanguard.

Dress reform, then, was seen by hydropaths as a basis for arguing for new freedoms for women. But the hydropathic goal of redefining woman's sphere, although it began with dress reform, did not stop there; the pages of the journal were sprinkled with less specific, but equally persuasive, women's emancipation issues.

Support for expanding women's influence sometimes expressed itself in articles that redefined women's roles in an empowering way, for example, by offering a wider range of life choices. This positive gender consciousness, defined as empowering women physically and to an extent socially, was manifested in diverse ways aimed at expanding women's opportunities and rewards. This was the case in "An Autobiography," which mentioned a "maiden lady" who

> was none the worse for living unmarried—in fact *she* was better. Celibacy is by no means the vice it is represented to be. . . . More especially is it virtuous in a *woman* to live *un*married. Society makes her dependent, an appendage, a thing; gives her half her rights only, and *that* grudgingly; places her interests, her hopes, her property, her name, her identity, in the power of the man to whom she surrenders.[122]

Throughout this narrative, value and credence are given to the choice not to marry and to the ensuing independence. Hydropaths, relying on the ideology of separate spheres and its concomitant emphasis on women's "unique nature," reflected an increased respect for women as women. Thus a legitimate role was created for women outside of marriage. Here, hydropaths echoed the reasoning of domestic feminists, who claimed that although women's special domain was the home and family, they still had virtues—moral superiority prime among them—that could be socially useful if they did not marry. In a similarly expansive and empowering vein, Austin, in "Thoughts in Spare Minutes," argued for women to take responsibility for those things closest to them, and to realize that "this is our right independent of legislative enactments. If the *desire* to grow is in us, there is *room* to grow."[123] This personal responsibility, she cautioned, is not *instead* of political activism but a necessary precursor to it. Women were encouraged to take control where feasible, but not to waver in their understanding of the basis of their power in overseeing their own and others' health.

Water-cure publications and practitioners were clearly in agreement rhetorically with and inferentially supportive of the women's rights movements' concerns. Direct discussion supporting suffrage is inferential and scant, although there was agreement that women needed social parity with men, but health was the decisive implement to be employed first and continuously in pursuing this goal. Practitioners supported feminist (i.e., more formal, women-organized) political activities, although separate endeavors for women and men were at times adjudged less satisfactory than efforts shared between the sexes. Hydropathic devotees were active in the women's rights movement, while practitioners largely focused on the more inclusive gender-conscious concerns articulated throughout this text. There was crossover among scattered individuals, but the practitioners' vision entailed improved living through right and healthful conditions of life, not formal politics.

The *Water-Cure Journal* did follow the activities and publications of exceptional women and women's rights activists in formal politics. For example, an ad for *The Una* appeared with some regularity. This magazine, devoted to the elevation of woman, was published in Providence, Rhode Island, by Paulina Wright Davis, a former lecturing companion of Gove Nichols.[124] In 1853 the *Phrenological Journal* had done a head-reading of Amelia Bloomer (the dress innovator), which was reprinted in the *Water-Cure Journal*. The journal took this opportunity to recommend *The Lily*, a feminist publication, to its readers.[125] Similarly, the lengthy book review of "Memoirs of Margaret Fuller Ossoli" praised her life and works, calling her "a choice spirit."[126] And while the women mentioned in the short article "Women Inventors" are not known by name, the journal was eager to point out that "eleven patents if we number rightly, have been granted within the past two years to ladies." Remarking that these inventors might not choose to "try their inventive skill in the household department," they suggested "let[ting] them try the locomotive engine, the steamship or the telegraph."[127] Always encouraging mental powers, the journal did not fail to mention physical ones as well. An 1847 filler told the story of a woman who had walked twelve miles in the snow to win a $500 bet made by an unbelieving male acquaintance.[128]

Encouraging words advising women to experiment and grow into their potential were repeated often in the journal. Another recurring call urged women to find pride and self-knowledge through the work they did, be it in a household or in a factory. Austin wrote a heartfelt article about her sense of pride not only in being a physician but also in being able to mend clothing. At first this may sound trivial, if not foolish, but Austin was encouraging women to take pride in woman's work, as they would in a (male) profession.[129]

Contributing authors to the journal, however, were not naive enough to think that placing the responsibility on women to develop a sense of pride was enough; women were not blamed for their life conditions and lack of opportunities. L. H. Bigarel, in "Working Girls," urged greater male respect for wage-earning women, saying, "Women, equally with men, live for a purpose. . . . Working girls are deserving of encourage-ment, and men ought to manifest their appreciation of their sterling qualities."[130]

An article by Holbrook, the editor of the journal, several months later took Bigarel's argument much further. In "Working Women," the plight of wage-earning women was starkly articulated, and in this case the clearly social and political realms were entered and critiqued:

> If there is one class of human beings on earth more abused than any other it is the working women. . . . Working men have a thousand advantages over working women. They have incomparably better opportunities for health, thought, development and education. They are paid higher wages for the same services, and are provided with schools, social entertainments, libraries, out-door sports, &c., of which women are deprived.[131]

Holbrook urged city dwellers to consider this situation and urged rural dwellers to welcome women farmers, since the experiment with women farming in Pekin, New York, had proved successful.

Urging women to farm was one of the more tangible responses seen in the journal's pages to the plight of working women in the 1860s. (And it may account in part for the keen eye kept on the southern states; their potential for farming probably appealed to the hydropathic leadership.) In "Woman as Farmer" Trall urged women who did not marry to farm—hygienically. He defined hygienic farming to be the cultivation of the earth "as it should be, as it must be to check the physiological degeneracy of the nations. [I am confident that] woman, as well as man, would find both pleasure and profit, both health and wealth, in tilling the ground."[132] Specifically, hygienic farming bore little resemblance to the standard raising of pigs and poultry, the fattening of beef and pork, the killing and eating of domestic animals, the making of butter and cheese, and the keeping of geese and ducks. Instead, Trall envisioned farming that yielded fruits, flowers, and grains that would, under women's auspices, "rapidly supersede hogs, tobacco, and whiskey, as the staple productions of rural districts."[133] Not only would farm work not be degrading, but it would serve the opposite purpose: the uplifting of womankind, and of humanity as well.

Trall's ultimate aspiration for his concept of hygienic farming was that it would be available to replace all other forms of wage labor then being performed by women.

> There are many thousands of wretched girls stitching their frail lives away in damp cellars and dingy attics, who would become . . . robust and blooming, and fit to be wives and mothers, if they were provided with the opportunity to earn their bread in the air and sunshine.[134]

Trall's enthusiasm for hygienic farming triggered supportive responses from some hydropathic followers, among them Delos Dunton, originator of a farming experiment in upstate New York. In 1864 he wrote "Items from 'Home of the Free,'" in which he argued for equal pay for women farmers.[135] This idea of hygienic farming by women had reached such popularity that in December of the same year a male reader, M.T.C. of Geneva, Kansas, offered 320 acres of prairie land and cash to start a women's farm.[136] (The longevity and success of these farming ventures are difficult to chart as it was their founding, not their operation, that received attention in the press.) The unabashed idealism of Trall's enthusiasm for hygienic farming reflects the extent to which values and goals ruled the world of hydropathy's strongest advocates. Concerned about existing factory conditions for working women, the zealous water-cure reformers chose instead to focus their concrete social-reform activism on the more idealistic concept of hygienic farming. Aware of social problems and injustices, they chose to create a social reality and world view that implemented their beliefs rather than work within the social climate they found so riddled with problems. Hygienic farming demonstrates that theirs was, to a large degree, a utopian vision. It further illustrates a clear point of divergence between the rhetoric of the leadership and the lived experience of most working-class women. While a few may have been able to relocate and leave all-things-familiar to pursue this vision, many more were tied to the seemingly unalterable circumstances of urban life.

As activities as diverse as dress reform and hygienic farming demonstrate, the hydropath's sense of expanding opportunities and life choices for women encompassed the personal, social, physical and, at

times, political realms. While urging women to become everything within
their capacity, the leaders identified the need for several substantial cultural and institutional innovations to expedite and implement their
philosophy. It is no wonder, then, that hydropathic writings conveyed a
certain ambivalence that reflected both the empowerment and powerlessness of women. For while the reformers' network could ease the way,
harsh economic and social strictures ruled in the larger culture. This
ambivalence is evident in "A Misfortune to Be a Woman." Arguing that it
is "a misfortune to be a woman, because woman is such a sufferer; and a
sufferer because she is a slave!" the anonymous author details the woes in
1864 of woman's daily role,[137] although she concludes in a positive and
hopeful tone: "To my sisters I would say, fear not to do and dare in the
cause of Truth and Righteousness; shrink not from following in the path
where duty leads, and strive ever so to live that while we well may say
'tis glorious to be a MAN, we may also add 'tis sweet, 'tis beautiful, 'tis
holy to be a WOMAN."[138]

Hydropathy, and its attendant reform network, provided women
with the philosophical and physiological base from which to struggle to
become full members of American society and at the same time implement the new vision of what constituted a desirable life. One was not
simply "inserted into" the ongoing social value system. Urging mental
competence, self-sufficiency, and social responsibility, water-cure
philosophy sought to render women the creators of their own futures.

Significantly, as empowering as these expanded opportunities and
choices were, they were self-limiting. Clearly, moral reform—including
health reform—offered one of the few ways for Victorian women to
exercise and experience power. But the moral reformers were "hamstrung
by their own self-definition. For as long as they couched their activities in
moral terms, other avenues of power lay beyond their reach."[139]

Hydropathy and Marriage

One innovative method by which a woman follower of hydropathy
could hope to integrate moral reformist ideals of opportunity and choice
into her personal life was through marriage to a like-minded man; this
need received journalistic support in the "Matrimonial Correspondence"
column. The holistic and empowering approach of water-cure philosophy
is typified in this search for ideal mates. Urging the interconnectedness of
the personal with the social, hydropaths created an alternative network
that offered private as well as institutional options for nineteenth-century
women. The popularity and success of the unions speak to the adherents'
sense of totality with the movement, and to their sense of isolation, for
seeking suitable partners through advertisements implies a dearth of like-
minded people in their hometowns. The column reflected the movement's
concern with women's and men's personal and emotional well-being, as

well as their political and social compatibility. Begun in the mid-1850s, the column corresponds chronologically with the height of reformist zeal as portrayed in the journal. By the late 1850s, the column had been abandoned and only an occasional, personally financed advertisement appeared.

During its heyday, "Matrimonial Correspondence" consisted of up to two dozen "personals" describing the writer and her or his criteria for a suitable partner. Letter No. 19, which appeared in March 1854, depicts a candid advertisement:

> I am nineteen years old; and a strong believer in the Water-Cure system, Temperance and *Woman's Rights*. I am in part vegetarian, eat flesh-meat occasionally, but care nothing about it. I drink cold water entirely, and bathe twice a day; do not think I can be called a slave to any bad habits. I do not wear the Bloomer costume. Phrenology and Physiology have always been favorite studies. . . . I understand Algebra, Chemistry, Natural Philosophy and Rhetoric, as well as sewing, washing, sweeping and cooking. I am of cheerful disposition, and enjoy a good joke, and am capable of giving one.
>
> Crazy Sabe[140]

Rosa Ann Ditch, of Rome, Ohio, seemed equally interested in common reform issues and personal harmony when she wrote:

> Now I am a farmer's daughter, under twenty-eight years of age; am not handsome, but rather plain looking. I can milk cows and make cheese to perfection. I can wash clothes and dishes, and make soap. I can make Graham bread, Graham pies and cakes; but I cannot look cross, nor can I scold. . . . As for dress, I will dress just as I have a mind to, in spite of all the men! I have an uncommon hatred for tobacco. . . . Now I don't want a tobacco-chewing, rum drinking husband; but I want a plain-looking, plain-spoken, pleasant and happy man; one that will love me, and whom I can love eternally.[141]

In the June 1854 issue of the journal the editor decided that, as a result of the lengthiness of individual letters and the dozens received each week, thereafter they would appear on the advertisement page under "Matrimonial" and would be financed by the writer.[142] Under this new format, "Irene of Massachusetts" got right to the point:

> Required: A man of intelligence, a follower of Jesus; a hydropath and vegetarian in principle; a friend to all the oppressed of every color and nation. . . . A cultivator of vegetable food in temperate climates (not California), of some free State in my own country would be greatly preferred.[143]

The letters written by male correspondents were not significantly different. R. Milo Wayland of Newport, Rhode Island, "wants a wife who is a Vegetarian, Hydropathic Bloomer, not over twenty-seven years of age; of mild disposition, honest, intelligent, fair health, constitution, education; no worshipper of custom as such."[144] The letter from "Harry," though, is noteworthy for its originality:

> A Heart to Let.—A heart with large chambers, well-furnished with Affection, and draped with Hope and Love. The title is warranted good and perfect, the terms are easy and payments few. It is strongly barred against tea, coffee, tobacco, alcohol, profanity and crime. Has had a tenant once, but now has left for worlds unknown. . . . Now, ladies, don't all speak at once.[145]

In December 1854 a written notice of the first successful unions appeared. As "Long Star" and "Duenna" wrote in: "You will oblige by noticing in your Journal, that No. 28 old series and No. 81 new series, have withdrawn, 'hand-in-hand,' from the list of Matrimonial Correspondents."[146] News of successful pairings appeared in the May 1855 and April 1856 issues as well. One such entry read:

> Messrs. Fowler & Wells,—You will withdraw "Tennessean," No. 92 and "Lucy Long," No. 61 new series. They have withdrawn hand in hand, and are most happily married. Please accept our thanks for your kindness in effecting our union. All who would marry happily let them marry phrenologically. . . . Success to the matrimonial department of your most excellent journal.[147]

In September 1856 "Agnes," "Ada Augusta," and "No. 200" withdrew their names after finding suitable mates. The last had "found that parity and perfection he was in search of."[148] These advertisements tellingly reveal the individual beliefs and preferences of hydropathic followers. Accepting some hydropathic rules and rejecting others, each created an individual system modeled, to a greater or a lesser degree, after the doctrine of the movement.

One other marriage occurred that deserves special mention. "A Wedding on Hydropathic Principles" took place between Dr. Allen G. Weed of New Jersey and Dr. Adeline M. Willis of Marion, Iowa. Classmates at Trall's Hygeio-Therapeutic College, they "have now united in hands, hearts, fortunes and *diplomas*."[149] The ceremony took place in the lecture room before the professors and students.

Conclusions

The hydropathic movement shared personnel and efforts with numerous other contemporary reform movements. In addition, because hydropathic philosophy and practices reflected these corollary reforms, the water-cure movement became a vital link in the national reform network and adopted into its tenets the beliefs promulgated in the vegetarian, physical education, temperance, and dress-reform movements.

Further, by encouraging dress reform, the movement took another step toward redefining traditional female roles. The adoption of reform dress complemented the reconceptualization of woman's physiology, intellectual abilities, and social roles. The writings of the movement's leadership also sanctioned several choices not usually offered to nineteenth-century women: choosing not to marry, acting as gender-conscious leaders, and experimenting with inventions and feats of strength. Also, the movement encouraged women to take pride in their daily responsibilities, changing perceptions of working women, and equal employment opportunities to young women through experimental farming.

Aware that social change and personal growth occur in the private as well as the public realm, the water-cure movement encouraged reform marriages through the journal's "Matrimonial Correspondence" column, which hoped to fulfill the emotional and intimate needs of one segment of its following. Here, women could advertise for their desired mate, thus taking the initiative in personal relationships and asserting their own values and needs.

This reform network fulfilled the humanistic philosophy and idealistic vision of hydropaths and thus served as a haven for social visionaries. Similarly, the hydropaths' emphasis on reforms strengthened their commitment to and conception of opportunities and choices available to women. Reform efforts encompassed the physical, social, political, and personal realms and stressed the necessity of women's full development—minimally encumbered by social restraints, although informed by a belief in, and adherence to, gender-specific attributes. Viewed in this context, the development among the female clientele at the cures of an identifiable network and enclave embodied both an extension of gender-specific spheres and the opportunity for autonomy and self-involvement and a supportive community.

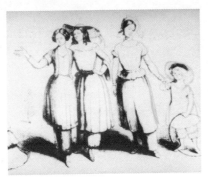

Chapter Five

Women at the Cures
Rest for the Weary Activist

As numerous nineteenth-century participants attested, water-cure establishments offered a physiological and psychological sanctuary. This was particularly true for women, whose ordained domestic role demanded that they nurture husband and family. The prospect of a respite during which *their* needs were paramount was attractive and exciting, and it could be justified by the medical nature of the sojourn.

Inspired by the ideology and community spirit of the hydropathic movement, some women closely connected with hydropathy chose to remain unmarried and share their lives with female companions; of these, some made their home in the communal living situations that existed at water-cure establishments.[1] This lure was particularly strong for women who were among the intellectual and social-reform leaders of their day. For these women, whose daily life demanded a strained balancing of social activism and personal relationships (sometimes evidenced in non-organic physical malaise), the cures served a particularly valuable role as communal sanctuary from the turmoil of public life. These women were among the few with a personal income that enabled them to go to the cures at will; they also enjoyed far greater mobility than most nineteenth-century women. Also, they operated out of a tradition of self-analysis that led them to write about their experiences.

The women discussed here, probably because of their activism and involvement in corollary social reforms, were, by and large, already familiar with the water-cure system. This is not to say that they were already "believers" in either the efficacy of water therapeutics or the regimen that awaited them. In this regard, then, the motivations and expectations of these exceptional women are indicative of the range of "callings" of average women. In many instances, for both famous and ordinary women, what began as a medical sojourn—or a recommended quest for the cures' general ambience, female clientele, or reform activities—*evolved into* an adoption of reform dress, altered diet, exposure to emancipationist thinkers, and self-determination.

As individual narratives have revealed, women hydropathic patients were, by and large, even before residence at a cure, an *informed* clientele; the ideological and political tone of the movement made it unlikely that a totally naive patron would arrive at the front step of a live-in cure. In some instances, a stay at a cure triggered gender-conscious (feminist) attitudes; in other cases, the decision to go to the cure reflected an already-held belief.

For social reformers, the cures had many attractions. Frequently physically and emotionally in need of respite from public life and often unmarried (hence unemcumbered by children), they were attracted by the peer nature of their fellow patients, the ready acceptance of reform ideologies, and the prospect of relief from physical malaise. Numerous establishments solicited a female clientele by advertising their ability to help sufferers from women's diseases. The Elmira Water Cure, for example, in 1863–1864 advertised as follows:

> Mrs. R. B. Gleason, M.D., gives her attention to the specific treatment of the Special Diseases of Females. Her large experience in this department of practice—her eminent success in the cure of many who have been confined to the bed for years, entitle her to public confidence and to the large practice she has already made.[2]

The list of noteworthy women who frequented the cures reveals the importance the establishments had as part of the larger social-reform and women's-support networks. A strong web of female companionship and activism was nurtured and flourished; lifelong relationships between women often began with a stay at a cure. For all women, the cures provided a legitimate destination away from their familial and domestic duties, since illness was considered a natural consequence of femaleness.

Except in a few cases, the cures did not provide an exclusively female setting. But women patients were treated in separate facilities, by female attendants, and lodged with female co-patients. The experience, then, when coupled with the emancipationist gender ideology, was conducive to fostering a sense of gender identity. Consequently, the nature of the female community that flourished at the cures is distinctive on several accounts.

Initially, women were attracted to the cures because the therapeutics they received emphasized the ability of nature to heal and the opportunity for each woman—not her physician—to control her own body. Once ensconced at a cure, women soon found that the other women there offered sympathy for their pain and a chance to discuss their fears.[3]

An even more pragmatic consideration, for married women, was an escape from the inevitability of childbearing.[4] While at the cures, women were spared pregnancies. Whether their often elongated stays were a premeditated calculation to avoid this duty or were a result of the alternatives they found at the cures is difficult to determine. But it is reasonable to credit a significant degree of the cures' popularity to a respite from pregnancy and its seemingly inevitable dangers.

Childrearing activities were similarly suspended, since at many cures children were admitted as patients but not as dependents of patients. At the Brattleboro, Vermont, Water Cure, for example, "Boarding schools grew up in the area to accommodate them, but while at the cure itself mothers had to resign themselves to a sweet interlude of childlessness."[5]

Harriet Beecher Stowe

This factor seems to have figured prominently in the stay of Harriet Beecher Stowe, who found relief from ten years of marriage and incessant childbearing during a long stay at Brattleboro.[6] Stowe went to Brattleboro in May 1846 exhausted from overwork, the birth of her fifth child, and the strains of living in poverty. She wrote in a personal letter before entering the cure: "[I am] sick of the smell of sour milk, and sour meat, and sour everything, and then the clothes *will* not dry, and no wet thing does, and everything smells moldy; and altogether I feel as if I never wanted to eat again."[7] Sensing her fragile state, congregants of the church of her husband, Calvin Stowe, paid her way and, as one of her biographers found, "Just the prospect of respite from her domestic chores raised Harriet's spirits."[8] Invigorated by the prospect of rest, but also feeling guilty, Harriet left Calvin at home alone in charge of their children. The therapies and social activities at the cure immediately began to broaden her limited world view, which had included "her brother, Henry Ward Beecher, beginning to thunder against the dance-hall and the theatre as the ante-chambers of sexual vice."[9] Harriet wrote Calvin:

> I am anxious for your health. Don't sit in your hot study without any ventilation . . . and, above all, do *amuse* yourself. . . . When you feel worried, go off somewhere and forget and throw it off. I wish you could be with me in Brattleboro and coast down hill on a sled, go sliding and snowballing by moonlight! I would snowball every bit of the *hypo* out of you![10]

Stowe remained at the cure for ten months, until March 1847. Temporarily rejuvenated by her fourteen months away from home, she conceived their sixth child on her return; this brought on another "neuralgic affection' of the eyes that all but blinded her for months."[11]

Calvin Stowe, disgruntled with his role of "housefather and nurse," himself exhausted from overwork, and feeling the need to escape the pressures of poverty, left for the Brattleboro Cure in June 1848 and was gone for fifteen months. Calvin's absence, tragically, coincided with the cholera death of their son Charley, in 1849.[12]

For Harriet, the months at the cure had been a vital reprieve that mended her weary body and exhausted spirit. Describing her daily routine, she wrote:

> The daily course I go through presupposes a degree of vigor beyond anything I ever had before. For this week, I have gone before breakfast to the wave-bath, and let all the waves and billows roll over me till every limb ached with cold and my hands would scarcely have feeling enough to dress me. After that I have walked til I was warm and come home to breakfast with such an appetite! . . . At eleven comes my douche . . . and after it a walk. . . . After dinner I roll ninepins or walk till four, then sitz-bath, and another walk until six.[13]

Stowe continued to advocate the use of water and in-home bathrooms in the years ahead, as evidenced in her essay "Our Houses—What Is Required to Make Them Healthful," which appeared in the *Water-Cure Journal* in 1865:[14]

> And now I come to the next great vital element for which "our house" must provide—"water water everywhere"; it must be plentiful, it must be easy to get at, it must be pure. . . . There should be a bath room to every two or three inmates, and the hot and cold water should circulate to every chamber.[15]

Aware that indoor running water was still not available in most homes, Stowe deemed its installation a goal for future planners. Four years later, Stowe wrote *An American Woman's Home: Or Principles of Domestic Science* with her sister, Catharine Beecher. They included a bathroom in the design of their "cottage" and counseled its frequent use.[16]

Stowe's water-cure experience, while it reflected her practice and advocacy of the system, was a one-time sojourn that helped her recover her strength but did not alter the demanding personal life to which she returned. A kindly intellectual reciprocity continued between Stowe and the hydropathic leadership in the years ahead, however, evidenced in the journal's chartings of her doings and the favorable reviews of her varied literary pursuits.[17]

Sexuality and Friendship

The supportive, nurturant, and homosocial nature of the cures was further enhanced by the overtly sensual and, possibly, sexual experiences that women encountered at the cures. Many water-cure therapies necessitated rubbing the patient, and these friction massages, when performed on a freshly bathed and rejuvenated body, probably had both very soothing and stimulating effects. There was, then, both a private and a public aspect to the sensuality at the cures. Private touching through massage, attendants' ministrations, bathing, drying, and wrapping were experienced in large open rooms where, photographs from the Dansville (New York) Water Cure reveal, dozens of women, sitting in tubs, wrapped in loose-fitting sheets and turbans, each experienced sensual pleasure not only from their own sensations but also from the ambience generated when relaxed, comfortable, stimulated, and soothed bathers shared a common room and a common experience.[18]

More specifically, certain water-cure processes could result in sexual release for women. Treatment of prolapsus uteri, dysmenorrhea (painful menstruation), ovaritis (an acute or chronic inflammation of the ovaries), barrenness, leucorrhea (commonly called "whites"), and hysteria ("depending upon the ovarian or uterine system") were all treated with "the local treatment of sitzbaths, vaginal injections, and the bandage, [which] must be used perseveringly."[19] T. L. Nichols in his treatise on the "Diseases of Women" urged the use of wet bandages "carefully and tightly applied" to the pelvic area. Nichols's therapeutics precluded overt masturbation, but "he did encourage patients to experience release of tension through stimulation of the 'pelvic' area."[20] To this end, vaginal injections were utilized to alleviate many of the above mentioned ailments.

In another instance, Nichols, writing in "The Curse Removed," elaborated on the causes of uterine disease, suggesting therapeutics for childbirth and pregnancy that could, clearly, have a sensual effect: "In bringing about a cure, it may be necessary to excite the action of the skin, by the wet sheet pack, and the douche. We support the falling womb with the wet bandage; we give tone by frequent sitz-baths and vaginal injections; in a word, we give health, and strength, and energy, to the whole system, and cure all its disorders."[21]

Such sensual sensations are a powerful force,[22] and when joined with the ambience of a female-centered retreat, shared understanding, trust, mutual nurturance, and exoneration from the stresses of married or family life, these sensual pleasures did translate into overt erotic activity between the women at the cures, although the extent of genital sex is impossible to determine. Richard von Krafft-Ebing, the pioneering nineteenth-century sex researcher, chronicled examples of same-sex eroticism at European cures. Framed though these cases are by his obvious contempt for non-heterosexual intercourse, they still clearly illustrate the same-sex bonds and attractions that originated and were acted on at the cures.[23]

In "Case 165" Krafft-Ebing chronicled what he termed the homosexual development of a Miss X, who in 1881, at the age of thirty-eight, had consulted him "on account of severe spinal irritation and obstinate sleeplessness, in combating which she had become addicted to morphine and chloral." Relatives reported that, before her illness, "she had neither had inclination for persons of the opposite nor those of her own sex."[24] Commencing in 1872 with the onset of her neurasthenia and hysterical symptoms (resulting from a fall), she demonstrated a "peculiar friendship for females, particularly young ladies; and she had a desire, and satisfied it, to wear hats and coats of masculine style."[25] In 1874 Miss X returned from a sojourn at a watering place and from that time forth "would associate only with ladies, [and] had a kind of love-relation with one or another. . . . This predilection for women was decidedly more than mere friendship, since it expressed itself in tears, jealousy, etc."[26] While at the watering place, a young lady, who Krafft-Ebing believes mistook Miss X for a man, fell in love with her. When this young lady married, the patient spoke of unfaithfulness and was depressed for a long time.

Despite Krafft-Ebing's thinly veiled moralism and disdain, he provides a sense of the potential for sexual contact at the cures. In fact, the woman just described in Case 165, also had a homoerotic relationship with Case 159, "and she wrote her affectionate letters like those of a lover to his beloved." Mrs. C of Case 159 was thirty-two years old, "feminine in appearance," married to an official, and described by her physician as "peculiar, obstinate, silent, quick-tempered, and eccentric." She had three children, but confided to Krafft-Ebing that she gladly avoided coitus, saying, "I should have preferred intercourse with a woman."[27] When she traveled to a water cure in 1878 (for neurasthenia) she met Case 165. Her husband reported developments on her return: "She was no longer a woman, no longer had any love for me and the children, and would have no more of marital approaches. She was inflamed with passionate love for her female friend, and had taste for nothing else."[28]

Her husband forbade her lover entrance into their house. Passionate love letters between the two women ensued with such expressions in them as "My dove! I live only for you, my soul." The relationship between the two women continued (without another catalogued visit to a cure) for five years, until 1882. Both women met early demises, Mrs. C from tuberculosis in 1885 and her love, Miss X, from "exhaustion" in 1889.[29]

In most instances it is difficult to determine the precise nature of the intimate contact between women who frequented the cures. Close female friendships were a socially acceptable form of emotional contact (and fulfillment) for women, whose rigid gender-role differentiation led to the emotional segregation of women and men. A variety of supportive networks and intimate bonds evolved from these close friendships, and countless passages from letters and diaries reflect women's intense feelings of love, concern, and sensuality for their female friends. Called, alternately, "the love of kindred spirits," "Boston marriage," and "sentimental friendship," these bonds often became lifetime commitments.[30]

What records exist render it impossible to assert either that these bondings were sexual or that they had no sexual component at all.[31] One historian, who relied on sources that prescribed behavior, did not examine the women's actual conduct but contended that nineteenth-century women had so internalized the "doctrine" of passionlessness that "these romantic friendships were love relationships in every sense except perhaps the genital. They might kiss, fondle each other, sleep together, utter expressions of overwhelming love and promises of eternal faithfulness, and yet see their passions as nothing more than effusions of the spirit."[32]

It is possible to assert that these women, most often, would not have defined themselves as lesbian. Contentions about the "passionlessness" of women hold that they may have avoided heterosexual sex for the following reasons: as a way to secure autonomy, as a result of the powerful proscriptions on female passion, through a fear or disdain for pregnancy and childbearing, or because of inadequate male attention to female pleasure.[33] The question whether this presumed passionlessness ruled in same-sex relationships is not settled, however. Since female sexuality was linked in the popular mind (and by definition) to reproduction, it is possible that neither the women themselves nor their contemporaries would have considered the relationships sexual.[34] In short, in considering the intimate "marriages" and sensual pleasures shared by nineteenth-century women who frequented the cures, analysts must avoid "labeling women lesbians who might violently reject the label, or, on the other hand, glossing over the significance of women's relationships by labeling them Victorian."[35]

The lack of precision encountered in defining the nature of the sexual contact among women at the cures and in applying the word lesbian to their relationships in no way obviates the "all-consuming emotional relationship [and] the seriousness or the intensity of the women's passions for each other."[36] What is indisputable is that women in "Boston marriages," married women whose central source of emotional (and possibly sensual) expression was with a romantic friend, and unmarried women seeking a "kindred spirit" used the cures to further their romantic attachments. The cures served to introduce women to one another, to support and rejuvenate a strained couple or individual from a "Boston marriage" in a stressful period in her life, or to provide a married woman the opportunity to form a new—or nurture an ongoing—romantic friendship.

The famed "Ladies of Llangollen," Lady Eleanor Butler and Miss Sarah Ponsonby of England, who eloped in the spring of 1778, were among many of these early "kindred spirits" who found enjoyment and peaceful haven together at a cure. Between 1794 and 1809, the two women went to Barmouth, England, for a "water excursion" to re-create a tour they had made together nineteen years earlier and to escape from financial problems.[37] A close friend of theirs, Anna Seward, also visited a cure (at Harrogate), an experience she found relaxing if somewhat unusual.[38] Similarly, Jane Austen sojourned in Bath, England, to take the mineral cure with her ailing father and gouty brother, Edward, in 1799. Her novel *Persuasion*, written in 1816, shows Bath in its decline.[39]

Catharine Beecher

Indicative of nineteenth-century American women who formed and maintained romantic friendships and commitments with other women through the cures, was Catharine Beecher, renowned teacher, writer on moral and religious topics, and advocate for women's education. A sufferer from "nervous excitability," which usually centered in the paralysis of one limb, she had tried "drugs, diets, carbonate of iron, with tartar emetic pustules on the spine[!], but she found no visible relief until she visited a water cure establishment."[40] In her *Letters to the People on Health and Happiness* (1855) Beecher praised the "inestimable benefits" of the water cure and recommended its use to her readers.[41] During the summer of 1847, a period of personal crisis for Catharine, Beecher joined her sister, Harriet Beecher Stowe, at the Brattleboro (Vermont) Water Cure, where the latter had been since May 1846. It was the summer when her colleague, William Slade, abandoned his work for women's education. Beecher, faced with the prospect of striking out on her own, retreated to the Brattleboro Cure, which was under the direction of Dr. Wesselhoeft. She hoped that her paralyzed limb would be aided by the water treatment; her usual therapeutics at Brattleboro entailed:

> At four in the morning packed in a wet sheet; kept in it from two to three hours; then up, and in a reeking perspiration immersed in the coldest plunge-bath. Then a walk as far as strength would allow, and drink five or six tumblers of the coldest water. At eleven A.M. stand under a douche of the coldest water falling *eighteen feet, for ten minutes*. Then walk, and drink three or four tumblers of water. At three P.M. sit half an hour in a *sitz*-bath of the coldest water. Then walk and drink again. At nine P.M. sit half an hour with the feet in the coldest water, then rub them till warm. Then cover the weak limb and a third of the body in wet bandages and *retire to rest*. This same wet bandage to be worn all day, and kept constantly wet.[42]

Although her paralytic condition was not significantly altered at the cure, Beecher continued to frequent various cures from 1843 throughout the 1850s for at least two months out of every year.[43] In part, the explanation for this lies in her interest in cultivating women's aid and companionship.

During her stay in Brattleboro, Beecher met Nancy Johnson, a Vermont resident not then a patient at the cure, who became Beecher's secretary. While there, she also cultivated the friendship of Delia Bacon, a former pupil, who became her steady companion in the years 1847 to 1850. The parallels in Beecher's and Bacon's lives were numerous, and their bond, while intensely caring, had a damaging effect that apexed in a public trial wherein Bacon accused her suitor (a minister) of misleading her as to his intentions and therefore disgracing her. The suitor denounced Bacon and discredited her by claiming she had been the aggressor in their ill-fated relationship. Much of this turmoil came about largely by activities on Beecher's part.[44] Bacon, while embroiled in legal machinations with her suitor, became an activist on behalf of women's education through Beecher's influence. Simultaneous with her involvement with Bacon, Beecher invited Johnson to accompany her to the cure (1847), a woman through whom the desire for a more positive "new life" was expressed.[45] Both Bacon and Johnson were attracted to the cures for treatment of maladies they shared with Beecher (lame feet) and, possibly, by a charismatic lure that she exercised in her romantic friendships.[46]

Johnson was a teacher whom Beecher urged to become a hydropath and whom she invited to take the cure at her expense.[47] In 1849 Beecher convinced Bacon, her first companion, to spend a month as her guest at the Round Hill Water Cure in Northampton, the cure that she had come to prefer. This was during the height of the public furor surrounding Bacon's trial. At Round Hill Beecher and Bacon partook of the water therapies, which greatly improved Beecher's nervous condition.[48] Beecher credited her cure to exercises and water-cure therapies and thereafter pursued both.[49] (Round Hill, under Dr. Halsted, emphasized motorpathy and specialized in the rejuvenation of paralyzed limbs. This probably accounts for Beecher's interest in Round Hill.) Bacon, meanwhile, was not vindicated in the trial, since her suitor was chastised only for "imprudent" behavior. After the publication of a book by Beecher discussing in detail the public trial of Bacon's "courtship," Bacon fled to England, where she worked on scholarly research projects for several years. In 1858, suffering from ever-increasing mental distress, she was brought back to America by her family, who placed her in an insane asylum; she died there in 1859.[50]

Beecher's early generosity toward Johnson led the latter, in 1848, to accept an offer to be Beecher's personal secretary during her labors on behalf of women's education. Beecher selected Burlington, Iowa, as the site of her school, but was beset with numerous financial and personnel problems, which once again triggered physical and mental exhaustion.[51] She persuaded Johnson to stay and run the newly established institution, while she retreated east once more to take the cure. After months of hardship and no aid from Beecher, Johnson abandoned the school, and she refused Beecher's offer to continue work with "the cause" on Beecher's return.

Beecher, on her way to Johnson, met Mary Mortimer in LeRoy, New York. For a third time she invited a woman friend to a cure, this time to spend the autumn with her at Round Hill Water Cure. Mortimer, like Beecher, suffered from a lame foot, and Beecher won her affection by supervising her hydropathic cure. Mortimer, in gratitude, remained in Milwaukee, the second site of Beecher's school, for the rest of her life. For six years, she nurtured the institution where Beecher had planned to retire and remained there long after Beecher had abandoned the project.[52]

Beecher, one of her biographers has noted, was an enthusiastic supporter of water cures because they were "centers of female culture [that] made it possible for women to escape the confines of their sick rooms and commune with sympathetic peers."[53] She lived, for varying lengths of time, at thirteen cures and, tellingly, after she no longer sought the cure's therapies, she continued to frequent them. Seeking proximity to her family and to a water cure when her health was weak before her death in 1878, she moved to Elmira, New York, to live with her brother, Thomas. Here, Beecher formed one last close friendship with a woman. This last friend is referred to only as "R," and little evidence remains to illuminate their relationship.[54]

Beecher was aware that her advocacy of the system had done much to popularize it. In *A Treatise on Domestic Economy* (1841) she described the skin as a purifying organ, which, through perspiration, cleansed the humors of the blood.[55] In this portrayal she followed, quite closely, the teachings of Priessnitz and his American popularizers. The goal of bathing, accordingly, was to rid oneself of this "conduit" perspiration, not to rid oneself of dirt or to seek sensual gratification. Also echoing hydropathic teachings, Beecher advocated cold bathing and vigorous rubbing with a towel. Beecher's book was actually one of the first popular endorsements of the system. Nine years later, in 1850, aware that "many persons were thus induced to resort to establishments of this description,"[56] Beecher wrote in the *New York Tribune* that the intervening years had enabled her to read more about, inquire about, and experience the water cure. She then explicated at great length the imperative use of water for preserving health and the guidance of a skilled physician who "is not only a scientist and experienced, [and] able to detect the true nature of the disease, but one who is careful and attentive in observing the effects of his prescriptions."[57] Beecher cautioned that in large establishments this could be difficult to achieve, causing patients to suffer from neglect. This was a noteworthy validation of the curative element resident in the healer–patient dyad; less attention was tantamount to neglect and was seen as inducing injury and retarding or preventing recovery. Other vital features of the water cure as expostulated in her *Tribune* essay were intelligent nursing carried out by trained personnel and the use of pure water, which facilitated the discharge of unhealthful humors and abnormal secretions.

Beecher admonished her readers throughout her article to be aware of those cures that were ill equipped and ill trained to care appropriately for patients. She concluded by contrasting Priessnitz's "heroic" brand of hydropathy with the moderate methods of Franke, a German author. She endorsed the more moderate system as safer and more efficacious, noting that heroic water cure originated among the "hardy, phlegmatic German race, and both the system, and the physicians who administer it, are not appropriately geared to the 'highly excitable temperment' of Americans, especially American women."[58] Beecher's preference for the more moderate system echoed the concern of the American hydropathic leaders—that all water processes be sensitive to the patient's "reactive powers." But her differentiation between systems was more pronounced than the American leaders, whose therapeutics and textual teachings emphasized moderation. This difference implies that she had at least a tangential concern about, or experience with, water-cure techniques that were dramatically and discomfortingly applied. She gave no further particulars.

Alice James

Other nineteenth-century women, many of them infirm from physical maladies that corresponded with demanding or frustrating social and personal roles, reveled in the simple medicine and female companionship available to them at the cures. Among them, Alice James, sister of Henry and William James, "like a great many other nineteenth-century women . . . was 'delicate,' 'high strung,' 'nervous,' and given to prostrations." James "had her first nervous breakdown at age 19, and her condition was called, at various points in her life, neurasthenia, hysteria, rheumatic gout, suppressed gout, cardiac complication, spinal neurosis, nervous hyperesthenia and spinal crisis."[59] One of her biographers has speculated that perhaps the immense success of her two brothers, one an author and the other a psychologist, immobilized her in a state of adopted invalidism, which enabled her to escape the necessity of serving others and attempting to define her own abilities. It also enabled her to maintain a sense of untapped potential.[60]

James's debility escalated rapidly, condemning her to a series of medical treatments that included a three-month stay at the Adams Nervine Asylum in Jamaica Plain, Massachusetts, in 1883. Not specifically a water cure, the asylum did utilize some tangentially related hydropathic therapies:

The Adams Nervine doctors advised her to rest, supervised her nutritional intake, gave her treatments of hot air, vapor baths, and massage. In 1883 the asylum acquired a popular new appliance called the Holtz Electrical Machine: hospital attendants applied its faradic and galvanic currents to Alice's nerves and muscles to relieve pain and stimulate normal functioning.[61]

James felt improved after the three-month stay, but no miracle cure occurred. Interestingly, her father, Henry James, Sr., after suffering what was termed a "vastation" (a laying waste), sought out doctors who prescribed rest, fresh air, and water cures. The elder James encouraged Alice to try these therapeutics, but the suggestion was not taken up.[62]

Alice James, in an endless struggle to alleviate her physical and emotional pain, found respite, love, and nurturance in the companionship of Katharine Peabody Loring, who became her soulmate from 1879 until James's death in 1892. Loring, as healthy as James was sickly, was the source of great joy and comfort to her companion. Theirs was not a proper "Boston marriage," however, since Loring kept house for her father in Beverly, Massachusetts, and cared for her sickly sister. The two women began to share a home together after James's cancer was diagnosed, and at that time Loring was taught a modified hypnosis by Dr. Lloyd Tuckey, an eminent British psychiatrist, which was used to put James to sleep and eliminated her sense of terror during the process.[63]

Despite James's deteriorating health and imminent death, she commented of the year 1891, which she had spent almost exclusively with Katharine, "This year has been the happiest I have ever known."[64] Although one biographical source on William James notes that his wife found the women's relationship "suspiciously lesbian," both Alice and her family regarded the bond with Katharine as the central source of joy and meaning in Alice's life.[65]

James's fleeting experiment with water processes served only as another temporary relief from her travails. The nature and extent of her invalidism rendered water cure an unlikely solution, since its adoption would have necessitated abandonment of the "patient" role, which she seemed unable to relinquish. Her death from organic causes (cardiac trouble and breast cancer) served as vindication for a lifetime of inorganic malaise.

Susan B. Anthony

It is likely that numerous women tried to use the water cure fleetingly, unsuccessfully, as James did, as a therapy that would cure them, while they remained passive patients. More patients, however, were notably aware of the active role required of them on commencing hydropathic treatment. One such patient, Susan B. Anthony, planned her travels to coincide with a stop at a cure in 1885. After months on the road speech-making, she resided at the Worcester Hydropathic Institute, which was run by her cousin, Dr. Seth Rogers.[66] The vigorous and spartan treatment that awaited her, while not relaxing, was invigorating and challenging.

> First thing in the morning dripping sheet; pack at 10 o'clock for 45 minutes, come out of that, take a shower followed by a sitz bath, with a pail of water at 75 degrees poured over the shoulders, after which a dry sheet, then brisk exercises. At 4 P.M., the program repeated, and then again at 9 P.M. My day is so cut up with four baths, four dressings and undressings, four exercisings, one drive and three eatings, that I do not have time to put two thoughts together.[67]

One has the distinct impression that this busy, physically demanding schedule suited Anthony, and others like her, quite well.

Jeannette Marks

Jeannette Marks, a noted author, professor at Mount Holyoke College, and "Boston marriage" companion of Mary Woolley (president of Mount Holyoke), sojourned at a cure in 1909–1910 for reasons quite similar to Anthony's twenty-four years earlier: Marks, too, was seeking to recuperate from the demands of public and professional life. After her visit to the Battle Creek (Michigan) Sanitarium, which Woolley financed, Marks continued "all of her life to follow a modified form of the Battle Creek regimen, eschewing meat or eating it very lightly, and speaking with disapproval of even such very mild stimulants as cocoa."[68] When Marks returned to Mount Holyoke, in South Hadley, Massachusetts, she brought with her a supply of corn flakes; to this Woolley added nuts, raisins, and whole-grain cereals. Marks's health and spirits held steady until 1912, when she considered going to Battle Creek again. She held off until the summer of 1914, when she returned shortly after her father's death.[69]

The Marks–Woolley "marriage" spanned fifty-two years, and Marks found relief from recurring nervous afflictions in the water processes and the life-style alterations advocated by John Harvey Kellogg's cure at Battle Creek. Portrayed by one biographer as continuously ill at ease in comparing her own achievements with Woolley's eminent career, Marks retreated frequently to the Battle Creek cure, where she formed strong attachments with women that, seemingly, stirred feelings of jealousy in Woolley.[70] Whether one accepts this interpretation or not, Marks's sojourns correspond with times of stress in their relationship and her attempts to reassert her individuality. It was a place where, within the woman's culture at the cures, she could receive the validation and rejuvenation she so needed.

The Marks-Woolley "marriage" has perhaps undergone more scru-

tiny than any other. A biographer of Woolley's shifted her focus to examine the women's lives together after she had assured herself that her two
subjects were not, blessedly, lesbian.[71] This interpretation has been
criticized as trivializing the intensity of the Marks–Woolley bond. As one
historian noted:

> Even if they did renounce all physical contact we can still argue
> that they were lesbians. Genital "proofs" to confirm lesbianism are
> never required to confirm the heterosexuality of men and women
> who live together for twenty, or fifty, years. Such proofs are not
> demanded even when discussing ephemeral love relations between
> adult women and men.[72]

If we could allow Marks and Woolley to determine their own iden-
tities, it is unlikely that they would refer to themselves as lesbians, despite
the widely known ritual in which one would kiss the other good night.
Proof of the unlikelihood of their categorizing themselves as lesbian lies
in Marks's authorship of two articles (and a potential book) that denounced
the unnaturalness of romantic friendships. "Unwise College Friendships,"
written in 1908 and unpublished, portrays love between women to be
"unpleasant or worse," an "abnormal condition." A later piece, "A Girl's
Student Days and After," also cautions against same-sex love, while a
1926–1927 contemplated book on homosexuality in literature would have
emphasized insanity and suicide within same-sex love.[73] Marks's self-
negating attitudes must be viewed within the context of changing American
views on the desirability of same-sex love, which in the twentieth century
began to stress pathological causation and to shun the favorable attitude
toward love between women that was so prevalent in the nineteenth
century.[74] It is possible that her sentiments reflected her fear of being
thought a lesbian; she may have assimilated the negative valuations that
came to be assigned to "Boston marriages" such as her own. Or such
sentiments may have been a deliberate "cover," given the growing emphasis on heterosexuality and suspicion of same-sex relationships.

Long-Term Stays

Women used sojourns at the cures to escape domestic or familial
routines, recover from physical and spiritual malaise, enjoy and secure
female companionship, and participate in a reform atmosphere that emphasized the importance of taking care of oneself, instead of others.
Further, through invalidism, "Women could also express affection for
one another. Whether acting as nurse or patient, the usual taboos against
intimacy between women were suspended when they cared for each
other's illnesses."[75] For these reasons, a stay at a cure had a profound
influence on women—so profound that in some instances what was in-

itially intended to be a relatively short recuperative visit blossomed into
many years of residence at a cure. Hattie B. L. Brown, first a patient and
later an attendant at "Our Home on the Hillside" in Dansville, New York,
personified this choice. She had never been well in her life and had been
pronounced incurable by more than one physician. Describing the sequence of events that led to her permanent residence at the cure, Brown
recalled:

> [I] came to the Hillside in 1883 as a helper. I found its atmosphere
> so kindly, its spirit so generous in every way in its care of its hel-
> pers, that I felt at home at once. . . . Under their teachings a new
> world was open before me. I became awakened in conscience to
> realize my personal responsibility in the matter of health of body
> and mind. . . . I finally went to live at Brightside as a companion to
> Dr. Harriet N. Austin, who was a glorious woman and a great help
> to me in many ways. You see I soon forgot that I ever was ill. . . . I
> owe my health, as well as my spiritual development along higher
> lines, to my associations with the Jackson family, with whom it has
> been my privilege to live and work during the past twenty-five
> years.[76]

Clara Barton

Austin apparently attracted a number of women with her skillful
medical management and endearing personal warmth. Clara Barton, founder of the American Red Cross, eventually established a permanent
residency in close proximity to Austin. Barton, worn and weary from
years of activity, stayed at the Dansville Water Cure in 1876 at the urging
of a friend. At his suggestion Barton wrote to the cure for publications
and received from them the fine volume *How to Treat the Sick Without
Medicine*. On its first page Barton found counsel that calmed her fears,
answered her questions, dispelled her doubts, and made her crooked
ways plain when she read *"worn out lives; bankrupt strength; quiet;
reserved force; rest; absolute rest."*[77] On reading the book, Barton felt as if
a "veil had been lifted—that I had been shown the way, and I should walk
therein. From that day I knew I should go to Dansville."[78] Barton continued to read voluminously and soon thereafter addressed a letter to
Harriet Austin asking to be received as a patient. Barton's self-esteem and
physical strength were at a low point, as she recalled: "I had so long felt
myself good for nothing worse than nothing, and a trouble to every one,
that it was with great diffidence I asked that privilege, and I asked no
more."[79]

Austin replied affirmatively "with sisterly kindness," and thus Barton arrived in Dansville in May 1876. Her sense of hope and joy reached
its peak: "I said to myself, it is Heaven, and here at last is the knowledge

and humanity that will permit me to rest if I need it, to recognize my necessities without shame, and perhaps come back a little into life. How strange it seemed to be out of my invalid home and once more in society."[80]

In addition to her sense of having found a home, Barton was singularly impressed with the size and vitality of the institution (about three hundred patients) as well as the caliber of patients: "I think I never saw together any group of people that combines the degrees of intellect, general intelligence, and culture as is collected here. The speech of each person one meets is kind, charitable, and refined."[81] By now a follower of hydropathic dietary and hygienic principles, Barton came to Dansville with an eye toward making the cure her home, which she did until she ventured forth to establish her own residence, which was

> just as near to this Institute and these people as I could possibly get, and thus I have remained, following every direction, heeding every suggestion, taking my breakfast of granula and milk, and fruit, religiously without change these four years—nay, almost five years from the commencement, and from that poor self-tortured writing sufferer of 5 or 6 years ago under God, through Dr. Jackson and his efficient associates, I am able to come here and tell you my little story.[82]

One of the "efficient associates" of Jackson's who held particular meaning for Barton was Austin, with whom she formed a close personal relationship. Under Austin's guidance, Barton experimented for a short while with the American costume. When speaking at the cure in 1880 (still a neighbor to it herself), Barton extolled Austin's pioneering efforts on behalf of dress reform to her listeners: "Ladies, the very freedom of *dress* we find so healthful and welcome has been wrought out in pain. Harriet Austin trod the pioneer paths with bleeding feet that we might walk on flowers. All thanks, all honor to her. Heaven's Blessing on a brave life!"[83]

Barton's testimony, for it is indeed that, to the efforts of Austin and Jackson reveals the sense of spiritual and physical rebirth she gained at the cure. Imploring her audience to *trust* and *obey* the principles of the cure, Barton reminded the women that no ordinary physician would ever treat them as effectively as Jackson and that when "men and women shall build monuments of gratitude to advanced thought, humanitarian effort, and useful lives, they will build one to him."[84]

Conclusions

Life at a cure provided a supportive and nurturant environment that fostered liaisons between women patients, female physicians and their patients, and the cure's female employees. In whatever capacity women participated, their sojourns at and affiliations with the cures were remembered positively and, in certain instances, became a central feature in their lives. A case in point is the female staff at the Dansville cure. In 1908 the Jackson Health Resort (the name it had adopted by that time) compiled a list of personnel and their years of service. Of the forty people listed who had been at the cure for more than ten years, twenty-four were women, not including any of the Jacksons.[85] This indicates women made up more than half the staff, suggests a sizeable female clientele, and confirms the generally familylike ambience of this cure. (These factors were operative notwithstanding the prevalence of weary businessmen who constituted a large percentage of the resorts' clientele.) For a good number of these women, their tenure at the cure involved more than simply earning a living. For some women employees, the cures became their home and family.

For all potential clients, including reform activists and professional women, the rhetorical lure of the cures promised restoration of health. It would be naive to think, however, that all patrons were drawn simply by an ideological position. Adherence to and basic agreement with water-cure philosophy figured to varying degrees in women's initial attraction to the cures, but other, less demonstrable factors were also operative. The freedom from pregnancy and the implied availability of abortive techniques (see Chapter Two, note 52) probably drew married women. For single women, women in "Boston marriages," and married women, the cures offered a pleasant atmosphere in which to escape one's daily routine, the stresses of work, and familial and personal relationships. Further, they offered gender-conscious camaradarie and a medically sanctioned, communal, sensual atmosphere. These features, while hardly articulated in advertising broadsides and journal articles, are evidenced—or perhaps implied—in the context of women's lives.

There was probably an evolution, then, from what may have attracted a woman to a cure (medical principles) to what endeared it to her so devotedly (social philosophy and communal feeling). What clients envisioned in the water cure, what they valued about it, and why they adopted it seem to reflect closely their initial expectations as well as their evolving sense of self-determination. There was probably another agenda, though, often unarticulated but discernible in the life experiences of individual women. For reform activists and professional women, the live-in cures offered freedom from public scrutiny and demands, a legitimate focus on oneself as opposed to one's labors and relationships, the opportunity to commune with like-minded residents, the respite from the isolation and demands of home, the prospect of companionship and new or rejuvenated relationships, and genuine physical restoration. It was, in essence, an equalizing experience; patients were united by common concerns, priorities, and goals. Women of various callings, activists and professionals prime among them, recalled the days, weeks, and months spent at the cures as the time that enabled them to relax and recuperate while they relished the invigorating reform atmosphere and the precious salve of female companionship. Medical therapeutics, in short, were a significant, but not the sole, asset of the cures. For some women, the cures accorded a life turning point: Genuine self-discovery through physical well-being meshed with social involvement through gender identification to create a magnificent sense of hope and strength. As one grateful former patient of Rachel Gleason's wrote to her years later:

> I was among the first to graduate from your care, where I was washed and cleansed from many a mental cloud as well as from physical ills, and restored to my friends, clothed with a new inspiration. How I was stimulated and nurtured by your precept and example, dear Mrs. Gleason, through that weary useless time. You were my physician, counsellor and friend. Whatsoever I am, whatsoever I have accomplished, I owe to the example of your useful, consistent life, Blessed among women.[86]

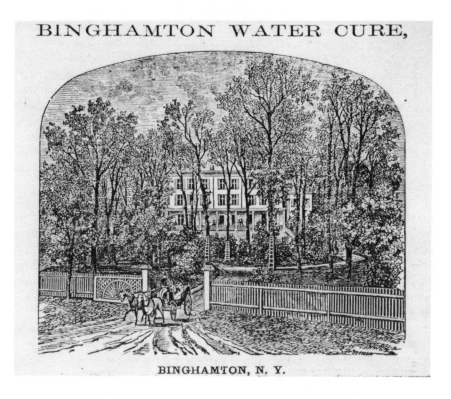

BINGHAMTON WATER CURE,

BINGHAMTON, N. Y.

Conclusion

Demise and Legacy
of the Water-Cure Movement

The water-cure movement lingered into the early 1900s, but its ideological popularity and national influence had begun to wane by the late 1860s. Beliefs in the perfectability of humankind coincided with and peaked at the same time as hydropathy. Hydropaths, like other contemporary reformers, believed that pointing the way to right living would usher in bodily perfection as a precursor to millennial and societal reformation. Reflecting cultural beliefs, they valued self-denial and self-control as mechanisms that led not only to spiritual and physical advancement but to economic rewards as well. The appeal of hydropathy emanated both from this philosophy, which echoed popular sentiment, and from its therapeutics, whose efficacy in large part resulted from a productive meshing of the human and hygienic elements implicit in successful medical care. Specifically, hydropathy emphasized the medical encounter as a primary healing tool; self-doctoring and right living as a means to self-determination; and adherence to water-cure philosophy for its medical-reform orientation, simplicity, and gender consciousness. Beginning in the 1860s, many critical components of hydropathy's appeal underwent significant changes, foreshadowing not only the dilution of the movement's potency but also its ultimate demise. This decline can be traced through theoretical, internal, and medical shortcomings.

Theoretical Failures

Theoretically, the harmonious universal vision that hydropathy posited became increasingly untenable because of the movement's ultimate inability to open the outer circle of explanation and integrate other

159

"truths." The reluctance of the hydropathic leadership to admit the inadequacy of its "peaceful vision" in a nation torn asunder by Civil War, experiencing rapid and unsettling urbanization and immigration, and facing an ever-increasing disparity between socioeconomic classes inevitably caused this message of societal betterment through personal health to fall far short of universal acceptance. The movement failed, in short, to provide inclusive answers for all of life's uncertainties. That hydropathy claimed to offer such a universal vision speaks to its idealism, insular logic, and narrow diagnosis of societal ills. (This final point was most poignantly demonstrated in its response to the Civil War.) In fact, the movement became increasingly antimodern, as can be seen in the emphasis on bucolic joys, the negative depictions of city living and working girls' lives, and the naive proposed solutions.

Hydropathic believers were ultimately forced to recognize that bodily perfection did not usher in societal reformation. Not only did right living not yield personal guarantees of health, longevity, and prosperity, but the irony of a nation at war with itself while proclaiming a belief in human perfectibility must have been powerful indeed. Twenty years of pointing the way to right living was impotent and inconsequential in the face of armed battle and issues of human worth. Not only the doctrines of the movement, then, but also the Civil War served as a huge disappointment for utopian thinkers.

Further, the self-denial and self-control that were such a pivotal aspect of the "good citizen," as embodied in hydropathic thought, gradually gave way to a far more self-indulgent, pleasure-seeking, consumer-oriented vision of the good life. The "good citizen" in this latter model was still measured by his or her contribution to the common good (which could, significantly, be "bought" through philanthropy instead of through personal example or one's own labor), although personal happiness and success increasingly correlated with conspicuous wealth, leisure-time distractions, and escape from drudgery.[1] In this context, an issue as simple as dress reform may have signaled an undesirable status leveling for some in a culture where clothing was increasingly used to signify class.

For men, the precise elements that made one an exemplary hydropathic follower may have impeded one's value on the open market: Restraint, moderation, and caution were not the assets with which fortunes were made in late-nineteenth-century urban America. The measure of the self-made man was no longer plodding restraint and labor but clever—and profitable—risk taking. This trend was suggested by the activities of the more flamboyant hydropathic physicians, who seemed almost frustrated by the austere tenets of the system and who sought their rewards outside the fold. As achievement and fulfillment for men were increasingly measured in terms of personal acquisitiveness, adherence to a system that promoted austerity and simplicity conflicted with the self-made man's ability to buy and display the rewards of his labor. Thus

personal achievement became increasingly detached from a physiological or spiritual component and focused anew on economic success and
the amassing of wealth.

For female followers of hydropathy, the homosocial bonding (same-
sex camaraderie and intimacy) fostered at the cures and the informal
politics that radiated from them became problematic. The female enclave
that flourished at the cures (among male co-patients) was a continuance
of the larger female support network that thrived in mid-nineteenth-century America. Thus the cures both reflected and perpetuated women's
homosocial relationships. One can hypothesize that sexual activities, in all
their real or imagined stages at the cures, may have contributed to the
demise in popularity of the cures among contemporaries who increasingly emphasized heterosocial (opposite-sex bonding, camaradarie, and
intimacy) bonding.[2] Given the increasing societal emphasis on
heterosociality, an environment that fostered intimate emotional and even
sensual relationships between women would be likely to fall into disuse.
This shift away from societally approved same-sex intimacy, therefore,
reflected a changing cultural perception of male and female natures, one
that made men and women less "social opposites" and more "ideal companions."[3] (Earlier, hydropaths had propounded a version of this companionate union, but at that time it was able to coexist with a special
female community.) It also corresponded, in the late nineteenth and
early twentieth centuries, with the development of a view of lesbianism
as deviant that was perpetuated by the early sexologists. There was a
marked and negative shift away from the romanticized or erotic perceptions of women's same-sex love held by earlier generations.[4]

From 1870 to 1920, then, this separate female sphere became increasingly devalued for the supposed threat it posed to relations between
the sexes. Further, women's influence became more *public* in these years,
thus affecting not only the informal nature of their political activism
(which continued but was joined by a far greater emphasis on bringing
about change in social policy) but also their gender-specific projects and
concerns. Since an "emancipationist" ideology, evidenced in expanded
opportunities and avenues of expression for women, was slowly gaining
ascendancy in the larger culture—embodied in women's colleges, the first
generation of regularly trained physicians, and women's activism on behalf
of political suffrage and labor activism—hydropathy's unique offering of
gender consciousness was somewhat overshadowed by equally articulate
activist constituencies.[5] Important to the lure of hydropathy, women's
instrumentality in these other public realms included but transcended
health and, at times, evinced more permissive sexual expression. In effect, one of the movement's unique aspects was usurped to a noticeable
degree by a variety of social-reform and feminist organizations that
eclipsed the hydropathic conception of women's influence. This move
into the gender-mixed public realm, while not new, was noteworthy for

its pervasiveness, its eventual undermining of gender-specific efforts, and its discrediting of same-sex bonding.

In short, as more and more activities solicited joint male and female participation, the existence of this female enclave may have seemed to some a vestige of the past and contrary to the new heterosociality. As one who traced this shift from homosociality to heterosociality and the decline in women's institutions observes: "The decline of feminism in the 1920s can be attributed in part to the devaluation of women's culture in general and of separate female institutions in particular. . . . Women gave up many of the strengths of the female sphere without gaining equally from the man's world they entered.[6]

This move for women into increasingly public (i.e., male) and more formal political realms reflected a less severe distinction in popular thought between the archetypical female and male character—dissimilarities were minimized and complementary aspects were emphasized.[7] While this resulted in arguable benefits to both women and men, one observable loss for women was the abandonment or minimization of women-only traditions, rituals, institutions, leisure-time activities, and health retreats.[8] This is particularly significant for hydropathic establishments, because among the main recreational "retreats" that gained in popularity while the gender-conscious water establishments waned were the heterosocial, more urban, working-class entertainments like vaudeville, dance-halls, and family amusement parks. In addition, the conspicuous leisure of elites found a new lure in gentrified water retreats.[9] This shift reflected not only a new delight in transcending daily drudgery but also a new-found desire to do so within a heterosocial context. This was accompanied by changing concepts of leisure time. In the later years of the nineteenth century Americans designed more formal, genteel leisure activities, and thus the concept of a "vacation" arose.[10] Watering places arose to meet the new demand for vacation sites, but they offered luxurious cuisine and entertainment antithetical to hydropathy's principles. These new spas, such as Grand Isle, Louisiana, and Eureka Springs, Arkansas, were overnight successes, catering to financially secure families seeking summer resorts. As did the water-cure establishments, these spas attracted a large female clientele. Whereas the cold-water cure legitimized the pursuit of women's (and men's) health, the elegant spas legitimized the new concept of leisure[11] and fostered a "new" concept of health that was far more passively oriented for the recipient. Because the fashionable watering places were located at mineral springs, the notion of healthful recreation was kept alive. Health, in the new context, could be derived from escape from routine tasks, inactivity, rest, and self-pampering. This flourishing new kind of leisure retreat of the Gilded Age diminished the use of cold-water cures. New watering places appealed to an American public relieved by the cessation of the Civil War. The emphasis on grand hotels, ample barrooms, gambling tables, and festive cotillions provided a more alluring prospect to many patrons than did the simple foods, country walks, and cold-water therapeutics available at hydropathic establishments; they appealed, in short, to growing trends toward conspicuous leisure and consumption. Directors of cold-water establishments, aware of the competition offered by the more luxurious watering places, modified some of their own accoutrements to parallel more closely those of the fashionable resorts. This occurred, quite noticeably, in the realm of activities. Several cures in Massachusetts and New York introduced billiards and dancing, open-air vaudeville and singing, bowling alleys, and charades.[12] It seems logical to assume that these innovations resulted from the successes gained at, and clientele lost to, the new centers of leisure activity.[13]

In short, the new fashionable watering places provided competition to the cold-water cures. As James A. Jackson commented in "Years of Uncertainty and Change, 1910–1929," his clientele dropped off considerably during these years. The automobile, he noted, played a vital role because people (particularly weary businessmen) "found relaxation nearer home by taking evening or weekend motor trips, and thus felt less need to visit the Sanatorium."[14] Quite possibly, Jackson's clientele shifted their business to the closer-to-home fashionable water resorts for the reasons cited. Also, the "new-found" appeal of the wilderness as a national treasure and physician-promoted emphasis on climatology legitimized the more luxurious watering places by stressing as attributes features long heralded by the cold-water cures.[15]

Thus, both the changing nature of American life and values (toward an increasingly class-distinct, acquisitive, consumer-oriented mode), reflected in the new concept of "escapist" vacationing, and a marked change in the social relations between the sexes (toward a stronger emphasis on heterosexual bonding) contributed to the demise of the hydropathic movement. For many late-nineteenth-century Americans, self-restraint in the marketplace, class leveling, and same-sex affinities were seen as not truly modern—nor desirable. This suggests that during the final stages of the movement the rhetoric of self-control and self-restraint propounded by hydropathic reformers was partly class based. As societal class distinctions intensified, the reformers' endorsement of the middling sorts against the decadent rich and the working class (the latter now seen as urban and somewhat disorderly) polarized.

Other forces of change within American society hastened the hydropathic decline. Among them were the increasing availability of in-home plumbing,[16] which rendered the cures' water supplies less unique; the decreased responsiveness of Americans in the 1860s to the admonitions of health reformers;[17] improvements in sanitation (which reduced disease); and waning interest in a restraint-oriented life regimen. The interplay among these factors was diverse and complex. Additionally, the nation's all-pervading concern with the Civil War (which caused a drop in subscriptions to the *Water-Cure Journal* and decreased attendance at the cures, thus causing concern with economic stability) and the questionable effect the leadership's neutral position had on the movement's reform credibility were contributors to the decline in popularity.

Internal Failures

Internal factors also contributed to the lessening of hydropathy's popularity and credibility. The elements of the medical encounter that had made hydropathy such a powerful therapeutic force—touch, communication, faith, and trust—while not drastically altered, began to change form. The communal context of the water-cure establishment, once such an asset in stimulating patient enthusiasm, possibly lost some of its appeal as a more private physician–patient relationship gained ascendancy. Further, as more and more establishments brought into service mechanical therapy (e.g., galvanism, electrochemical vapor baths, and exercise equipment), the emphasis shifted from the physician–patient dyad to the machine–patient dyad. This change, coupled with a marked deemphasis on water as the primary healing agent, which had necessitated washing, wrapping, and rubbing, subsumed the efficacy that resulted from therapeutic touch. With it were lost the rapport and sympathy that emanate from intimate contact, but never from a machine.[18] This gradual, yet identifiable, transition away from physician–patient intimacy undermined one of hydropathy's greatest assets.

Hydropathy's extreme emphasis on patient autonomy also undermined the physician's role. The hygienic physician was a teacher, not an irreplaceable sage, and by educating their clientele to care for themselves, hydropaths gradually contributed to their own loss of importance. As the editor of the journal wrote in March 1864: "The Hygienic physician soon teaches his patient to be independent of him, and so runs his own business down; while the Drug doctor leaves his patients more ignorant and more sickly than he finds him, and so works his own business up."[19] Moreover, hydropaths worsened their situation by not limiting the number of practitioners who competed for the available patients. Remember also that in many instances, among domestic self-doctors, physicians did not play *any* role save that of educating author. For home doctorers and cure frequenters who did utilize physician expertise, this is not to say that after one consultation a patient would no longer need a physician's advice or that new clientele would not arise. But the cycle of repeated consultation, physician omnipotence, and patient dependency was replaced by a model that fostered patient control and responsibility. This was not, ultimately, helpful to the live-in cures, which owed much of their efficacy to the healer–patient dyad. And among home self-doctorers, who often used older literature, the texts' directives remained plausible regardless of the leadership's instrumentality or vibrancy.

As has been shown, what hydropathy offered was a systemic panacea, with water and hygienic principles as the primary agents. However, the hydropathic establishments and practitioners did not hesitate to embrace other innovations, many of which included complementary reforms, but some of which actively contradicted the hydropathic written word. This erratic, and at times conflicting, conglomerate of therapeutics gradually diluted the original, unique emphasis on the curative powers of cold water. This shift in emphasis was reflected in the late 1850s when establishments began using new names and new forms of therapy. Most often, the name change involved dropping (or adding to) "Water Cure" and putting in its stead "Hygienic Institute."[20] The Mount Prospect Water-Cure became the Mount Prospect Medical Institute of Binghamton, and inebriate asylum; the Elmira Water Cure became the Gleason Sanitarium and then the Gleason Health Resort; the Dansville Water-Cure became the Jackson Sanatorium and later the Jackson Health Resort; and the Round Hill Water Cure became a summer resort hotel for the well-to-do.[21] In a sense, hydropathy's flexibility, and the leadership's unwillingness to exact theoretical and behavioral consistency, although it contributed to the appeal of the movement, also contributed to its demise.

This trend away from pure hydropathic principles was exemplified in Trall's *The Hygienic System* (1872), which argues against the use of drugs and in favor of the water cure, but, importantly, not as a panacea. Thus "did one of the two introducers of water-cure into America in the 1840's and the leading exponent of the practice for many years gradually change into an exponent of hygienic medication."[22] Another reason for the shift away from strict hydropathic principles was the relative lack of solid texts, such as existed in France and Germany. There was a dearth of material (after the initial writing flurry of the 1840s to 1870s, with the exception of two texts by John Harvey Kellogg,) until Simon Baruch's *The Principles and Practices of Hydropathy, A Guide to the Application of Water in Disease* was published in New York in 1898. John Harvey Kellogg's *Rational Hydrotherapy* (1901) was the next significant work, although both Baruch and Kellogg emphasized the use of water in conjunction with other therapeutics.[23]

The April 1885 issue of the *Herald of Health* (formerly the *Water-Cure Journal*) demonstrated the movement's refusal to function as a systemic vision or therapy, the unwillingness of the leadership (in the person of M. L. Holbrook as editor) to take a strong theoretical position on what constituted the "good life" via health-care practices, and the lack of new literature on the subject by hydropathic theorists. The issue as a whole had a tone of noncommittal "consumer choice" about it. A note on the editorial page disclaimed advocacy or condemnation of any of the articles therein: "The PUBLISHER does not hold himself as indorsing [*sic*] every article that may appear in THE HERALD. He will allow the largest liberty of expression, believing that by so doing this magazine will prove to be more useful and acceptable to its patrons."[24]

The emphasis was on a presentation of options and education, in articles such as "How to Give Massage" from the *Homeopathic News*, numerous pieces on impure public water supplies, and "Health in Workshops," which enumerated industrial hazards. There were some familiar strains in articles on domestic tranquillity and reform dress for women.[25] Conspicuously absent were any feature-length, or even direct, references to water therapies. In fact, "Pure Water," a "filler" admonished, could be procured only through distillation, not through nature. And in answer to a query on beer drinking, formerly taboo, it was discouraged on the ground that one lost tone, not on the basis that alcohol was evil. One last example of the divergence from earlier positions was the reminder that weak eyes could be treated with direct massage; no mention was made of water, whereas formerly the eye bath had been advocated.[26] Unlike the advertisements in issues of previous decades, those in April 1885 proclaimed the marvels of diverse gadgetry. Finally, the lack of substantive writing was exemplified in the "Current Literature" section, which listed only one text, on brain exhaustion; and the sole literary advertisement was for Rachel Brooks Gleason's *Talk to My Patients*, which in 1885 was roughly forty years old.[27]

The issue radiated a sense that the journal was no longer on the cutting edge of social reform but, rather, on the outside looking in on issues of sanitation and general hygiene. Further, its contents hestitated to alienate any readers; it postured noncommittally and reflected, rather than created, cultural concerns. In an analogy that would have been unthinkable thirty years earlier, its self-description modestly contended: "The cause of public and personal hygiene is making rapid strides, and a health journal is now considered quite the thing to have in every family, as much so as a newspaper, a fashion magazine, or a farm journal."[28] Even the goals of the publication, while still comprehensive, had become more diffuse: "Its aim is to promote human health, temperance, a wholesome, natural way of living, the breaking off of all bad habits, and a happy cheerful life, and teach parents how to rear healthy, beautiful children."[29] Although these differed little from the goals of thirty years earlier, the note of surety that one need only follow the leadership in the quest for the "good life" had dissipated. The promisory command "Wash And Be Healed" had ceased to exist. The hygienic self-doctorer *had become* his or her own physician, thus undermining the leadership's potency.

The hydropathic leadership, in fact, experienced two irreversible blows in the discrediting of the Nicholses and the death of Shew at age thirty-nine. These two events interrupted the continuity and credibility of the movement's leadership. The Nicholses' "expulsion" came in 1856 when Trall, trying to quiet outside criticism of their links with free-love advocates, denounced them on the basis of their medical credentials, reliance on experiential expertise, and the ensuing invalidity of their writings within hydropathy.[30] This attack on the Nicholses, two of the most respected practitioners within the movement, probably did more to discredit hydropathy's leadership—and emphasis on experiential expertise, and self-doctoring through hydropathic texts for home use—than it did to calm outside criticism and restore the public's confidence. Further, it revealed a basic conservatism toward issues outside the "acceptable" reform fold—in this case, the Nicholses' position against legalized marriage. This ugly infighting followed the untimely death of Shew by only a few months. Although his death was not attributable to water-cure therapeutics (it was due, in fact, to his work years before as a photographer, which had brought him into contact with mercury, iodine, and bromine), his ill health could not be helped by cold-water therapeutics.[31] Shew's death in 1855 created concern among his followers over who would fill his strong leadership role,[32] and Trall's expulsion of the Nicholses left the once-hearty leadership depleted and splintered. In the decades to come, the leaders increasingly abdicated strong theoretical positions; this failure can be traced as much to personality differences as to their collective inability to embrace innovations originating in scientific medicine.

Medical Failures

In the *Water-Cure Journal*, hydropathic leaders rebutted the charges of quackery and incompetence leveled against them by allopaths and responded to allopathic ridicule of the Hydropathic College and also allegations about the water cure's waning popularity.[33] The publishers were aware that these charges had taken their toll; an 1859 article pointed out that allopathy's negative attitude toward hydropathy was causing difficulties in securing subscriptions,[34] and the journal issued challenges to the allopathic community to debate the efficacy of the two systems.[35] Serialized articles such as "To Allopathic Physicians," running from October 1856 through July 1858, argued the merits of the two systems and in inflammatory prose solicited an allopathic response.[36]

Allopathic medical journals did their utmost to discredit the water cure, thereby legitimizing hydropathy's concern with the allopathic portrayal of the system. In the early years, however, there seems to have been little congruence between allopathy's estimation and the view of the general populace. Articles appeared in the *Medical News* such as "The Rising Humbug—Hydropathy" (April 1843); "Victim of Hydropathy—Death of Sir Francis Burdett" (April 1844); "Hydropathy and Its Evils" (May 1849); and the *Boston Medical and Surgical Journal*'s "Hydropathy Coming Down" (1850).[37] Rausse's *Errors of Physicians and Others in the Practice of Water-Cure* (1849), when combined with the allopathic journal articles, provided a significant body of literature on which those unconverted to hygienic principles could base their dissent.[38]

In addition, graduates of medical schools were warned against false systems, which hang like hideous parasites upon the regular practice of medicine, including homeopathy, hydropathy, thomsonianism, eclecticism, mesmerism, and the pseudo-therapeutics of some of the disciples of modern spiritualism, which were the constant reliance of an easily deluded and superstitious people.[39]

Had the allopaths confined themselves to diatribes, both the responses of the hydropathic leadership and the movement's eventual fate might have been different, but they acted on tactics designed to ensure a more secure economic and social position for themselves.[40] In addition to the legislative and educational standards repeatedly implemented and rescinded during the middle years of the nineteenth century, medical societies aimed at excluding all nonallopathic practitioners were established, beginning with the formation of the American Medical Association (AMA) in 1848. The founding constitution of the AMA stipulated that admission could be offered to all "regular" physicians,

> excluding all Homeopathic, hydropathic, chronothermal and botanic physicians, and also all mesmeric and clairvoyant pretenders to the healing art, and all others who at any time or on any pretext claim peculiar merits for their practices not founded on the best system of physiology and pathology, as taught in the best schools in Europe and America.[41]

Local societies followed suit. A committee of the Philadelphia Medical Society, for example, distinguished in 1851 between graduates of allopathic and sectarian medical schools and declared that only the allopaths could be called physicians. Because of this exclusion, Philadelphia never attracted hydropathic practitioners since they could not be admitted as members of a county society.[42]

Hydropathic leaders were clearly aware of the implications of this strategy. Articles in the journal criticized and lamented allopaths' attempts to establish boards of examiners, who would be empowered to decide who could and could not practice medicine.[43] In addition to their exclusion from medical societies, water-cure doctors were not selected to serve on medical councils, on boards of health in cities, in cholera hospitals, or at police stations. In effect, hydropaths were systematically excluded from participating in the ever-broadening field of public health (an interest they clearly held dear, as exemplified in the April 1885 journal issue)—an ironic fate for a group that had pioneered in hygienics. A particularly poignant twist is that the expelled T. L. Nichols was chief organizer of the Society of Public Health in New York in the mid-1850s. The group's goals were to educate, enlighten, influence legislation, and, most ironically, since Nichols and his followers could not foresee that this would exclude them, "to elevate the standard of medical education and practice, so that the highest duty of the physician shall be the preservation of public health, and his greatest care the prevention rather than the cure of diseases."[44]

As two historians observed of the hydropathic role in national and municipal medical affairs, "They were completely ignored."[45] This exclusion from mainstream medical-care delivery gradually served to push hydropathy into a background role, as American society relied more and more heavily on municipal services and on licensing and professional affiliation. Here, a second component of hydropathic philosophy contributed to the demise of the movement. The unwillingness (albeit theoretically consistent with hydropathic philosophy) of the early leadership to distinguish between degree-trained practitioners and those who came to practice the water cure through experience or a "calling" left hydropathic practitioners, in the decades to follow, unable to compete with the "professional" regulars. In an increasingly complex society in which people turned to experts to guide them in realms that had previously been considered obvious enough to master for oneself, "scientific" approaches became the hallmark of innovative reform. This was such a widespread phenomenon (circa 1880–1920) that not only scientific medicine but also charity, law, journalism, teaching, management, public administration, housekeeping, childrearing, and social work all became duly professionalized through claims of special scientific knowledge and expertise.[46]

It can be argued, in fact, that scientific innovations were the new cultural panaceas for a nation that was experiencing major upheavals in nearly every aspect of life. Foremost among them was immigration, which ballooned between 1870 and 1890 to include 8 million newcomers. Many were from the older European sources, but they were joined by arrivals from southern and eastern Europe, who brought with them customs and religions alien to the Anglo-Saxon population. Further changes included a statistical shift away from the predominance of farm labor toward urban, industrial employment; reduced isolation through innovations in transportation and communication; and machinery and technology that made work more productive and dramatically changed people's ways of life. In economic life, fortunes were made and lost overnight, while at least half of all workers earned barely enough for subsistence, and nonagricultural workers experienced a 7 percent to 12 percent unemployment rate. If turn-of-the-century America was feast or famine for workers, it was ideal for business. At this time, 5 percent of the population received about one-third of the nation's personal income, and it was during these decades that monopoly capital took root, thus making the business model the one to be emulated.[47]

Scientific medicine both reflected and promulgated the belief that it, along with social research conducted by reform-oriented clubs and associations, could bring order and efficiency to the institutions that seemed to be faltering under the burden of coping with the complexities of modern times. It also offered tangible hope for relieving America's health concerns, since "if there was still disease—hookworm, tuberculosis, typhoid—medical science would soon find cures, as it already had for diphtheria and smallpox."[48] Medical science became, in short, a prime organizing principle for a nation in flux. The AMA reorganized and modernized so that it could be the leader of this new energy and professionalism. This, along with significant medical innovation, greatly enhanced the status of physicians. Consequently, membership in the AMA, which increased from 8,400 in 1900 to 70,000 in 1910 and to 60 percent of the profession in 1920, reflected the new-found credibility of scientific medicine.[49]

An important source of power for the American medical profession at this time was the medical lobby, which successfully linked issues such as sanitation laws, improved status for military physicians, and higher standards for education directly with the concerns—and expertise—of the AMA.[50] As a result, the 1898 AMA convention identified the need for uniform sanitary laws and pushed for the establishment of a national Department of Health, which, it was argued, should be headed by a physician. This marked the beginning of a long partnership between the interests and projects of public health and the medical profession (embodied in the Legislative Committee of the AMA and the medical lobby), which sought "to promote and preserve the public health and the material and moral welfare of the medical profession."[51]

Thus the improved status of public health as a profession also operated to improve the status of physicians. During the 1890s a cadre of new doctors transformed public health into a distinct field of medicine, which, by 1912, had its own professional school in the Massachusetts Institute of Technology. Advances in public health included diagnostic tests for cholera in 1892, experiments with diphtheria vaccine, reporting of tuberculosis information, and an infant mortality rate that lowered dramatically between 1885 and 1915.[52]

The improved status of the AMA and the public-health advances profoundly affected those who could not gain membership in the group. By defining inclusive criteria such as a course of study in an accredited institution, adherence to the techniques of regular medicine, and disavowal of experiential expertise, AMA members asserted themselves as educated, scientific professionals. By definition, those without the criteria to belong to the association were perceived as illegitimate competitors.[53]

Essentially, this alliance between public health and scientific medicine signaled the institutionalization of the belief that every empirical practitioner was to be phased out and replaced by the scientific physician-researcher.[54] Cases in point are the closings or mergers of homeopathic, eclectic, and irregular schools between 1906 and 1910,[55] and the deluge of philanthropic funds awarded to select medical schools and aimed at remedying poor medical education. These factors further solidified scientific medicine as the only legitimate modality.[56]

The legitimacy that accrued to, and the substantial breakthroughs accomplished by, those who pursued scientific medicine may account in part for the number of physicians trained at Elmira and Dansville who later pursued a regular medical education. Being modern and reform oriented now hinged on the adoption of scientific principles and methods of study. Increasingly, scientific investigative techniques, which signaled the abandonment of an allopathic "system analysis," gained credibility for the freedom of inquiry it offered and the quantifiable advances it produced. Hydropaths had similarly relinquished their systemic approach with their abandonment of water as the primary curative agent, but, unlike the regulars, they had not sought an alternative model (e.g., scientific investigation) through which to offer their therapeutics to the public.

Hydropathy, no longer existing under that rubric, was transformed into the loosely generalizable notion of hygienic living. But even hygienic living had become professionalized through the efforts of the AMA and the public health experts. Hydropathy's ready availability, emphasis on self-help, affordability, and now, without water as the prime conduit, nonmystical nature conflicted with the growing cultural fascination with expertise, the ability to purchase varying levels of goods, and the mystique inherent in the germ theory of disease—at least among cross-sections of the middle and upper classes. In an even more nebulous vein, the modern scientist, personified in the university-trained physician, came to be seen as possessing traits formerly attributed to sectarian health reformers: innovation, flexibility, and farsightedness. Similarly, medical scientists asserted that their truths (objectively arrived at) could point the way to right living, a position formerly taken by the hydropaths. A distinct divergence between the new scientific medicine and the earlier sectarian healing systems, however, was that this new specialized knowledge was not available to all but only to the few who had access to—or economic resources to purchase—the benefits of scientific medicine.

For women in late-nineteenth-century America, the desire to pursue a scientific medical education was a logical outgrowth of female participation in antebellum health reform;[57] scientific medicine had become the means through which to create a better society. Echoing rationales presented by the earlier health reformers, scientifically inclined women emphasized women's particular predisposition to nurture and their own vital mission of educating all women to care for their own body. Gender-conscious concerns such as these, and the value still ascribed to women-only institutions, were still satisfied, as the existence of women's hospitals exemplifies. Further, scientifically trained women doctors, while admittedly constricted by virtue of their emphasis on women's concerns, their exaggerated concept of womanhood, and their rationale's minimal applicability to other, less clearly "feminine" tasks,[58] were nonetheless presenting an ideology compatible with pursuing scientific medicine. Neither gender consciousness nor the sense of mission was sacrificed in the process; in fact, by pursuing scientific medicine, women could participate on the cutting edge of medical innovation. In short, several of the once-unique offerings of hydropathy (and all of medical sectarianism), including its "place for women," had been usurped or minimized by shifts in medical and cultural opportunities and priorities.

Shifts in philosophy within the regular medical profession in mid- and late-nineteenth-century America also served to blur the once distinctive differences between the two sects. Advances in antisepsis, bacteriology, and pathology, and an emphasis on hygiene and preventive therapeutics, brought allopathic and scientific perceptions of health closer to hydropathic and hygienic views.[59]

Mid-century hydropaths, conversely, stubbornly refused to integrate or endorse noteworthy scientific advances. A case in point is their early stance against vaccination[60] and vivisection—postures they were hard put to rectify given the tenets of hydropathic philosophy, lack of access to the necessary research facilities, and an unwillingness to integrate newer "truths." This revealed the leadership's inability to embrace certain efficacious advances offered by allopathy and scientific medicine, a particularly self-limiting view given their noted adoption of often contradictory, debatably efficacious, and faddish therapeutics.

The hydropathic leadership's refusal to sanction demonstrable scientific advances probably contributed to the decreased credibility and popularity of the movement. Also, advances in which hydropaths chose not to, or were not able to, participate included the increased specialization of medical practice; the germ theory of disease (via Pasteur and Koch, circa 1876), which within two decades isolated typhoid, malaria, leprosy, tuberculosis, cholera, tetanus, diphtheria, and the plague and began offering vaccinations; advances in anesthesia; X ray; modern surgery; clinical laboratory methods; and the increasing centrality of the hospital.[61] In the popular imagination these innovations combined to produce general faith in the sciences that had discovered the X ray, radioactivity, telegraphy, the telephone, celluloid film, the portable camera, movies, airplanes, and automobiles.[62]

Beyond this, the real benefits to be gained from modern surgical techniques and immunization, as the two major advances of biomedicine over folk medicine, increasingly determined patients' choice of a physician. The dynamics of the medical encounter (a realm in which hydropaths had excelled) became subsumed to considerations of the kind and nature of disease and the therapeutics offered, not the personal preference of the patient for a particular practitioner.[63] Indeed, people's choices and options in health-care settings and relationships changed and expanded. One fascinating possibility is that the communal, peer-oriented nature of the water-cure establishment, and the "talking cure" it offered, was gradually replaced by the private psychotherapeutic relationship.[64] In fact, Sigmund Freud, writing in *An Autobiographical Study*, noted that in the early years his limited treatment modalities often made him wonder if referring his patients to a water-cure would not be most efficacious.

> Anyone who wanted to make a living from the treatment of nervous patients must clearly be able to do something to help them. My therapeutic arsenal contained only two weapons, electrotherapy and hypnotism, for prescribing a visit to a hydropathic establishment after a single consultation was an inadequate source of income.[65]

Seemingly, over time, the intimacy, comfort, and symptomatic relief experienced at a cure could be found within the more expert and individual-centered therapeutic relationship.

The myriad theoretical, internal, and medical factors that coalesced to diminish the congruence of the hydropathic world view included changes in women's culture, in their private and familial lives, in societal expectations of women, and in opportunities open to them. In addition, American attitudes about health science changed, as did hydropathy's actual "offerings." Also radically altered were notions of expertise, individualism, and consumerism, all of which contributed to the demise of hydropathy.

Hydropathy's Legacy

The medical legacy of the nineteenth-century water-cure movement can be found in hydrotherapy. As two chroniclers of the movement summarized:

> Thus did hydropathy, . . . a system which claimed to cure all diseases by use of cold water, . . . finally become transformed to hydrotherapy, a series of both cold and hot water treatments in one form or another used in connection with other types of treatments and no longer claimed as a cure-all.[66]

Hydrotherapy, as we know it today, consists of exercises performed in water, "hot and cold packings, baths of hot and cold water, hot air and steam baths, sitz, spinal and foot baths, wet and dry bandages or compresses, etc."[67] Few texts of modern hydrotherapy credit Priessnitz and the nineteenth-century hydropathic movement as their precursors, although Dr. Sidney Licht's *Medical Hydrology* (1963) discusses the therapeutic uses of water, explores spas and hydrotherapy, and covers the Kneipp (cold-water) treatment.[68] Other hydrotherapeutic texts clearly reflect the early hydropathic influence, although credit is not given. For example, Bolton and Goodwin's *An Introduction to Pool Exercises* (1967) illustrates the importance of water in treating locomotor disability as well as chronic rheumatism and arthritis, while Moor et al.'s *Manual of Hydrotherapy and Massage* (1964) discusses "the use of water in any of its three forms, solid, liquid, or vapor, internally or externally, in the treatment of disease or trauma."[69] Hydrotherapy has been adopted by scientific medicine, as evidenced in texts such as Baruch's *An Epitome of Hydrotherapy for Physicians, Architects and Nurses* (1920); Morison's *On Cardiac Failure and Its Treatment, with Special Reference to the Use of Baths and Exercises* (1927); the *Proceedings of the International Congress on Rheumatism and Hydrology* (1938); Duffield's *Exercise in Water* (1976); Campion's *Hydrotherapy in Pediatrics* (1985); and in numerous medical articles.[70]

Demonstrably, hydropathy has survived as hydrotherapy, but there are other, less overt remnants of the water-cure movement. Modern hygiene has benefited from the hydropaths' (and other sectarians') emphasis on frequent bathing, disdain of drug therapy, and belief in disease prevention through self-regulated, reasonable living habits, diet, and exercise.

The hydropathic movement demonstrates that people's choices about health care have personal and social, as well as medical, content—a point also evidenced in our contemporary (and somewhat analogous) fascination with physical fitness. National enthusiasm for running, aerobics, improved "natural" dietetics, and self-improvement programs speaks to our "new-found" fascination and commitment to health. An integral part of this revival entails utilizing the comfort and physical well-being that water treatment provides in exercise, relaxation, and therapy. The virtual industry that has arisen around jacuzzis, spas, hot tubs, saunas, immersion float tanks, bottled drinking water, swimming facilities, and water resorts harkens to its nineteenth-century antecedents.[71]

Beyond the retention of these features of water cure is a valuable lesson: American health-care recipients, now as then, are insisting through the self-appointed adoption of these life-style revisions that health and sickness should be assessed more comprehensively and that contemporary medicine is too specialized, reductionalistic, and impersonal.[72] In short, our current trends have parallels in the nineteenth century. In both eras many Americans have expressed dissatisfaction with standard medical practice and pursued a high, seemingly idealistic level of well-being and fulfillment.[73] In both eras the near-obsessive concern with physical fitness and health has corresponded with a highly competitive, industrial life in which one's fitness was yet another competitive asset that improved job performance and individual advancement.

Finally, the pursuit of limitless personal fulfillment, well-being, and meaning through health may compensate for a belief that other, far larger aspects of one's life (future potential well-being and secure relation-ships within the local and global communities) are *not* controllable or ordered. Health and bodily perfectionism might be, in short, the ultimate metaphors for self-determination and choice amid cultural uncertainty and upheaval; they do indeed yield a self-directed, life-giving, empower-ing vision. Now, as then, health may be one of the few arenas in which a utopian, perfectionist ideal can be sought and—for given moments—realized.

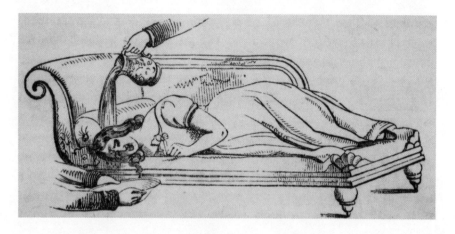

Notes

Introduction

1. See Paul Starr, *The Social Transformation of American Medicine* (New York: Basic Books, 1982), p. 99, for a discussion of the percentage of irregular practitioners in the nineteenth century.

2. See Harry B. Weiss and Howard R. Kemble, *The Great American Water-Cure Craze: A History of Hydropathy in the United States* (Trenton, N.J.: Past Times Press, 1967).

3. For information on the format, popularity, and circulation size of the *Water-Cure Journal*, see *Water-Cure Journal* 11, no. 6 (June 1851): 150; *Water-Cure Journal* 14, no. 6 (December 1852): 129–130; and *Water-Cure Journal* 29, no. 1 (January 1860): 9.

4. Gerald Grob, "The Social History of Medicine and Disease in America: Problems and Possibilities," *Journal of Social History* 10, no. 4 (June 1977): 391–410; and Ronald L. Numbers, "The History of American Medicine: A Field in Ferment," in *The Promise of American History: Progress and Prospects*, ed. Stanley I. Kutler and Stanley N. Katz (Baltimore: Johns Hopkins Press, 1982). Both provide excellent historiographical surveys of major interpretive junctures in medical history.

5. Supporters of this hypothesis include Evelyn M. Kitagawa, "On Morality," *Demography* 14, no. 4 (November 1977): 381–389; John B. and Sonja M. McKinlay, "The Questionable Contribution of Medical Measures to the Decline of Mortality in the United States in the Twentieth Century," *Health and Society*, Summer 1977, pp. 405–429; Abdel R. Omran, "Epidemiologic Transition in the United States: The Health Factor in Population Change," *Population Bulletin* 32, no. 2 (Washington, D.C.: Population Reference Bureau, 1977); and Thomas McKeown, *The Role of Medicine: Dream, Mirage, or Nemesis* (Princeton: Princeton University Press, 1979).

6. Indicative of this interpretation are William B. Walker, *The Health Reform*

Movement in the United States, 1830–1870 (Baltimore: Johns Hopkins University Press, 1955, Dissertation Abstracts International); Stephen Nissenbaum, *Sex, Diet, and Debility In Jacksonian America: Sylvester Graham and Health Reform* (Westport, Conn.: Greenwood Press, 1980); Ronald L. Numbers, *Prophetess of Health: A Study of Ellen G. White* (New York: Harper & Row, 1976); Gerald Carson, *Cornflake Crusade* (New York and Toronto: Holt, Rinehart, Winston, 1957); and James Whorton, *Crusaders for Fitness: A History of American Health Reformers, 1830–1920* (Princeton: Princeton University Press, 1982).

   7. Charles E. Rosenberg, "The Therapeutic Revolution: Medicine, Meaning and Social Change in Nineteenth-Century America," *Perspectives in Biology and Medicine,* Summer 1977, pp. 485–506, esp. p. 499.

   8. See Starr, *Social Transformation of American Medicine.*

   9. See M. Dena Gardiner, *The Principles of Exercise Therapy* (London: Bell, 1957); Herman Kamentz, "History of American Spas and Hydrotherapy," in *Medical Hydrology,* ed. Sidney Licht (Baltimore: Waverly Press, 1963), pp. 160–188; and Sidney Licht, ed., *Medical Hydrology* (Baltimore: Waverly Press, 1963).

   10. Weiss and Kemble, *Great American Water-Cure Craze,* and Jane Donegan, *Hydropathic Highway to Health: Women and Water-Cure In Antebellum America* (Westport, Conn.: Greenwood Press, 1986).

   Donegan's book focuses largely on New York State, on hydropathy's appeal to women as guardians of family health, as patients, and as medical practitioners. She concentrates on the treatment of women in pregnancy and childbirth and the pivotal role of dress reform in changing women's status. Her text is a valuable contribution.

   This book, *Wash and Be Healed: The Water-Cure Movement and Women's Health,* examines those same features and explores the movement's ideology and social vision, the viability and efficacy of hydropathic therapeutics and hygienic doctrine, specific Massachusetts cures, the conversion aspect of hydropathy, the role choices opened to women through hydropathic philosophy, the homosociality and intimacy among women at the cures, the use of the cures by women activists, the cross-class appeal of "home" vs. physicians' hydropathy, the larger reform network radiating to and from the movement, and its relationship with and contributions to orthodox medicine. Also see Susan E. Cayleff, "Wash and Be Healed:" The Nineteenth-Century Water-Cure Movement, 1840–1900; Simple Medicine and Women's Retreat," doctoral dissertation, Brown University, 1983, which was listed in 1983 through the University of Michigan dissertation service.

   11. See Guenter B. Risse, Ronald L. Numbers, and Judith Walzer Leavitt, *Medicine Without Doctors: Home Health Care in American History* (New York: Science History Publications, 1977); Regina Morantz, "Making Women Modern: Middle Class Women and Health Reform in Nineteenth-Century America," *Journal of Social History* 10, no. 4 (June 1977): 490–507; and Regina Morantz, "Nineteenth-Century Health Reform and Women: A Program of Self-Help," in Risse, Numbers, and Leavitt, *Medicine Without Doctors,* pp. 73–93.

   12. See Marshall Scott Legan, "Hydropathy in America: A Nineteenth-Century Panacea," *Bulletin of the History of Medicine* 45, no. 3 (May–June, 1971): 267–280; Weiss and Kemble, *Great American Water-Cure Craze;* and Kamentz, "History of American Spas and Hydrotherapy," pp. 160–189.

   13. See Ronald L. Numbers and Rennie B. Schoepflin, "Ministries of Healing: Mary Baker Eddy, Ellen G. White, and the Religion of Health," in *Women*

and Health in America, ed. Judith Walzer Leavitt (Madison: University of Wisconsin Press, 1984), pp. 376–389; Numbers, *Prophetess of Health;* Morantz, "Making Women Modern"; John B. Blake, "Health Reform," in *The Rise of Adventism, Religion and Society in Mid-Nineteenth-Century America,* ed. Edwin S. Gaustad (New York: Harper & Row, 1974), pp. 30–49; Carson, *Cornflake Crusade;* Nissenbaum, *Sex, Diet and Debility;* Richard W. Schwarz, *John Harvey Kellogg, M.D.* (Nashville, Tenn.: Southern Publishing, 1970); and Richard H. Shryock, "Sylvester Graham and the Popular Health Movement, 1830–1870," *Mississippi Valley Historical Review* 18, no. 2 (1932): 172–173.

14. See Kathryn Kish Sklar, *Catharine Beecher: A Study in American Domesticity* (New York: Norton, 1976); Kathryn Kish Sklar, "All Hail to Pure Cold Water!" in Leavitt, ed., *Women and Health in America,* pp. 246–254; and Anna Mary Wells, *Miss Marks and Miss Woolley* (Boston: Houghton Mifflin, 1978).

15. Morantz, "Nineteenth-Century Health Reform and Women," p. 81.

16. See Blake, "Health Reform"; Numbers, *Prophetess of Health;* and Sklar, *Catharine Beecher.*

17. Legan in particular, in "Hydropathy in America," seems ambivalent about the social, cultural, and (particularly) medical value of the cold-water cure when he refers to hydropathy as one of many "aberrations [that] achieved the status of cults or schools of medical doctrine" (p. 267).

18. Henry Burnell Shafer, *The American Medical Profession, 1783 to 1850* (New York: Columbia University Press, 1939), pp. 96–97.

19. This discussion was largely informed by Rosenberg's "Therapeutic Revolution," pp. 485–506.

20. In fact, one historian commented, "Throughout the period, harmful drugs made the presence of the physician a dubious advantage in much medical care." See William G. Rothstein, *American Physicians in the Nineteenth-Century: From Sects to Science* (Baltimore: Johns Hopkins University Press, 1972), p. 186.

21. See Frederick C. Waite, "The First Medical Diploma Mill in the United States," *Bulletin of the History of Medicine* 20 (November 1946): 495–504; and Charles W. Eliot, *Harvard Memories* (Cambridge: Harvard University Press, 1923), for further information on the poor standards in allopathic medical schools.

22. See Barbara Ehrenreich and Deirdre English, *For Her Own Good: 150 Years of the Experts' Advice to Women* (Garden City, N.Y.: Doubleday Anchor, 1978), Chaps. 2 and 3, "The Rise of the Experts," pp. 33–98; Chaps. 4–7, "The Reign of the Experts," pp. 101–265; Vern Bullough and Martha Voght, "Women, Menstruation and Nineteenth-Century Medicine," *Bulletin of the History of Medicine* 47, no. 1 (1973): 66–82; Carroll Smith-Rosenberg and Charles Rosenberg, "The Female Animal: Medical and Biological Views of Woman and Her Role in Nineteenth-Century America," *Journal of American History,* June 1973 to March 1974, pp. 332–357; and John S. Haller and Robin M. Haller, *The Physician and Sexuality in Victorian America* (Urbana: University of Illinois Press, 1974).

23. One case in point is the male midwife who later became the obstetrician. See Susan Cayleff, "The Eradication of Female Midwifery," Master's Thesis, Sarah Lawrence College, 1978.

24. Where women had once controlled childbearing, herbal medicines, and abortion, the schooled physician now competed for the same clientele (although at times different services were offered). Refuting arguments charging them with lack of experience (many medical students had not seen a delivery by the time

they graduated) and immodesty in attending female patients, physicians argued that all childbearing was a medical event requiring physician intervention. For information on women's roles as healers in seventeenth-, eighteenth-, and nineteenth-century America, see Starr, *Social Transformation*, pp. 49–51, and Chap. 1, "Medicine in a Democratic Culture, 1760–1850," wherein he chronicles the demise of women's central role as health-care providers; Zoila Acevedo, R.N., "Abortion in Early America," *Women and Health* 4, no. 2 (Summer 1979): 159–166; Ehrenreich and English, *For Her Own Good;* Cayleff, "Eradication of Female Midwifery"; and Richard W. Wertz and Dorothy C. Wertz, *Lying-in: A History of Childbirth in America* (New York: Free Press, 1977).

25. See Charles Meigs, *Females and Their Diseases* (Philadelphia: Lea and Blanchard, 1848); Carroll Smith-Rosenberg, "Puberty to Menopause: The Cycle of Femininity in Nineteenth-Century America," in *Clio's Consciousness Raised: New Perspectives on the History of Women*, ed. Mary Hartman and Lois W. Banner (New York: Harper & Row, 1974), pp. 23–53. See also Ann Douglas Wood, "The Fashionable Diseases: Women's Complaints and Their Treatment in Nineteenth-Century America," *Journal of Interdisciplinary History* 4, no. 1 (Summer 1973): 25–52; G. J. Barker-Benfield, *The Horrors of the Half-Known Life: Male Attitudes toward Women and Sexuality in Nineteenth Century America* (Harper & Row, 1976); Ehrenreich and English, "The Dictatorship of the Ovaries," in *For Her Own Good*, pp. 120–125; and Haller and Haller, *Physician and Sexuality*.

26. Robert N. Bellah, Richard Madsen, William M. Sullivan, Ann Swidler, and Steven M. Tipton, *Habits of the Heart: Individualism and Commitment in American Life* (Berkeley: University of California Press, 1985), esp. pp. 27–51.

27. Barbara Welter, in "The Cult of True Womanhood, 1820–1860," *American Quarterly* 28 (Summer 1966): 151–174, characterized these counterbalancing traits as piety, purity, submissiveness and domesticity. Juxtaposed with the corresponding male traits they present a stark example of the "social opposite."

28. Carroll Smith-Rosenberg, in "The Female World of Love and Ritual: Relations between Women in Nineteenth-Century America," *Signs* 1 (1975): 1–29, first identified this web of female nurturance, cooperation, and commitment to others. It too compares dramatically with the male hierarchical model of competition and individualism.

29. Carol Gilligan, *In a Different Voice: Psychological Theory and Women's Development* (Cambridge: Harvard University Press, 1982), posits that the [male] "developmental litany intones the celebration of separation, autonomy, individuation, and natural rights" (p. 23). Women, conversely, are concerned with relationships and responsibilities to others (p. 17); the separate-sphere ideology in mid-nineteenth-century America championed these dichotomous pursuits for women and men.

30. See Smith-Rosenberg, "The Female World"; and Lillian Faderman, *Surpassing the Love of Men: Romantic Friendship and Love between Women from the Renaissance to the Present* (New York: Morrow, 1981), esp. "Kindred Spirits," pp. 157–178, "New Women," pp. 178–190, and "Boston Marriage," pp. 190–203. Nancy F. Cott, *The Bonds of Womanhood: "Woman's Sphere" in New England, 1780–1835* (New Haven: Yale University Press, 1977); and L. C. Taylor and C. Lasch, "Two 'Kindred Spirits': Sorority and Family in New England, 1839–1846," *New England Quarterly* 36 (March 1963): 23–41, discuss woman's sphere and female bonding in the eighteenth through the mid-nineteenth century.

31. Rosalind Rosenberg, "In Search of Woman's Nature, 1850-1920," *Feminist Studies* 3, nos. 1 and 2 (Fall 1975): 141-155, argues that religious activity and the reform movements associated with it enabled women to transcend their confining domestic sphere without rejecting their female identity; the idea of womanhood had come to encompass spiritual leadership as well as domestic nurturance. Also see Anne M. Boylan, "Women in Groups: An Analysis of Women's Benevolent Organizations in New York and Boston, 1797-1840," *Journal of American History* 71, no. 3 (December 1984): 497-523; and Paula Baker, "The Domestication of Politics: Women and American Political Society, 1780-1920," *American Historical Review* 89, no. 3 (June 1984): 620-647.

32. Women "moral reformers" devoted efforts to the double standard of sexual morality; the victimization of prostitutes; childrearing; Christian benevolent work; antislavery efforts, and health issues. See Cott, *Bonds of Womanhood*, pp. 7-8, 132-135, 141-146, 149-151, 154-157, 178-182, 194; Rosenberg, "In Search of Woman's Nature"; Morantz, "Making Women Modern"; and Morantz, "Nineteenth-Century Health Reform and Women."

33. Sarah Stage, *Female Complaints: Lydia Pinkham and the Business of Women's Medicine* (New York: Norton, 1979), "The Age of the Womb," pp. 64-88.

34. Marian Lowe, "The Dialectic of Biology and Culture," in *Woman's Nature: Rationalizations of Inequality*, ed. Marian Lowe and Ruth Hubbard (New York: Pergamon Press, 1983), pp. 39-62, provides an excellent essay that posits that women's physicality (strength, size, etc.) and intellectual ability have been constructed by cultural beliefs and then invoked as the justification for prescribed social roles.

35. Ehrenreich and English, *For Her Own Good*, pp. 69-98, 101-140, argue that physicians hoped to assign woman to her appropriate place in the scheme of things by pointing out "the true nature of woman, the sources of her frailty, and the biological limits of her social role" (p. 116).

36. See Edward H. Clarke, *Sex in Education, or a Fair Chance for the Girls* (Boston, 1873). Gardner, writing in the *History of the Art of Midwifery* (New York, 1852), speaks of "the natural incapacity of females in the practice of obstetrics." Also see Mary Roth Walsh, *Doctors Wanted: No Women Need Apply: Sexual Barriers in the Medical Profession, 1835-1975* (New Haven: Yale University Press, 1975), pp. xiv-xv.

37. Alexander Walker, *Woman Physiologically Considered, as to Mind, Morals, Marriage, Matrimonial Slavery, Infidelity and Divorce*, vol. 3, *The Anthropological Works of Alexander Walker* (New York: Henry G. Langley, 1844), p. 35.

38. Thomas Addis Emmett, *The Principles and Practice of Gynecology*, 3d ed. (Philadelphia: Henry C. Lea's Son, 1884), p. 22.

39. John Wiltbank, *Introductory Lecture for the Session 1853-54* (Philadelphia: Edward Grattan, 1854), p. 7, as quoted in Smith-Rosenberg, "Puberty to Menopause," p. 24.

40. For information on the medical management of these critical junctures, see Smith-Rosenberg, "Puberty to Menopause"; J. Delaney et al., *The Curse: A Cultural History of Menstruation* (New York: Dutton, 1976); Bullough and Voght, "Women, Menstruation and Nineteenth-Century Medicine"; Cayleff, "Eradication of Female Midwifery"; John Duffy, "Anglo-American Reaction to Obstetrical Anesthesia," *Bulletin of the History of Medicine* 38 (1964): 32-44; Charles Rosenberg, "And Heal the Sick: The Hospital and the Patient in Nineteenth Century

America," *Journal of Social History* 10, no. 4 (June 1977): 428–448; and Wertz and Wertz, *Lying-In*.

41. Haller and Haller, in *Physician and Sexuality*, charge nineteenth-century physicians with "concealing their punitive moralism in the guise of medical prognosis" (p. 84). Wood, in "Fashionable Diseases," and Barker-Benfield, in *Horrors of the Half-Known Life*, characterize these therapeutics as hostile attempts to control women. This charge of "punitive moralism" surfaces repeatedly in historical interpretation when specific therapeutics for women's diseases are discussed, particularly hysteria, neurasthenia, ovarian insanity, masturbation, and sexual surgery. Smith-Rosenberg, emphasizing the results of these beliefs in "Puberty to Menopause," p. 33, claimed that these physicians' beliefs "served as an absolute biological justification for woman's restricted role." Morantz, in "Perils of Feminist History," refutes these charges and attributes the therapeutics to the low degree of medical knowledge in the era.

42. Coronaro, who lived in the extravagant style of the Italian upper class, suffered general malaise, which triggered his desire to reform his wayward health habits. See Luigi Coronaro, *Discourses on a Sober and Temperate Life Wherein Is Demonstrated by His Own Example, the Method of Preserving Health to Extreme Old Age* (New York: Mahlon Day, 1833; originally published in Italy in 1558).Note: Blake's "Health Reform" was most helpful in providing this chronology of texts and personalities.

43. See E. Smith, *Compleat Housewife; or, Accomplish'd Gentlewoman's Companion*, 4th ed. (London: J. and J. Pemberton, 1729); William Buchan, *Domestic Medicine; or, The Family Physician* (1769); and John Wesley, *Primitive Physic* (England, 1747). Also see Blake, "Health Reform," pp. 31–32, where he discusses the importance of these texts.

44. Samuel Thomson, *New Guide to Health Prefixed by a Narrative of the Life and Medical Discoveries of the Author*, 2d ed. (Boston: E. G. House, 1825); Blake, "Health Reform," pp. 31–33; and Richard H. Shryock, "Empiricism vs. Rationalism in American Medicine 1650–1950," *American Antiquarian Society Proceedings* 79 (April 1969): 129–131.

45. Frederick C. Waite, "American Sectarian Medical Colleges Before the Civil War," *Bulletin of the History of Medicine* 19 (1946): 149.

46. Alex Berman, "The Thomsonian Movement and Its Relation to American Pharmacy and Medicine," *Bulletin of the History of Medicine* 25 (1951): 519.

47. Ibid., p. 524; and Thomson's *New Guide*, 3d ed.

48. Waite, "American Sectarian," p. 149.

49. Blake, "Health Reform," pp. 33–34; and Waite, "American Sectarian," pp. 14–20. By 1861 the primary Eclectic degree-granting school had awarded nearly 200 degrees, approximately one-third going to women. See John B. Blake, "Women and Medicine in Ante-Bellum America," *Bulletin of the History of Medicine* 39, no. 2 (March–April 1965); 99–123, esp. p. 117.

50. See Samuel Hahnemann, *Organon of the Art of Healing* (New York: Boericks and Tafel, 1876); and J. Laurie *Homeopathic Domestic Medicine* (New York: William Radde, 1848), pp. iii–iv. The exact dosages, once compounded, were so infinitesimal that numerous historians have noted they might not have cured, but "neither did they harm." See Shryock, "Empiricism vs. Rationalism," p. 119.

51. One school alone, The Homeopathic Medical College of the State of

New York, by 1860 had produced roughly 750 to 760 physicians. See Waite, "American Sectarian," p. 29.

52. Calling allopathy "the *destructive* art of healing," the homeopathic physician J. S. Douglass, in *Practical Homeopathy* (Milwaukee, Wisc: Lewis Sherman, 1894), went on to observe that "large doses produce diseases—small ones cure them" (pp. xii–xiii).

53. See Hahnemann, *Organon*, p. 32, wherein he derides the allopaths' use of evacuative therapeutics as well as their use of opium.

54. See Martha Verbrugge, "The Ladies' Physiological Institute of Boston and Vicinity: Self-Improvement and Social Activism in the Late Nineteenth Century," paper delivered at a "Women in the Health Professions Conference," Boston College, November 15, 1980.

55. Blake, "Health Reform," p. 35.

56. See Nissenbaum, *Sex, Diet, and Debility*; Shryock, "Sylvester Graham and the Popular Health Movement"; Walker, *Health Reform Movement in the United States*; John R. Betts, "Mind and Body in Early American Thought," *Journal of American History* 54, March 1968, pp. 787–805; and Blake, "Health Reform."

57. See Sylvester Graham, *Lectures on the Science of Human Life*, 2 vols. (Boston: Marsh, Capen, Lyon and Webb, 1839); Shryock, "Sylvester Graham," p. 174; and Blake, "Health Reform," p. 37. Graham admonished his listeners against culinary gluttony, believed that the stomach was the center of the system, and advocated the use of only whole grain bread, unbolted. This belief eventually produced the "graham cracker," which was a dietary mainstay in hygienic households.

58. See Shryock, "Sylvester Graham," p. 176.

59. Morantz, "Making Women Modern," p. 497.

60. *New York Herald of Health* 6 (1865): 97, as cited in Shryock, "Sylvester Graham," p. 176.

61. See William A. Alcott, *The House I Live in; or the Human Body; For the Use of Families and Schools*, 4th ed. (Boston: George W. Light, 1839). The entire book analogizes the human body to a house; it was written to educate children on physiology and anatomy. Also see William A. Alcott, *The Laws of Health or, Sequel to 'The House I Live in'* (Boston: John P. Jewett, 1860).

62. Blake, "Health Reform," p. 42.

63. See William A. Alcott, *The Young Wife, or Duties of Woman in the Marriage Relation* (Boston: George W. Light, 1837), wherein the wife is instructed to be her husband's helpmate. In the text submission is delineated as the husband's responsibility as well as the wife's, and wives are instructed to enforce sobriety in their home. Also see William A. Alcott, *The Use of Tobacco: Its Physical, Intellectual and Moral Effects on the Human System*, 3d ed. (Boston: Bela Marsh, 1848), pp. 1, 6, which proselytizes the interconnectedness of vices.

64. William A. Alcott, *The Young Woman's Book of Health* (New York and Auburn, N.Y.: Miller, Orton and Mulligan, 1855), p. 104.

65. Blake, "Health Reform," p. 42.

66. William A. Alcott, *Health Journal and Independent Magazine* 1 (1843): 29; as quoted in Shryock, "Sylvester Graham," p. 178.

67. Elizabeth Shafer, "Phrenology's Golden Years," *American History Illustrated* 8, no. 10 (February 1974): 36.

68. See: O. S. Fowler and L. N. Fowler, *The Illustrated Self-Instructor in Phrenology and Physiology* (New York: Fowler and Wells, 1855); J. Gaspar Spurzheim, *A View of the Philosophical Principles of Phrenology* (London: Treutell, Wurtz and Richter, 1860); and George Combe, *A System of Phrenology* (Boston: Marsh, Capen and Lyon, 1838).

69. C. R. Jones, "Orson Squire Fowler, Practical Phrenologist," *Old-Time New England* 57, no. 4(1967): 105–106. Fowler's presses owned the *Water-Cure Journal*, acquired in 1848, among other publications. Also see Shafer, "Phrenology's Golden Years."

70. Shafer, "Phrenology's Golden Years," p. 41.

71. See Combe, *System of Phrenology;* and Shafer, "Phrenology's Golden Years," p. 41.

72. Shafer, "Phrenology's Golden Years," p. 42.

73. See O. S. Fowler, *Self-Culture and Perfection of Character* (New York: Samuel R. Wells, 1868); O. S. Fowler, *Sexual Science* (Philadelphia: National Publishing, 1870); and Jones, "Orson Squire Fowler," p. 109.

74. Jones, "Orson Squire Fowler," p. 109; original source not cited.

75. See Chapter One. See also Weiss and Kemble, *Great American Water-Cure Craze*, pp. 18–32.

Chapter One

1. David J. Hufford, "Folk Healers," in *Handbook of American Folklore*, ed. Richard M. Dorsson (Bloomington: Indiana University Press, 1983), pp. 306–313, defines a health system as print oriented, not dominating the cultural mainstream enough to be official, possessing a combination of elements arranged in more or less orderly relationships to form a whole, reflecting a consensus among a number of people, as well as an individual's collection of health-related information and attitudes that varies somewhat from the group's views–practices (p. 307). As Isaiah Berlin posits in *The Hedgehog and the Fox: An Essay on Tolstoy's View of History* (New York: Touchstone Books, Simon & Schuster, 1953), the attractiveness, viability, and limitations of people who "relate everything to a single central vision," versus those who "pursue many ends, often unrelated and even contradictory," lends insight into the attractiveness and adoption of hydropathy by so many. It offered, in short, that "single central vision" (p. 1).

2. David Sobel, "Introduction," in *Ways of Health*, ed. David Sobel (New York: Harcourt Brace Jovanovich, 1979), pp. 223–230, identifies these elements as the common therapeutic features that unorthodox healers tend to maximize (p. 228), as does Wilbur H. Watson, *Black Folk Medicine: The Therapeutic Significance of Faith and Trust* (New Brunswick, N.J.: Transaction Books, 1985); and Leon Eisenberg, "Disease and Illness: Distinctions between Professional and Popular Ideas of Sickness," a modified version of a manuscript that appeared in *Research and Medical Practice: Their Interaction*, Ciba Foundation Symposium no. 44 (Amsterdam: Elsevier/Excerpta Medica/North Holland, 1976), pp. 3–23, wherein Eisenberg argues that symptomatic relief is the commonest outcome for most episodes of illness under medical care, which he attributes to the social dynamics of the medical encounter. Similarly, Dolores Krieger, writing on "Therapeutic Touch: The Imprimatur of Nursing," *American Journal of Nursing*,

May 1975, pp. 784–787, found that the laying-on of hands (defined as the placing of hands for about 10 to 15 minutes on or close to the body of an ill person by someone who intends to help or to heal that person) quantifiably increased hemoglobin levels in sick persons. (Increased hemoglobin levels increase the blood's capacity to carry oxygen to tissues, which does, in fact, accelerate the healing process.) The process of therapeutic touch is not affected by the subject's "faith," although the healer "must have some belief system that underlies his actions" (p. 786). Krieger differentiates between "simple touch," which, she posits, instills a sense of well-being and being cared for, and therapeutic touch.

The efficacy of hydropathic therapeutics most likely benefited from a combination of therapeutic touch, simple touch, and physician presence, features that became deemphasized in technological medicine.

3. See Joel Shew, M.D., ed., *Water-Cure Journal* 1, no. 1 (December 1, 1845): Masthead.

4. Hilary Graham's, "Providers, Negotiators, and Mediators: Women as the Hidden Carers," in *Women, Health, and Healing toward a New Perspective*, ed. Ellen Levin and Virginia Olesen (New York: Tavistock, 1985), pp. 25–62, highlights the informal, unpaid work that women do to protect and promote the health of others.

5. See T. K. Young, "Sweat Baths and the Indians," *Canadian Medical Association Journal* 119, no. 5 (September 9, 1978): 406–408; Anonymous, "The Sweat Lodge: The Purification Ritual of the Native Americans," *Horizons*, Fall 1983, p. 23; and Leonard E. Barrett, "Healing in the Balmyard: The Practice of Folk Healing in Jamaica, W.I.," in *American Folk Medicine*, ed. W. Hand (Berkeley: University of California Press, 1976), pp. 285–300, which describes the herbal bath ritualistically administered. Similarly, *Curanderos*, Hispanic folk healers, will often place a container of water under the bed of a sick person, believing that during the course of the ritual ceremony the sickness will leave the body and enter the water, which is then disposed of, thus ridding the patient of the ailment. And in the treatment of *susto* (fright sickness) among Hispanics, sickness is "swept out" of the body by using medicinal branches and water. See Arthur J. Rubel, "The Epidemiology of a Folk Illness: *Susto* in Hispanic America," *Ethnology* 3 (1964): 268–283, esp. pp. 277, 279.

6. Herman Kamentz, "History of American Spas and Hydrotherapy," in *Medical Hydrology*, ed. Sidney Licht (Baltimore: Waverly Press, 1963), pp. 160–189.

7. E. S. Turner, *Taking the Cure* (London: Michael Joseph, 1967), p. 9.

8. Ibid., p. 17.

9. John Floyer, *Psychrolusia, or History of Cold-Bathing* (London, 1702); and Harry B. Weiss and Howard R. Kemble, *The Great American Water-Cure Craze: A History of Hydropathy in the United States* (Trenton, N.J.: Past Times Press, 1967), p. 2.

10. Weiss and Kemble, *Great American Water-Cure Craze*, p. 2.

11. Tobias Smollett, *An Essay on the External Use of Water* (Baltimore: Johns Hopkins University Press, 1935), reprinted from *Bulletin of the Institute of the History of Medicine*, 3, no. 1 (January 1935), original edition appeared in 1752, originally quoted in Friedrich Hoffman, *Operaomnia physicomedica*, 6 vols. (Geneva, 1748), 5:140.

12. Ibid., pp. 77–81.

13. John Wesley, *Primitive Physic, or an Easy and Natural Method of Curing Most Diseases* (London: Thomas Trye, 1747); and James Currie, *Medical Reports, on the Effects of Water, Cold and Warm, as a Remedy in Fever and Other Diseases, Whether Applied to the Surface of the Body, or Used Internally* (Philadelphia: J. Humphreys, 1808); and R. T. Trall, *Hydropathic Encyclopedia: A System of Hydropathy and Hygiene in Eight Parts: Designed as a Guide to Families and Students, and a Text-Book for Physicians*, 2 vols. (New York: Fowler and Wells, 1850), pp. 46–51.

14. Benjamin Rush, *Directions for the Use of the Mineral Water and Cold Baths at Harrowgate Near Philadelphia* (Philadelphia, 1786); and John B. Blake, "Health Reform," in *The Rise of Adventism: Religion and Society in Mid-Nineteenth-Century America*, ed. Edwin S. Gaustad (New York: Harper & Row, 1974), p. 44.

15. Rush, *Directions for the Use*.

16. John Bell, *On Baths and Mineral Waters* (Philadelphia, 1831); and Kamentz, "History of American Spas," p. 171.

17. Blake, "Health Reform," p. 44.

18. Francis Graeter, ed. and trans., *Hydriatics: Or Manual of the Water Cure, Especially as Practiced by Vincent Priessnitz in Grafenberg*, comp. from the writings of Charles Munde, Dr. Oertel, Dr. Bernhard Hirschel, and other eyewitnesses and practitioners, 3d ed. (New York: William Radde, 1843); Captain Claridge, "History of Vincent Priessnitz," *Water-Cure Journal* 1, no. 4 (January 15, 1846): 49–52 (Priessnitz had cured Claridge); Captain Claridge, *Hydropathy: or the Cold Water Cure as Practiced by Vincent Priessnitz at Graefenberg, Silesia, Austria* (London: James Madden, 1842); Joel Shew, *Hydropathy, Or, the Water Cure: Its Principles, Modes of Treatment, &c.* (New York: Wiley and Putnam, 1845); and Weiss and Kemble, *Great American Water-Cure Craze*, p. 4. According to Hufford, in "Folk Healers," this personal revelation, or "conversion" to belief in a healing system, is common among those who become healers in their adult life; "disorder and illness, often a period of great stress, a crisis; inspiration, sometimes accompanied by mystical experiences; some help and input from an 'expert'; revitalization which is generally stable over time provided that some social support is available" (p. 311).

19. Priessnitz's methods and all water-cure philosophy were ably disseminated in America by the *Water-Cure Journal*, which was the best-circulating and longest-lasting publication of the water-cure movement. It is reasonable to assume that nearly all the articles appearing anonymously in the journal were written by its current editors. Twenty other journals have been identified. See Weiss and Kemble, *Great American Water-Cure Craze*, pp. 25–29, 35, 77, 82–84, 118, 135, 139, 172, 178–181, 185, 212, 220. In addition, some cures had "in-house" publications. Articles in the *Water-Cure Journal* emphasized the contribution of Priessnitz to American hydropathy: Claridge, "History of Vincent Priessnitz," pp. 49–52; Joel Shew, M.D., "Priessnitz and Grafenberg Improved Upon," *Water-Cure Journal* 10, no. 4 (October 1850): 143–145; J. W. DeForest," Reminiscences of Grafenberg, No. 2," *Water-Cure Journal* 26, no. 3 (September 1858): 40; Joel Shew, M.D., "Life and Character of Vincent Priessnitz," *Water-Cure Journal* 32, no. 1 (July 1861): 4–5; and "The Pioneers of Health Reform," *Herald of Health* 5, no. 1 (January 1865): 17–18.

20. Graetor, ed., *Hydriatics;* see esp. "The Water Cure, According to Priessnitz," p. 70.

21. Turner, *Taking the Cure*, p. 145; and re the number of patients at Grafenberg in 1839, see Graeter, *Hydriatics*, p. 69; in that same year Priessnitz answered 1,632 letters.

22. *Water-Cure Journal* 1, no. 5 (February 1, 1846); and Weiss and Kemble, *Great American Water-Cure Craze*, p. 5.

23. Weiss and Kemble, *Great American Water-Cure Craze*, p. 17.

24. Graeter, *Hydriatics*, pp. 79-80; Claridge, *Hydropathy;* and Turner, *Taking the Cure*, p. 152.

25. Graeter, "Treatment of Single Diseases: Weak Digestion, Debility of The Stomach," in *Hydriatics*, pp. 105-106.

26. Weiss and Kemble, *Great American Water-Cure Craze*, p. 6.

27. Robert May Graham, M.D. *Graefenberg; or, a True Report of the Water-Cure, with an Account of Its Antiquity* (1844); and Weiss and Kemble, *Great American Water-Cure Craze*, p. 10.

28. "Pioneers of Health Reform," p. 17.

29. Claridge, *Hydropathy*, esp. "Hydropathic Method of Curing Disease," pp. 193-203; "Priessnitz's Genius in Detecting Diseases—Cases of Cures, &c.," pp. 181-193; "The Crisis," pp. 92-96; "The Hydropathic Treatment," pp. 73-85; and "Drugs," pp. 85-92. See also Shew, *Hydropathy*, pp. 164-165; and "Crisis," in *Hydropathic Encyclopedia*, pp. 59-67. Weiss and Kemble, *Great American Water-Cure Craze*, pp. 7-8 and 11, discuss these features and Priessnitz's adoption of them from their true originators.

30. Claridge, *Hydropathy*, p. 193.

31. John King, M.D. *Observations on Hydropathy, or, The Cold Water Cure . . . as Witnessed by the Author during His Residence at Graefenberg, Silesian Austria* (London: Madden, 1835).

32. John Gibbs, *Letters from Graefenberg, in the Years 1843, 1844, 1845, 1846; with the Report . . . of the Enniscorthy Hydropathic Society* (London: Charles Gilpin, 1847): and Weiss and Kemble, *Great American Water-Cure Craze*, 7, 8, 11.

33. See the following articles in the *Medical News:* "The Rising Humbug—Hydropathy" (April 1843); "The Water-Cure, a Hydropathic Ballad" (September 1843); "Victim of Hydropathy—Death of Sir Francis Burdett" (April 1844); and "Hydropathy and Its Evils" (May 1849). Also see "Hydropathy Coming Down," *Boston Medical and Surgical Journal* 42 (1850): 533-534. See also Marshall Scott Legan, "Hydropathy in America: A Nineteenth-Century Panacea," *Bulletin of the History of Medicine* 45, no. 3 (May–June 1971): 279-280.

34. "The New York Observer on Water-Cure," *Water-Cure Journal* 3, no. 5 (March 1, 1847): 78.

35. Frank Luther Mott, *A History of American Magazines* (New York: Appleton, 1930), 1:441. Also see Legan, "Hydropathy in America," p. 278.

36. Legan, "Hydropathy in America," pp. 271-272.

37. Shew, *Hydropathy*, p. 136.

38. "Pioneers of Health Reform," p. 18.

39. Trall, *Hydropathic Encyclopedia*, esp. "Philosophy of Water-Cure," pp. 3-4.

40. Ibid., p. 4.

41. *Water-Cure Journal* 3, no. 4 (February 15, 1847): 62; and Blake, "Health Reform," pp. 44-45.

42. "Pioneers of Health Reform," p. 18.

43. For information on the format and popularity of the *Journal,* see *Water-Cure Journal* 11, no. 6 (June 1851): 150; *Water-Cure Journal* 14, no. 6 (December 1852): 129–130; and *Water-Cure Journal* 29, no. 1 (January 1860): 9.

44. See Mott, *History of American Magazines,* 1:441.

45. *Herald of Health* 4, no. 1 (July 1867): 1, an inference that the goal of 100,000 by 1860 had not been reached.

46. See "To Our Lady Friends," *Water-Cure Journal* 20, no. 6 (December 1855): 121; *Water-Cure Journal* 34, no. 5 (December 1862): 128; *Water-Cure Journal* 9, no. 2 (February 1867): 99, enumerates prizes given for securing new subscribers.

47. See *Water-Cure Journal* 1, no. 1 (December 1, 1845); *The Hygienic Teacher and Water-Cure Journal* 34, no. 1 (July 1862); *Herald of Health* 3, no. 1 (January 1864); and *Herald of Health* 5, no. 1 (January 1865).

48. *Herald of Health* 3, no. 3 (March 1864); *Herald of Health* 3, no. 4 (April 1864); *Herald of Health* 3, no. 6 (June 1864); *Herald of Health* 4, no. 1 (July 1864); and *Herald of Health* 4, no. 5 (November 1864). Weiss and Kemble, *Great American Water-Cure Craze,* p. 25, mention Whitemarsh, without any initials, in conjunction with Shew. No further information is available on him.

49. See *Water-Cure Journal* 1, no. 1 (December 1, 1845); *Herald of Health* 3, no. 4 (April 1864); and *Herald of Health,* 1866 and 1867, which was the first year with M. L. Holbrook as editor. Weiss and Kemble, *Great American Water-Cure Craze,* p. 28, claim the editorship is not cited after 1849. I found occasional references past this date.

50. "Pioneers of Health Reform," pp. 17–18.

51. Turner, *Taking the Cure,* p. 162.

52. Sidney Licht, "What Is a Spa?" in Licht, ed., *Medical Hydrology,* p. 439. By definition these contained a significant chemical content that flowed naturally from the ground. The six ions often found in mineral waters are sodium, calcium, magnesium, chloride, bicarbonate, and sulfate.

53. Kamentz, "History of American Spas," p. 172. Also see Edna Ferber, *Saratoga Trunk* (Cleveland: Forum Books, World, 1946), wherein the female protagonist sojourns to the mineral waters to recover from a bereavement.

54. The Editor, "Mineral Springs," *Herald of Health* 4, no. 4 (October 1864): 130.

55. A. L. Wood, "Answers to Correspondents. Saratoga Mineral Waters," *Herald of Health and Journal of Physical Culture* 8, no. 3 (September 1866): 136.

56. Indicative texts include Trall, *Hydropathic Encyclopedia*; James Caleb Jackson, *How to Treat the Sick Without Medicine* (Dansville, N.Y., 1874); Thomas L. Nichols, An Introduction to the Water-Cure (New York: Fowler and Wells, 1850); Roland S. Houghton, "Hygiene and Hydropathy," *Water-Cure Journal* 10, no. 2 (August 1850): 33–40; "What Is Disease?" *Water-Cure Journal* 23, no. 6 (June 1857): 13–14; and An Essay on Sources at the end of this text.

57. Eric J. Cassell, "The Nature of Suffering and the Goals of Medicine," *New England Journal of Medicine* 306 (March 18, 1982): 639–645, identifies the dual obligation of the medical profession as the relief of suffering (and no further inducement to suffering) and the cure of disease (p. 639). Also see David Barnard, "Comfort," *Medical Humanities Rounds* 3, no. 3 (Galveston, Texas: Institute for the Medical Humanities, November 1985).

58. Weiss and Kemble, *Great American Water-Cure Craze,* pp. 20–24, give further elaboration on these texts.

59. James Caleb Jackson, untitled article, *Water-Cure Journal* 4, no. 6 (December 1847): 359–360.

60. Joel Shew, *Hydropathic Family Physician* (New York: Fowlers and Wells, 1854), pp. iii, 307–310.

61. Eisenberg, "Disease and Illness" p. 16.

62. K. Calestro, "Psychotherapy, Faith Healing, and Suggestion," *Journal of Psychiatry* 10 (June 1972): 84, as quoted in Stephen H. Allison and H. Newton Malony, "Filipino Psychic Surgery: Myth, Magic, or Miracle," *Journal of Religion and Health* 20, no. 1 (Spring 1981): 48–62, esp. p. 55.

63. Allison and Malony, "Filipino Psychic Surgery," p. 55, establish the linkage to other forms of healing that utilize faith between healer and patient.

64. See Brian Inglis, "Osteopathy and Chiropractic," *Fringe Medicine*, 1964, pp. 94–127, esp. p. 120.

65. Raymond Cunningham, "From Holiness to Healing: The Faith Cure in America, 1872–1892," *Church History*, September 23, 1974, pp. 499–513.

66. See R. Laurence Moore, "The Spiritualist Medium: A Study of Female Professionalism in Victorian America," *American Quarterly* 27, no. 2 (May 1975): 200–221.

67. R. T. Trall, "Professional Matters: Clairvoyance," *Water-Cure Journal* 15, no. 5 (May 1853): n.p.

68. Thomas L. Nichols, *Esoteric Anthropology* (Port Chester, N.Y., 1854), p. 266.

69. Trall, *Hydropathic Encyclopedia*, p. 4.

70. "Water-Cure Catechism," *Water-Cure Journal* 21, no. 3 (March 1856): 54–55.

71. Mrs. M. L. Shew, *Water-Cure For Ladies* (New York, 1844).

72. Jackson, *How to Treat the Sick*, p. 9.

73. Ibid., pp. 24–25, 28. Also see Mary G. Nichols, *The Sick Cured Without Medicine!* (Worcester, Mass., n.d.).

74. R. T. Trall, "Topics of the Month. The Philosophy of Our System," *Water-Cure Journal* 28, no. 5 (November 1859): 73.

75. E. Gervis, "Hemorrhage from Leech-Bites," *Water-Cure Journal* 3, no. 1 (January 1847): 25–26. Reprinted from the *London Lancet*.

76. "Swallowed a Leech," *Water-Cure Journal* 9, no. 3 (March 1850): 89. Reprinted from the *Sunday Dispatch*.

77. A.E.H., "Water-Cure at Home," *Water-Cure Journal* 11, no. 2 (February 1851): 45.

78. E. Potter, "Isn't It Murder?" *Water-Cure Journal* 14, no. 5 (November 1852): 116.

79. Ibid.

80. "On a Doctor," *Water-Cure Journal* 7, no. 4 (April 1849): 126.

81. Anonymous, *Water-Cure Journal* 10, no. 6 (December 1850): 245.

82. "The Doctor's 'Occupation Gone'—A Healthy Country," *Water-Cure Journal* 16, no. 5 (November 1853): 110.

83. F. B. Perkins, "Self-Government in Diet and Doctoring," *Water-Cure Journal* 8, no. 3 (September 1866): 105–106.

84. Nichols, *Esoteric Anthropology*, p. 286.

85. Nichols, *Introduction to the Water-Cure*, p. 34.

86. See Harold Donaldson Eberlein, "When Society First Took a Bath," in *Sickness and Health In America*, ed. Judith Walzer Leavitt and Ronald Numbers

(Madison: University of Wisconsin Press, 1978), pp. 331–341, reprinted from *Pennsylvania Magazine of History* 67 (1943): 30–48. See also Chapter Two, note 63.

87. See Advertisement, "Shower and Other Baths," *Water-Cure Journal* 2, no. 2 (June 15, 1846): 32. Jacqueline S. Wilkie, "Submerged Sensuality: The Evolution of American Attitudes towards Bathing," Ms., Central Michigan University, Mount Pleasant, 1984), p. 2 (lent by the author prior to publication). A modified version of this paper appeared as "Submerged Sensuality: Technology and Perceptions of Bathing," *Journal of Social History* 19, no. 4 (1986): 649–664. Wilkie cites May N. Stone, "The Plumbing Paradox: American Attitudes toward Late Nineteenth-Century Domestic Sanitary Arrangements," *Winterthur Portfolio*, 1979, pp. 283–309. Also see James S. Duncan, ed., *Housing and Identity: Cross Cultural Perspectives* (New York: Holmes and Meier, 1982); and Eberlein, "When Society First Took a Bath."

88. Wilkie, "Submerged Sensuality," pp. 3–4, citing Arthur Channing Downs, Jr., "Andrew Jackson Downing and the American Bathroom," *Historic Preservation* 34 (October–December 1971): 32–34; and "Model Cottages," *Godey's Ladies Book* 62 and 63 (1861).

89. Wilkie, "Submerged Sensuality," pp. 7–8.

90. Anonymous, "A Sermon on Cleanliness: Cleanliness Is Next to Godliness," *Water-Cure Journal* 10, no. 1 (July 1850): 14.

91. See Jackson, *How to Treat the Sick;* Joel Shew, *Children Their Hydropathic Management* (New York: Fowler and Wells, 1852); Trall, *Hydropathic Encyclopedia;* and Nichols, *An Introduction to the Water-Cure.*

92. Mary Gove Nichols, *Experience in Water-Cure: A Familiar Exposition of the Principles and Results of Water Treatment, in the Cure of Acute and Chronic Diseases, Illustrated by Numerous Cases in the Practice of the Author; with an Explanation of Water-Cure Processes, Advice on Diet and Regimen, and Particular Directions to Women in the Treatment of Female Diseases, Water Treatment in Childbirth and the Diseases of Infancy* (New York: Fowler and Wells, 1850), pp. 13–14.

93. Ibid., p. 14.

94. Ibid.

95. Ibid., p. 15.

96. Ibid.

97. Ibid.

98. Ibid., pp. 15–16.

99. Ibid, p. 16.

100. Weiss and Kemble, *Great American Water-Cure Craze,* p. 24.

101. Gove Nichols, *Experience in Water-Cure,* p. 16.

102. Ibid.

103. Ibid., p. 17.

104. "The Water-Cure Processes Illustrated," *Water-Cure Journal* 8, no. 1 (July 1849): 1–7.

105. Joel Shew, "The Wet Bandage," *Water-Cure Journal* 18, no. 6 (December 1854): 123–124; G. H. Taylor, "Bathing," *Water-Cure Journal* 21, no. 3 (March 1856): 49–50; "A Rubber Sheet," *Water-Cure Journal* 29, no. 2 (February 1860): 18; and S. O. Gleason, "Fomentation," *Water-Cure Journal* 34, no. 2 (August 1862): 43–44. Parts III, IV, and V of E. P. Miller, M.D., "How to Bathe," ap-

peared in the *Herald of Health and Journal of Physical Culture* 9, nos. 1, 2, and 6 (January, February, and June 1867).

106. See Cassel, "The Nature of Suffering and the Goals of Medicine."

107. Harriet Penfield, "A Remarkable Cure," *Water-Cure Journal* 1, no. 8 (March 15, 1846): 123, in a letter written on February 7 from Lorain County, Ohio.

108. Ibid.

109. Carrie May, "A Wet-Sheet Pack," *Water-Cure Journal* 23, no. 1 (January 1857): 24.

110. Nichols, *An Introduction to the Water-Cure*, p. 35.

111. E. P. Miller, *Dyspepsia: Its Varieties, Causes, Symptoms, And Treatment by Hydropathy and Hygiene* (New York: Miller, Haynes 1870), pp. 68–69.

112. R. T. Trall, *Digestion and Dyspepsia; A Complete Explanation of the Physiology of the Digestive Process with the Symptoms and Treatment of Dyspepsia and Other Disorders of the Digestive Organs* (New York: S. R. Wells, 1873), p. 7.

113. Ibid.; for information against the use of tobacco and tight lacing, see pp. 64–74.

114. Ibid., pp. 86–87.

115. Ibid., p. 14.

116. R. T. Trall, *The New Hydropathic Cook-book; with Recipes for Cooking on Hygienic Principles* (New York: Fowler and Wells, 1856), p. 19.

117. Ibid.; see the Index.

118. Miller, *Dyspepsia: Its Varieties, Causes, Symptoms*, p. 74.

119. Mrs. Julia A. Pye, *Invalid Cookery: A Manual of Recipes for the Preparation of Food for the Sick and Convalescent; to Which Is Added a Chapter of Practical Suggestions for the Sick Room* (Chicago: Knight and Leonard, 1880), unnumbered page in preface.

120. Joseph Scott, "Experience in Water-Cure," *Water-Cure Journal* 14, no. 5 (November 1852): 106.

121. For information on water-cure processes in surgery and wounds, see Joel Shew, M.D. "Water-Cure in Surgery—No. V: Broken Bones," *Water-Cure Journal* 15, no. 2 (February 1853); and J. A. Spear, "Water Treatment in Wounds," *Water-Cure Journal* 9, no. 4 (April 1850): 120. Hydropathic management of other ailments are discussed throughout the text.

122. Gove Nichols, *Experience in Water-Cure*, pp. 37–39.

123. For a full discussion of these factors, see James H. Cassidy, "Why Self-Help? Americans Alone with Their Diseases 1800–1850," in *Medicine Without Doctors*, ed. Guenter B. Risse, Ronald L. Numbers and Judith Walzer Leavitt (New York: Science History Publications, 1977), pp. 31–48.

124. Ronald L. Numbers, "Do-It-Yourself the Sectarian Way," in Risse, Numbers, and Leavitt, eds., *Medicine Without Doctors*, pp. 49–72.

125. Roy M. Anker, "Popular Religion and Theories of Self-Help," in *Handbook of American Popular Culture*, ed. M. Thomas Inge (Westport, Conn.: Greenwood Press, 1980), 2:287–316.

126. In fact, one's ability to be mentally and socially (i.e., economically) productive was intrinsically tied to one's physical health. American interest in physical fitness valued self-improvement because it had an impact on social

productivity and advancement. See John R. Betts, "Mind and Body in Early American Thought," *Journal of American History* 54 (March 1968): 787–805; and Joan Paul, "The Health Reformers: George Baker Windship and Boston's Strength Seekers," *Journal of Sport History* 10, no. 3 (Winter 1983): 41–57, which delineates the favorable connection between physical self-discipline and health.

127. "Professional Matters," *Water-Cure Journal* 16, no. 2 (August 1853): 43.

128. Ibid.

129. "Facts in Domestic Practice of Water-Cure," *Water-Cure Journal* 1, no. 2 (May 15, 1846): 189.

130. Ibid.

131. Ibid.

132. Joel Shew, M.D. "A Word to Water Patients on Household Treatment," *Water-Cure Journal* 9, no. 4 (April 1850): 104–105.

133. Ibid.

134. Ibid., p. 105. The "particulars" range from age, sex, and occupation to specific questions re difficulty in urination, asthmatic history, eating habits, respirations per minutes, night sweats, medications taken, practice of the solitary vice, and, for women, menstrual histories. In all, about 60 health-related areas are probed. Shew does suggest that a fee proportionate to one's income be paid for such advice.

135. Anonymous, "A Case of Home Treatment in Water-Cure," *Water-Cure Journal* 10, no. 1 (July 1850): 29.

136. Ibid.

137. "Prospectus for 1851," *Water-Cure Journal* 11, no. 1 (January 1851): 24.

138. A.E.H., "Water-Cure at Home," *Water-Cure Journal* 11, no. 2 (February 1851): 45.

139. Mrs. Jane V. Hull, "Home Practice in Water-Cure," *Water-Cure Journal* 11, no. 3 (March 1851): 72.

140. Ibid.

141. Solomon Freez, "Interesting Cases in Home Practice," *Water-Cure Journal* 11, no. 6 (June 1851): 147–148. *Note:* Elsewhere, an M.D. named Solomon Frease appears. It is difficult to determine if this is the same individual.

142. An Ex-Druggist, "Domestic Practice of Hydropathy," *Water-Cure Journal* 12, no. 2 (August 1851): 39.

143. Joel Shew discussed the domestic care of these problems. Re wounds and hemorrhages, see *Water-Cure Journal* 17, no. 3 (March 1854): 73–75; Re choking, see *Water-Cure Journal* 17, no. 5 (May 1854): 97–98.

144. See "Home Voices: Extracts from Letters" in the following issues of the *Water-Cure Journal:* 18, no. 1 (July 1854): 4–5; 19, no. 1 (February 1855): n.p.; 10, no. 4 (October 1855): 89; 12, no. 4 (April 1857): 84; 24, no. 1 (July 1857): 17.

145. Anonymous from Unionville Centre, Pennsylvania, "Home Voices: A Village Supplied with the Journal," *Water-Cure Journal* 20, no. 4 (October 1855): 89.

146. Ibid.

147. Ibid.

148. James Caleb Jackson, "Sick-Headache," *Water-Cure Journal* 33, no. 6 (June 1862): 121–122.

149. See "Nurses for the Sick," *Water-Cure Journal* 20, no. 6 (December 1855): 124; W. T. Vail, M.D. "Domestic Practice—No. 2," *Herald of Health* 4, no. 5 (November 1864): 150–152; J. H. Hero, "Errors in Home Practice," *Water-Cure Journal* 20, no. 5 (November 1855): 102; Howard Johnson, M.D., "Domestic Practice of Hydropathy," *Water-Cure Journal* 8, no. 6 (December 1849): 185; and E. P. Miller, M.D. "Hygienic Home Treatment of Diseases," *Herald of Health* 9, no. 4 (April 1867): 193–194.

Chapter Two

1. Jemima Pringle, "Wellington Square, C. W. Voices of the People," *Herald of Health* 3, no. 1 (January 1864): 40.

2. Ibid.

3. Ibid.

4. Ibid.

5. "I," "Extract from a Letter Written by a Woman at a Water-Cure, to a Friend," *Water-Cure Journal* 19, no. 3 (March 1855): 60.

6. Ibid.

7. Mary Jenks, "Astonishing Cure!" *Water-Cure Journal* 15, no. 5 (May 1853): 113.

8. Ibid.

9. Ibid.

10. Ibid.

11. Anonymous, *Water-Cure Journal* 4, no. 1 (July 1, 1847): 223.

12. Ibid.

13. Fanny B. Johnson, "An Old-Time Patient of Father Jackson's," quoted in William D. Conklin, *The Jackson Health Resort* (Dansville, N.Y.: privately printed, 1971), pp. 24–25.

14. See "Mrs. Wright's Lectures to Ladies on Anatomy, Physiology, and Health," *Water-Cure Journal* 2, no. 1 (June 1846): 11–12.

15. *Boston Quarterly Review*, April 1842, quoted in Samuel Gregory, *Facts and Important Information for Young Women on the Subject of Masturbation: With Its Cause, Prevention, and Cure* (Boston, 1857), reprinted in Charles R. Rosenberg and Carroll Smith-Rosenberg, eds., *Sex, Marriage and Society: The Secret Vice Exposed! Some Arguments Against Masturbation* (New York: Arno Press, 1974), p. 11. Gove, not yet married to Nichols, was referred to as Mrs. Gove. Throughout this text, she is referred to as Gove Nichols. Also see Chapter Three.

16. (A Physician), *Licentiousness and Its Effects upon Bodily and Mental Health* (New York: Graham, 1844), quoted in John S. Haller and Robin M. Haller, *The Physician and Sexuality in Victorian America* (Urbana: University of Illinois Press, 1974), pp. 94–102.

17. See R. T. Trall, M.D. "The Solitary Vice," in *Sexual Physiology: A Scientific and Popular Exposition of the Fundamental Problems in Sociology* (London: Health Promotion, 1861), p. 234.

18. R. T. Trall, *Pathology of the Reproductive Organs; Embracing All Forms of Sexual Disorders* (Boston: B. Leverett Emerson, 1863), p. 70.

19. Ibid., p. 129.

20. Ibid., pp. 131–132.

21. Ibid., pp. 132–134. Also see "Spermatorrhea," *Water-Cure Journal* 31, no. 5 (May 1861): 73–74.

22. Mary Gove Nichols, *Experience in Water-Cure:* Trall, *A Familiar Exposition of the Principles and Results of Water Treatment, in the Cure of Acute and Chronic Diseases, Illustrated by Numerous Cases in the Practice of the Author,* etc. (New York: Fowler and Wells, 1850); p. 73.

23. Trall, *Sexual Physiology,* p. iv.

24. Ibid., p. iii.

25. Ibid., pp. 57–58.

26. Ibid., p. 59; see also Chap. 5.

27. Ibid., p. 69; see also Chap. 6.

28. Ibid., p. 133; see also Chap. 9.

29. Ibid., p. 245; see also Chap. 14.

30. Ibid., p. 248.

31. Nancy F. Cott, "Passionlessness: An Interpretation of Victorian Sexual Ideology," *Signs* 4 (1978): 219–236, argues that passionlessness offered self-preservation and social advancement for women.

32. Trall, *Sexual Physiology,* pp. 201–204; see also Chap. 12. Also, an article in the *Herald of Health* 8, no. 1 (July 1866): 23–24, argued that feeble women should bear children only once every five years.

33. Trall, *Sexual Physiology,* p. 202.

34. Ibid., pp. 205–206.

35. Ibid., pp. 209, 211.

36. Ibid.

37. Ibid., p. 213.

38. Ibid.

39. Ibid., p. 214.

40. Ibid., pp. 226, 228.

41. Ibid., p. 217.

42. Ibid., p. 233; see also Chap. 14.

43. Gove Nichols, *Experience in Water-Cure,* pp. 74–75.

44. Joel Shew, M.D., "Pregnancy and Childbirth," *Water-Cure Journal* 2 , no. 5 (August 1, 1846): 72. Shew went on to describe the successful delivery of the woman's child.

45. Mrs. O.C.W., "Childbirth—a Contrast," *Water-Cure Journal* 11, no. 4 (April 1851): 88.

46. Ibid.

47. Ibid.

48. "Water-Cure Mothers and Water-Cure Babies Have Little Need of Doctors," *Water-Cure Journal* 16, no. 2 (August 1853): 36.

49. Joel Shew, M.D., "Twelve Cases in Midwifery with Details of Treatment," *Water-Cure Journal* 11, no. 3 (March 1851): 64. Also see *Water-Cure Journal* 11, no. 5 (May 1851), for the second half of "Twelve Cases."

50. T. L. Nichols, M.D., "The Curse Removed," *Water-Cure Journal* 10, no. 5 (November 1850): 167–173.

51. "Bathing to Be Practiced during the Time of Menstruation—Treatment in Suppressed and Painful Menstruation," *Water-Cure Journal* 1, no. 3 (January 1, 1846): 43–45.

52. Trall, *Pathology of the Reproductive Organs,* esp. "Female Diseases," pp. 140–162. For further information on the hydropathic response to menstruation, see *Water-Cure Journal* 1, no. 2 (December 15, 1845): 28; and *Water-Cure Journal* 1, no. 3 (January 1, 1846): 43–45. *Note:* "Suppressed menstruation" was often a code term for induced abortion. Although Trall and others directly discussed the means for inducing abortion elsewhere, the usage of the term in this context could be taken to imply that abortion could be accomplished employing these means; the suggested applications of water were nearly identical.

53. Trall, *Pathology of the Reproductive Organs,* p. 50.

54. "Case of Bathing in Advanced Age" (From the Editor's Note Book) *Water-Cure Journal* 4, no. 3 (September 1847): 268.

55. Ibid.

56. Mary S. Gove, "Case of Uterine Haemorrhage," *Water-Cure Journal* 1, no. 4 (January 14, 1846): 55.

57. Mercy P. Howes, "Female Weakness—Case of Mrs. Howes," *Water-Cure Journal* 3, no. 6 (March 15, 1847): 87.

58. See P. H. Hayes, M.D. (Wyoming, NY) "Prolapsus Uteri," *Water-Cure Journal* 15, no. 6 (June 1853): 127–128, esp. p. 128; and P. H. Hayes, M.D., "Prolapus Uteri—No. II," *Water-Cure Journal* 16, no. 2 (August 1853): 34.

59. Hayes, "Prolapsus Uteri—No. II," p. 34.

60. See E. S. Turner, *Taking the Cure* (London: Michael Joseph, 1967).

61. Joel Shew, M.D. and F. D. Peirson, M.D., eds., "Water in Barrenness," *Water-Cure Journal* 4, no. 2 (August 1847): 240–241.

62. "Accidents and Emergencies," *Water-Cure Journal* 11, no. 1 (January 1851): 20.

63. For further examples of the use and efficacy of water in treating nervousness and insanity, see *Water-Cure Journal* 4, no. 2 (August 1847): 247; and Rev. J. B. Thorp, of Frankfort, Kentucky (via Fowler and Wells) "Water vs. Insanity," *Water-Cure Journal* 27, no. 4 (April 1859): 56. In this case, John Stroehors, of Covington, Kentucky (1858), became insane from pecuniary embarrassment and was taken to the Western Lunatic Asylum in Hopkinsville. His caretaker, A. Montgomery, *"poured cold water freely upon his head,* which *instantly* quieted him." Stroehors became well and was restored to reason within three months; he credited the water application with his cure (p. 56). John H. Kellogg in 1902 recommended a combined rain douche, horizontal jet, and multiple-circle douche for neurasthenia and other nervous disorders. See J. H. Kellogg, *Rational Hydrotherapy* (Philadelphia: F. A. Davis, 1902).

64. L. Reuben, M.D., "Imaginary Diseases," *Water-Cure Journal* 9, no. 4 (April 1850): 120.

65. Ibid.

66. Trall, *Pathology of the Reproductive Organs,* p. 197.

67. See R. T. Trall, "Allopathic Midwifery," *Water-Cure Journal* 9, no. 4 (April 1850): 121–123; and B.S. (Connecticut), "Bleeding during Pregnancy," *Water-Cure Journal* 22, no. 4 (October 1856): 89.

68. Trall, *Pathology of the Reproductive Organs,* pp. 169–170; and Ellen H. Goodell, M.D., "The Cause of Female Diseases," *Herald of Health* 4, no. 3 (September 1864): 95–96.

69. Ivan Illich, in *Medical Nemesis* (New York: Pantheon, 1976), cautions that the more inclusive the definition of health, medical claims and possible

intervention increase proportionately. In the case of hydropathy, essentially all aspects of human behavior and societal organization were seen as health issues.

70. Mary Gove Nichols, "Education. A Letter from Mrs. Gove Nichols," *Water-Cure Journal* 14, no. 1 (July 1852): 13.

71. "Our Mothers Are the Best Reformers," *Water-Cure Journal* 14, no. 1 (July 1852): 19–20.

72. R. Roxana, "Physical Development the Duty of Mothers," *Water-Cure Journal* 14, no. 3 (September 1852): 58–60.

73. Theodosia, "Advice to Weakly Females," *Water-Cure Journal* 14, no. 3 (September 1852): 62–63.

74. "Prospectus for 1851," *Water-Cure Journal* 11, no. 1 (January 1851): 24. Other subheadings in the Prospectus for the year were "Hydropathy," "Philosophy of Health," "Reforms," "To Invalids," "To Those in Health," "Water-Cure at Home," and the fees of subscription.

75. See A Mother, "To Mothers," *Water-Cure Journal* 10, no. 4 (October 1850): n.p.; Joel Shew, "For Mothers. A Short Case," *Water-Cure Journal* 18, no. 6 (December 1854): 129; "Thank God for Water," *Water-Cure Journal* 23, no. 2 (February 1857): 36. Also see Joel Shew, *Children, Their Hydropathic Management in Health and Disease; A Descriptive and Practical Work, Designed as a Guide for Families and Physicians* (New York: Fowler and Wells, 1852); "Hydropathy for Infants," *Water-Cure Journal* 9, no. 4 (April 1850): 115–117; "Rearing Children Physiologically. Rules for Thoughtless Parents," *Water-Cure Journal* 31, no. 2 (February 1861): 15–16; and "The Child's Pocket Etiquette. In Ten Commandments," *Herald of Health and Journal of Physical Culture* 6, no. 5 (November 1865): 153.

76. See "Daisy Has Left Us," in *The Sibyl—For Reforms*, ed. Dr. Lydia Sayer Hasbrook (Middletown, N.Y.: February 1, 1860), pp. 692–693.

77. "A Good Mother," *Water-Cure Journal* 6, no. 6 (December 1848): 153.

78. Rachel Brooks Gleason, "Letters to Ladies," *Herald of Health and Journal of Physical Culture* 10, no. 1 (July 1867): 11–14.

79. Rev. O. B. Frothingham, "Women at Home," *Herald of Health and Journal of Physical Culture* 9, no. 6 (June 1867): 262–266.

80. Rachel Brooks Gleason, "Letters to Ladies. Society," *Herald of Health and Journal of Physical Culture* 10, no. 3 (September 1867): 117–120; and Mollie Bryant, "Visiting the Sick," *Hygienic Teacher and Water-Cure Journal* 34, no. 5 (November 1862): 109–110.

81. "Scissorings. How to Heal a Longing for Divorce," *Water-Cure Journal* 31, no. 6 (June 1861): 87; and "Married Life," *Water-Cure Journal* 32, no. 2 (August 1861): 41.

82. Louisa Bell, "The Paternal Headship," *Water-Cure Journal* 32, no. 3 (October 1861): 78.

83. F.G., "How to Keep a Husband," *Herald of Health and Journal of Physical Culture* 9, no. 2 (February 1867): 76–77.

84. Ellen H. Goodell, M.D., "Responsibilities of Fathers," *Herald of Health and Journal of Physical Culture* 6, no. 3 (September 1865): 72–73.

85. Rev. Henry Ward Beecher, "How to Choose a Wife," *Herald of Health and Journal of Physical Culture* 10, no. 6 (December 1867): 273–275.

86. See Mary Roth Walsh, *Doctors Wanted: No Women Need Apply; Sexual Barriers in the Medical Profession, 1835–1975* (New Haven: Yale University Press, 1977); and An Essay on Sources, this text; see also Regina Markell Morantz-

Sanchez, *Sympathy and Science: Women Physicians in American Medicine* (New York: Oxford University Press, 1985).

87. Martin Kaufman, "The Admission of Women to Nineteenth-Century Medical Societies," *Bulletin of the History of Medicine* 50, no. 2 (Summer 1976): 251–260. Kaufman studied records of the Massachusetts and Pennsylvania Medical Societies and the (national) American Medical Association to reach his conclusions.

88. Walsh, *Doctors Wanted*, pp. xiv–xv, 106–108.

89. Elizabeth Blackwell, *Pioneer Work in Opening the Medical Profession to Women* (New York: Schocken, 1977), Introduction. Also see Regina M. Morantz, "Feminism, Professionalism, and Germs: The Thought of Mary Putnam Jacobi and Elizabeth Blackwell," *American Quarterly* 34, no. 5 (Winter 1982); 459–478; and Morantz-Sanchez, *Sympathy and Science*.

90. Thomas Woody, *A History of Women's Education in the United States*, vol. 2 (New York: Octagon Books, 1974), pp. 322, 360; and Virginia G. Drachman, *Hospital with a Heart: Women Doctors and the Paradox of Separatism at the New England Hospital, 1862–1969* (Ithaca: Cornell University Press, 1984).

91. John B. Blake, "Women and Medicine in Ante-Bellum America," *Bulletin of the History of Medicine* 39, no. 3 (March–April 1965): 100.

92. Regina M. Morantz, "Making Women Modern: Middle Class Women and Health Reform in Nineteenth-Century America," *Journal of Social History* 10, no. 4 (June 1977): 490–507, offers insights into the motivations of women pursuing health reform. Barbara Ehrenreich and Deirdre English, in *For Her Own Good: 50 Years of the Experts' Advice to Women* (Garden City, N.Y.: Doubleday Anchor Books, 1978), pp. 65–66, when speaking of women's adoption of reform sects in general, charted exclusion, bad experiences as patients, or philosophical beliefs as the motivating factors. I contend that in the case of women water-curers, the order of these factors would be reversed, and exclusion from allopathy would play a minimal role. Ehrenreich and English also note that women aspiring to be allopathic physicians were critiquing allopathic therapeutics and the propriety/morality of the physician–patient relationship. Ibid., pp. 61–63.

93. Blake, "Women and Medicine," p. 117.

94. T. L. Nichols, M.D., "Medical Education. The American Hydropathic Institute," *Water-Cure Journal* 12, no. 3 (September 1851): 66.

95. M. S. Gove Nichols, "Woman the Physician," *Water-Cure Journal* 12, no. 4 (October 1851): 74.

96. Ibid., p. 75.

97. See the announcement of "The Ladies Medical Missionary Society," Secretary Mrs. Sarah J. Hale, *Water-Cure Journal* 13, no. 3 (March 1852): 62–63; "More Persecution—Fun Ahead," *Water-Cure Journal* 14, no. 1 (July 1852): 24; and "A Step Backward," *Water-Cure Journal* 26, no. 4 (October 1858): 57.

98. "A Step Backward," p. 47.

99. "Female Physicians," *Water-Cure Journal* 29, no. 3 (March 1860): 45.

100. Huldah Allen, M.D., "Hygienic Nurses," *Herald of Health* 3, no. 3 (March 1864): 95; and "Qualifications of a Nurse," *Water-Cure Journal* 33, no. 6 (June 1862): 136.

101. M. L. Holbrook, M.D., "Topics of the Month. Shall Women Be Doctors?" *Herald of Health and Journal of Physical Culture* 10, no. 2 (August 1867): 81–82.

102. Ibid., p. 82.

103. See the *Water-Cure Journal* at the following issues: 13, no. 5 (May 1852): 113; 18, no. 1 (July 1854): 14; 21, no. 5 (May 1856): 109; 26, no. 2 (August 1858): 26-27; 27, no. 5 (May 1859): 74-75; 31, no. 5 (May 1861): 65-67; and 33, no. 5 (May 1862): 109.

104. See the ads in *Water-Cure Journal* 22, no. 6 (December 1856): 136. Williamsburg is spelled Williamsburgh in these advertisements.

105. Numerous water-cure schools other than the American Hydropathic Institute opened and survived for varying lengths of time. See Harry B. Weiss and Howard R. Kemble, *The Great American Water-Cure Craze: A History of Hydropathy in the United States* (Trenton, N.J.: Past Times Press, 1967), pp. 33–40.

106. "Letter from Miss Coggswell, M.D.," *Water-Cure Journal* 22, no. 3 (September 1856): 60.

107. Adaline M. W. Weed, M.D., "Water-Cure Travel on the Pacific Coast," *Water-Cure Journal* 31, no. 3 (March 1861): 40.

108. Paula Baker, in "The Domestication of Politics: Women and American Political Society, 1780-1920," *American Historical Review* 89, no. 3 (June 1984): 620-647, argues that the social service work of women's organizations was based on an ideology of domesticity that expanded the environs of "the home" into the public realm. We must expand our definition of politics to include women's use of *in*formal channels, which would embrace voluntary activities, protest movements, and lobbying. These efforts were as much a part of the nineteenth-century political system as was balloting (p. 647). (Viewed thus, women's doctoring was expressive of a private and public politically informal feminism.)

109. Mrs. McAndrew, "Mrs. McAndrew to Female Physicians," *Water-Cure Journal* 27, no. 3 (March 1859): 38.

Chapter Three

1. See Whitney R. Cross, "Utopia Now," in *The Burned-Over District: The Social and Intellectual History of Enthusiastic Religion in Western New York, 1800-1850* (Ithaca: Cornell University Press, 1982); and E. C. Atwater and L. A. Kohn, "Rochester and the Water Cure," *Rochester History* 32, no. 4 (1970): 1-24.

2. Three water-cure establishments were for women only: Dr. Amelia W. Lines (Williamsburg, Brooklyn), Dr. Mary Ann Case (Norwich, N.Y.), and W. Shepard (Columbus, Ohio). Ads appeared for these establishments in the following issues of the *Water-Cure Journal:* 22, no. 6 (December 1856): 136; "Water-Cure For Ladies," 24, no. 2 (August 1857): 46, 46; Shepard's Columbus, Ohio Cure; and "Personal Matters," 24, no. 1 (July 1857): n.p., which mentions Mrs. Lines's (of the Brooklyn cure) move to Plainfield, New Jersey, "in order to recruit [i.e., strengthen] after three years' severe and incessant professional labor."

3. "Dr. S. O. Gleason," Gleason papers, no date, from the Chemung County Historical Society, unnumbered. *Note:* The use of a hyphen in the names of individual cures (e.g., Elmira Water-Cure) was erratically employed, although most often omitted. Therefore, throughout the text, cure names appear without the hyphen. The notes retain the original, varying punctuation.

4. Of the cures studied in depth, all advertised in the *Water-Cure Journal* with some regularity. A list by establishment (see below) will serve as further reference to their location, facilities, staff, gender composition, and longevity. Also see Jane B. Donegan, *Hydropathic Highway to Health: Women and Water-*

Cure in Antebellum America (Westport, Conn.: Greenwood Press, 1986), p. xv, who notes the numerical preponderance of men and the difficulty in arriving at exact percentages. Testimonials signed by former patients are another source that illuminates the gender percentages. See *Water-Cure Journal* 34, no. 1 (July 1862) re Our Home (slightly more men than women) and earlier advertisements for Our Home and Round Hill House that report a slight to significant predominance of men. Ratios varied from 3:1 (men to women) to 4:3 to roughly equal. There were other places where the gender ratio was comparable. For example, in the larger cures, about half or slightly fewer of the attending staff was female; this supports our premise since attendants were most often assigned on a same-sex basis. It is difficult to extract firm numbers on this point, but it is not essential to our thesis to assert firm gender proportions for we do not maintain that cures were female centers numerically.

Binghamton, New York: *Water-Cure Journal* 11, no. 3 (March 1851): 76; 11, no. 6 (June 1851): 159, 13, no. 5 (May 1852): 120; 20, no. 3 (September 1855): 68; 23, no. 6 (June 1857): 140–141; 24, no. 3 (September 1857): 68; 25, no. 6 (June 1858): 94; 32, no. 2 (August 1861): 44; 34, no. 2 (August 1862): 45. *Herald of Health* 4, no. 3 (September 1864): 112; 9, no. 2 (February 1867): 101.

Elmira, New York: *Water-Cure Journal* 13, no. 5 (May 1852): 120; 14, no. 6 (December 1852): 138; 15, no. 2 (February 1853): 47; 16, no. 5 (November 1853): 116; 17, no. 4 (April 1854): 93; 18, no. 2 (August 1854): 32; 18, no. 6 (December 1854): 135; 20, no. 3 (September 1855): 68; 23, no. 5 (May 1857): 116–117; 25, no. 3 (March 1858): n.p.; 27, no. 4 (April 1859): n.p. *Herald of Health* 4, no. 3 (September 1864): 112.

Dansville, New York: *Water-Cure Journal* 17, no. 6 (June 1854): 137; 20, no. 1 (July 1855): 20–21; 21, no. 6 (June 1856): 139; 23, no. 5 (May 1857): 116–117; 26, no. 6 (December 1858): 94; 27, no. 2 (February 1859): 29; 27, no. 6 (June 1859): 91; 28, no. 5 (November 1859): 78; 28, no. 6 (December 1859): 93; 30, no. 6 (December 1860): 93; 32, no. 1 (July 1861): 21; 32, no. 5 (November 1861): 117.

Springfield, Massachusetts: *Water-Cure Journal* 7, no. 6 (June 1849): 176; 11 no. 2 (February 1851): 48, 53.

Athol, Massachusetts: *Water-Cure Journal* 10, no. 6 (December 1850): 242–243; 13, no. 5 (May 1852): 115, 119; 19, no. 3 (March 1855): 49; 20, no. 2 (August 1855): 43; 25, no. 6 (June 1858): 94.

Worcester, Massachusetts: *Water-Cure Journal* 12, no. 4 (October 1851): 95; 12, no. 6 (December 1851): 139; 13, no. 5 (May 1852): 120; 19, no. 6 (June 1855): 137; 23, no. 6 (June 1857): 140–141.

Northampton, Massachusetts, Round Hill House: *Water-Cure Journal* 12, no. 6 (December 1851): 139; 17, no. 6 (June 1854): 137; 18, no. 1 (July 1854): 18; 19, no. 4 (April 1855): 91; 20, no. 1 (July 1855): 19; 20, no. 4 (October 1855): 92; 24, no. 3 (September 1857): 68; 29, no. 2 (February 1860): 30.

Northampton, Massachusetts, Water Cure: *Water-Cure-Journal* 1, no. 5 (February 1, 1846): 79; 2, no. 12 (November 15, 1846): 189–190.

5. "Mount Prospect Water Cure, Binghamton, Broome County, N.Y.," in *A Documentary History of Broome County*, vol. 1, ed. Frederick Wallace Putnam (Binghamton, N.Y., n.p., 1926).

6. I visited the site of the former Elmira Water Cure in October 1981 and traveled the same roads that carriages with arriving passengers would have taken. The area, at that time, was essentially undeveloped and quite stunning.

7. "Our Chief Remedy—Water," *Herald of Health and Journal of Physical Culture*, March 1869. Reprinted as "Elmira Water Cure," *Chemung County Historical Journal*, December 1966, p. 1539.

8. "Hydropathic Establishment on Round Hill," *Daily Hampshire Gazette*, April 20, 1847, p. 1.

9. "Marking Another Milestone . . . Our Seven Hundredth Forgotten Facts about Springfield," *Shopping News* (from the vertical file on Water-Cure at Springfield City Library, Springfield, Mass., n.d.).

10. "Round Hill Water Cure Establishment, Northampton, Massachusetts," *Northampton Herald*, May 16, 1847.

11. Untitled, *Daily Hampshire Gazette*, June 26, 1855, p. 2.

12. *Binghamton City Directory* (Binghamton, N.Y., 1861–62), pp. 19–20.

13. "Northampton Water Cure," *Daily Hampshire Gazette*, June 8, 1847, p. 3.

14. David Ruggles, "Water-Cure Establishment," Letter to the Editor, October 26, 1846 *Water-Cure Journal* 2, no. 12 (November 15, 1846): 189. A third establishment existed in Northampton, the Northampton Water-Cure Infirmary, two miles west of Round Hill, which was "obliged to decline a much larger number of applications than they have patients under treatment. Several ladies have left the Brattleboro Infirmary and gone to Northampton for a thorough cure." See "COMMUNICATED," *Water-Cure Journal* 1, no. 1 (December 1, 1845): 79.

15. These photographs are in the possession of the Chemung County Historical Society, Elmira, New York.

16. Photographs of the cures from the late nineteenth century, as well as patients' letters home, lend further insight into the clientele. See William D. Conklin, *The Jackson Health Resort* (Dansville, N.Y., 1971), distributed privately by the author, which contains several photographs of the cure and its patrons.

Ann Douglas, *The Feminization of American Culture* (New York: Avon Books, 1977), defines feminized culture as the development of sentimental mass culture due to the conflation of women's and clergy's influence. In this context I use it to describe a feminized cultural milieu (the cures) that stressed an emancipationist approach more than a sentimentalist one; it was a context in which an empowering vision of womanhood reigned, but one that relied heavily on social constructions of woman's nature.

17. Excerpt of a letter from Isabella Waite in Milledgeville, Georgia, to her husband, William (in Savannah), as reprinted in the *Water-Cure Journal* 2, no. 6 (August 15, 1846): pp. 91–93.

18. "Elmira Water Cure," *Sunday Telegram*, August 31, 1952, p. 63, as quoted from *Elmira Weekly Supplement of 1873*.

19. "Raze Landmark," *Elmira Star Gazette*, November 24, 1959, n.p.; and "'Water Cure' Is Monument to Gleasons," *Sunday Telegram*, January 9, 1955, pp 6–8, re Mark Twain stopping there and his wife's use of the cure.

20. "Famous Health Resort Here Comes from Very Small Beginning," *The Telegram*, August 5, 1923, n.p., quoted in 1877 from Beecher.

21. "Elmira Owes the Existence of Famous Health Resort, Located On East Hill to Both Dr. and Mrs. Silas O. Gleason," *The Telegram*, August 5, 1923 (copy of a clipping lent by granddaughter Ada Gleason, p. 3 of 3 typed); "Sixtieth Year of Gleason Health Resort, Story of Institution's Great Development,"

Elmira Star Gazette, June 1, 1912 (copied from a clipping lent by Ada Gleason Bush, p. 2 of 2 typed); and Evelyn Giammichelle and Eva Taylor, "Elmira Water-Cure: Silas and Rachel Gleason and Their 'Tavern for the Sick,'" *Chemung Historical Journal,* December 1966, pp. 1535–1541.

22. See Theodore Stanton and Harriet Stanton Blatch, *Elizabeth Cady Stanton,* 2 vols. (New York: Arno Press, 1969), pp. 172–173.

23. Laura Elizabeth [Howe] Richards and Maud [Howe] Elliott, *Julia Ward Howe, 1819–1910,* vol. 1 (Boston and New York: Houghton, 1916), p. 118.

24. Ibid.

25. Maria Waterbury, "Journal—1872," *Seven Years among the Freed Men* (Chicago: n.p., 1891). The *hot* baths and meat eating reflect the abandonment of doctrinaire principles.

26. Ibid.

27. Ibid.; see also "Elmira Famous Health Resort," p. 3.

28. Adele A. Gleason, *In Memoriam 1820–1905 Rachel Brooks Gleason,* booklet, n.d. (lent by Ada Gleason Bush).

29. "Round Hill Water Cure Retreat," *Daily Hampshire Gazette,* May 30, 1848, p. 2.

30. Ibid.

31. *Round Hill Water Cure and Motorpathic Institute, Northampton, Massachusetts* pamphlet, Forbes Library, Northampton, Mass., n.d.

32. Ibid., pp. 3, 4, 5.

33. Ibid., p. 1.

34. See *Water-Cure Journal* 27, no. 3 (March 1858): 38; *Hygienic Teacher and Water-Cure Journal* 34, no. 3 (October 1862): 79. The cost per year had increased to $1.50 by 1865; see *Water-Cure Journal* 4, no. 5 (November 1847): 323.

35. Joel Shew, M.D. "To Cheapen Water-Cure," *Water-Cure Journal* 18, no. 4 (October 1854): 75–76.

36. See *Water-Cure Journal* 2, no. 12 (November 15, 1846): 178; "Topics . . . Dollars and Cents," *Water-Cure Journal* 33, no. 2 (February 1862): 33. Shew tells patients in the *Water-Cure Journal* 9, no. 4 (April 1850): 104–105, to write water-cure physicians for diagnosis and treatment.

37. See "Scrofula," *Water-Cure Journal* 2, no. 12 (November 15, 1846): 178l.

38. See Joel Shew, M.D. "A Word to Water Patients on Household Treatment," *Water-Cure Journal and Herald of Reforms* 9, no. 4 (April 1850): 104–105, esp. p. 105.

39. "Salaries of Professional Men," *Water-Cure Journal* 26, no. 3 (September 1858): 48. The byline at the close of the article is *Life Illustrated.*

40. Ibid.

41. R. T. Trall, "Topics . . . The Contract System vs. Fees," *Herald of Health* 3, no. 2 (February 1864): 61.

42. R. T. Trall, "Topics . . . Medical Fees," *Herald of Health* 3, no. 3 (March 1864): 101–102.

43. J. C. Jackson, "Considerations for Commonfolks—No. 2," *Water-Cure Journal and Herald of Reforms* 9, no. 6 (June 1850): 170. Indicative of his pro-laboring-class sentiment and his commitment to economic accessibility, Jackson had a "$3 Standing Offer to Poor Invalids" to whom he would send 6 copies of *Laws of Life* for one year, plus a Prescription for Home Treatment. In return, the

recipient would send him $3 and the names of six people who would agree to pay the postage on the six papers and read them. This was a value of roughly $10–$12. See *Water-Cure Journal* 31, no. 6 (June 1861): 94.

44. Jackson, "Considerations for Commonfolks," p. 170.

45. Ibid.

46. Putnam, *A Documentary History*, n.p.

47. Ibid.

48. (Elmira) *Sunday Telegram*, July 21, 1946, p. 63.

49. *The Gleason Health Resort* (Syracuse, N. Y.: Mason Press, 1898[?]), p. 20.

50. *The Gleason Health Resort, Elmira, New York*, brochure lent by Georgianna Palmer, dated August 25, 1955, p. 12.

51. William D. Conklin, *The Jackson Health Resort* (Dansville, N.Y.: privately printed, 1971), p. 249.

52. "Easthampton Water-Cure," *Water-Cure Journal* advertisement, n.d.; and Harry B. Weiss and Howard B. Kemble, *The Great American Water-Cure Craze: A History of Hydropathy in the United States* (Trenton, N.J.: Past Times Press, 1967), p. 133

53. "Marking Another Milestone."

54. "Springfield Water Cure," *Springfield City Directory, 1851–52*, pp. 108–109.

58. "Northampton Water Cure," *Daily Hampshire Gazette*, June 8, 1847, p. 3.

56. See *Historical Statistics of the United States, Colonial Times to 1970*, Bicentennial ed., 2 vols. (Washington, D.C.: U.S. Bureau of the Census, 1975); Series D 705–714, "Farm Laborers—Average Monthly Earnings with Board, by Geographic Divisions, 1818–1948," p. 163. Original source: Stanley Lebergott, *Manpower in Economic Growth: The American Record Since 1800*, tables A-23 and A-24, pp. 257ff.

57. *Historical Statistics*, Series E 123–134, "Wholesale Prices of Selected Commodities: 1800 to 1970—Con.," p. 209.

58. Ibid.; Series E 52–63, "Wholesale Price Indexes (Warren and Pearson), by Major Product Groups: 1749 to 1890," p. 201. The list of "all commodities" included farm products, foods, hides and leather products, textile products, fuel and lighting, metals and metal products, building materials, chemicals and drugs, house furnishing goods, spirits, and miscellaneous.

59. Ibid.; Series D 718–721, "Daily Wage Rates on the Erie Canal: 1828 to 1881," p. 164.

60. For example, a farm laborer in New England in 1880 earned (with board) $13.94 per month, or $167 annually. Ibid.; Series D 705–714, "Farm Laborers," p. 163.

61. Ibid., Series E 52–63, "Wholesale Price Indexes," p. 201.

62. Ibid.; Series D 728–734, "Daily Wages of Five Skilled Occupations and of Laborers, in Manufacturing Establishments: 1860–1880," p. 165. Other skilled trades listed here include blacksmiths, carpenters, engineers and machinists.

63. Ibid.; Series D 739–764, "Average Annual Earnings per Full-Time Employee, by Industry: 1900–1970—Con.," p. 167.

64. Ibid.; Series D 913–926, "Military Annual Pay Rates, 1865–1970," p. 176.

65. Rosalyn Baxandall, Linda Gordon, and Susan Reverby, *America's Work-*

ing Women: A Documentary History—1600 to the Present (New York: Vintage, 1976), pp. 41, 406–407.

66. Ibid., p. 55. When comparing male and female wages, they likely paid out proportionate amounts. A man's pay might be spent on housing, food, miscellaneous costs, and support of others. A woman's might be distributed in much the same way, unless housing is provided, and/or monies are sent home to family.

67. Ibid., pp. 55, 56.

68. Ibid., p. 83.

69. Johnson, "An Old-Time Patient," p. 24.

70. George Rosen, *Fees and Fee Bills: Some Economic Aspects of Medical Practice in Nineteenth-Century America* (Baltimore: Johns Hopkins University Press, 1946), pp. 21–22. Rosen provides a clear tabulation of medical costs using account books kept by physicians or patients, and fee bills issued by medical societies.

71. Ibid., pp. 43–45.

72. Ibid., pp. 85–88.

73. R. T. Trall, *Herald of Health* 3, no. 3 (March 1864): 101–102.

74. Rosen, *Fees and Fee Bills*, pp. 85–88.

75. R. T. Trall, *Herald of Health* 3, no. 3 (March 1864): 101–102.

76. Gunther B. Risse, Ronald L. Numbers, and Judith W. Leavitt, *Medicine Without Doctors: Home Health Care in American History* (New York: Science History Publications, 1977), discuss the economic aspects of home health care in nineteenth-century America.

77. E.B.H., "Glen Haven Water Cure," *The Sybil—For Reforms* 3 (November 1, 1858): 450. The letter was addressed to Mrs. Hasbrouck.

78. Ibid.

79. William S. Lawyer, ed., *Binghamton: Its Settlement, Growth and Development and the Factors in Its History 1800–1900* (Binghamton, N.Y.: Century Memorial Publishing, 1900), p. 414.

80. Putnam, *Documentary History*, n.p.

81. Gender consciousness was used in the nineteenth century both to limit and to emancipate women. Here I use the term in the positive sense, meaning that sensitivity and cognizance of gender issues was employed to expand opportunities for and self-definitions of women.

82. Giammichelle and Taylor, "Elmira Water Cure" "Famous Health Resort Here"; "Elmira Famous Health Resort"; and "Dr. S. O. Gleason," Gleason papers.

83. "Mrs. Rachel Brooks Gleason," loose page from Chemung County Historical Society.

84. Gleason, *In Memoriam Rachel Brooks Gleason*, p. 3.

85. "Dr. S. O. Gleason."

86. See Charles E. Rosenberg, "Social Class and Medical Care in Nineteenth-Century America: The Rise and Fall of the Dispensary," in *Sickness and Health in America: Readings in the History of Medicine and Public Health*, ed. Judith Walzer Leavitt and Ronald L. Numbers, (Madison: University of Wisconsin Press, 1978), pp. 157–171.

87. Ibid., pp. 160–161.

88. Ibid., pp. 158–159.

89. Ibid., p. 163.

90. "Elmira Water Cure," p. 63.

91. "History of the Water Cure: Gleason Health Resort Established June 1, 1852," *Sunday Telegram*, June 8, 1947, p. 40.

92. Thomas E. Byrne, "Chemung County 1890–1975: Health Care . . . Bigger and Better," in *Chemung County Historical Society*, (Elmira, N.Y.: Chemung County Historical Society, 1976), p. 459.

93. "Mrs. Rachel Brooks Gleason."

94. Conklin, *Jackson Health Resort*, pp. 282–290.

95. The Dansville Cure's central role in dress-reform activity is evidenced in a *Dansville Herald* June 22, 1859, article reprinted from the Cure's *Letter Box*. Probably written by Harriet Austin, it is forcefully in favor of dress reform and criticizes comments made by the press deriding it as "unsexing" women. A similar piece appeared in the *Dansville Herald*, April 27, 1859. Conklin, *Jackson Health Resort*, pp. 156–168, 136a, 137, discusses the commotion Jackson and women from the cure stirred in the New York papers in March 1868 when they went to hear a Dickens's presentation in reform dress.

96. See Schwarz, *John Harvey Kellogg, M.D.*, p. 24; Weiss and Kemble, *Great American Water-Cure Craze*, chap. 7; and Conklin, *Jackson Health Resort*, pp. 139–141, 153–154. Also instructive is the note from Dr. John H. Kellogg in Battle Creek, Michigan, on the 75th Anniversary Celebration, written to Jackson: "I trust your work is in every way prospering. There are many still here who do not forget that Battle Creek Sanatarium owes its beginning very largely to your work in Dansville" (p. 79).

97. Conklin, *Jackson Health Resort*, pp. 37–38, 313–315.

98. Ibid., p. 22, for further elaboration on the speakers.

99. Ibid., p. 348.

100. Ibid., p. 64.

101. Ibid., pp. 77–78.

102. Lilley B. Caswell, *Athol, Massachusetts, Past and Present* (Athol: Athol Transcript Company, 1899), p. 197; and William Lord, *History of Athol* (Somerville, Mass.: Somerville Printing Company, 1953), esp. "Professional Men," pp. 570–573.

103. See "A Historical Landmark: The Southard House," *Athol Transcript* 50, no. 37 (August 10, 1920): 1; Caswell, *Athol, Massachusetts*, pp. 196–199; J. Clarence Hill, "Dr. Joseph Lord, First of Long Succession of Athol Medicos," *Athol Daily News* 59, no. 16 (October 20, 1949): 10; and *Athol Almanac*, June 1886.

104. *Athol Almanac*, June 1886.

105. Caswell, *Athol, Massachusetts*, pp. 198–199.

109. Obituary for J. H. Hero, *Worcester West Chronicle* 33, no. 4 (January 13, 1898): 4.

107. J. H. Hero, "Errors in Home Practice," *Water-Cure Journal* 20, no. 5 (November 1855): 102. Westboro appears spelled both ways. For a silly and somewhat hostile exchange about the laying capacity of Hero's hens, as reported in the local *Greenfield Republic*, see "Water Cure Hens," *Water-Cure Journal* 13, no. 5 (May 1852): 115.

108. Obituary for J. H. Hero, p. 4.

109. Ibid.

110. Dr. James Oliver, "The Old Doctors of Athol and the Water Cure," *Athol Transcript*, January 3, 1896.

111. *Water-Cure Journal*, volume number unknown, p. 143; For information

on Dr. E. Snell and (his partner) Jasper Severance of the Springfield Water-Cure, see "Marking Another Milestone"; and "Springfield Water Cure," pp. 108–109.

112. "Water-Cure Establishment," *Daily Hampshire Gazette*, October 13, 1846. For information on Dennison's medical experiences in Ireland, see "Round Hill Water Cure Establishment." *Note:* Different sources use two spellings of Dennison's name, *Dennison* is used more frequently than *Denniston*.

113. Hall was described as "one of the most successful medical practitioners in this part of the Commonwealth, as well as a thorough student in all that pertains to his profession." See "Round Hill Water Cure," *Daily Hampshire Gazette*, November 16, 1847, p. 3. Woodward, from his days at the Worcester asylum, advocated water as a sedative therapy among mentally disturbed patients—hydropaths advocated this approach generally.

114. "Round Hill Water Cure Retreat," *Daily Hampshire Gazette*, May 30, 1848, p. 3. This time, Hall is aided by Dr. G. T. Dexter. The ownership had also undergone slight revision: J. A. Cummings and C. A. Hall were now listed as proprietors, as were Clark, of U. S. Hotel, and a newcomer, Alfred Randall.

115. "Dr. E. E. Denniston's Water Cure, At Springdale, Northampton, Mass.," *Daily Hampshire Gazette*, May 30, 1848, p. 3; and Weiss and Kemble, *Great American Water-Cure Craze*, p. 129.

116. "Round Hill Water Cure Retreat," p. 2.

117. Ibid.

118. Untitled, *Daily Hampshire Gazette*, June 26, 1855, p. 2.

119. "Letters from Round Hill—No. 2. Entertainment at the Water-Cure," *Daily Hampshire Gazette*, August 27, 1861, p. 1.

120. M. G. Kellogg, memoir dictated to Clara K. Butler, October 12, 1916; Ellen G. White to Edson and Willie White, February 6, 1873; J. H. Kellogg, "Hygieo-Therapy and Its Founder," p. 92, as quoted in Ronald L. Numbers, *Prophetess of Health: A Study of Ellen G. White* (New York: Harper & Row, 1976), pp. 66–67, 123–124.

121. See Weiss and Kemble, *Great American Water-Cure Craze*, pp. 35–38; *Water-Cure Journal* 31, no. 3 (March 1861): 45; *Herald of Health* 5, no. 5 (May 1865): 131.

122. Numbers, *Prophetess of Health*, notes the dubious value of some hydropathic diplomas. Other sects had similarly discreditable records; see Frederick C. Waite, "The First Medical Diploma Mill in the United States," *Bulletin of the History of Medicine* 20 (November 1946): 495–504.

123. Officers for 1849 were President Shew; and Vice-Presidents Freeman Hunt, Brooklyn, New York; S. O. Gleason, Glenhaven, New York; L. N. Fowler, Denniston, Massachusetts; and Dr. Bedortha, New York. Directors were Trall; C. H. Meeker, New Jersey; E. A. Kittredge, Massachusetts; M. W. Gray, Massachusetts; Dr. R. Wesselhoeft, Vermont; Dr. Philip Roof, New York; and Henry Foster, New York. Secretary was S. R. Wells (of the publishing house), New York. N. Houghton, New York City, served as treasurer and Trall was chairman of directors. See *Water-Cure Journal* 7, no. 5 (June 1849): 186–187. It was decided that directors should collect data of the society; share this information with the public; publish a periodical; hold an open clinic for the poor of New York at least two hours one day per week; give lectures and free advice to the poor, and provide a free ten-part lecture course on hydropathy. See "American Hydropathic Society Constitution," sect. E, ibid., p. 186.

124. Ibid., pp. 186–187.

125. In this second society, Shew was president, Drs. B. Wilmarth and Hubbard Foster, vice-presidents, and Drs. T. L. Nichols and L. Reuben, secretaries. See *Water-Cure Journal* 10, no. 1 (July 1850): 14.

126. See T. L. Nichols, "American Hydropathic Convention," ibid., p. 15.

127. Ibid.

128. See "Proceedings of the American Hygienic And Hydropathic Association," *Water-Cure Journal* 11, no. 6 (June 1851): 137–138.

129. See Weiss and Kemble, *Great American Water-Cure Craze*, pp. 39–40.

130. See *Water-Cure Journal* 3, no. 8 (April 15, 1847): 127; see also Ruggles's obituary, written by Dr. Seth Rogers of the Worcester Water Cure, which appeared in *Water-Cure Journal* 9, no. 2 (February 1850): 54.

131. Putnam, *Documentary History*, vol. 1, n.p.

132. *Sunday Telegram*, July 21, 1946, p. 63, quoted from Brigham, *Elmira Directory, 1863–1864*.

133. "Elmira Water Cure," *Sunday Telegram*, August 31, 1952, p. 63, quoted from *Elmira Weekly Gazette Supplement of 1873*.

134. Ibid.

135. Mrs. R. B. Gleason, M.D., *Hints to Patients*, 1889, pamphlet from the Chemung County Historical Society, p. 4.

136. The S. Weir Mitchell Rest Cure has, retrospectively, attained notoriety. Ann Douglas Wood's interpretive essay "The Fashionable Diseases: Women's Complaints and Their Treatment in Nineteenth-Century America," *Journal of Interdisciplinary History* 4, no. 1 (Summer 1973): 25–52, criticizes Mitchell's cure for its paternalistically based and physically passive program, which, she argues, embodied the height of therapy-turned-social-moralism and control. Ehrenreich and English, *For Her Own Good*, pp. 131–133, argue similarly. Regina Markell Morantz, in "The Perils of Feminist History," *Journal of Interdisciplinary History* 4, no. 4 (Spring 1974): 649–660, contends that Mitchell's rationale and hence justifiability have been distorted.

137. *Gleason Health Resort*, p. 9; and "Sixtieth Year of Gleason Health Resort."

138. "Sixtieth Year of Gleason Health Resort," p. 2.

139. Conklin, *Jackson Health Resort*, p. 144, as quoted from a letter by James C. Jackson to A. O. Bunnell, published in the *Dansville Advertiser*, September 7, 1876.

140. "Easthampton Water Cure," *Water-Cure Journal*. no vol., no date, p. 143; and Weiss and Kemble, *Great American Water-Cure Craze*, p. 133.

141. "Springfield Water Cure," pp. 108–109.

142. "Round Hill Water Cure Retreat," p. 3.

143. Ibid., p. 2.

144. *Round Hill Water-Cure and Motorpathic Institute*, p. 3.

145. Ibid., p. 2.

Chapter Four

1. *Water-Cure Journal* 11, no. 2 (February 1851): 45.

2. *Water-Cure Journal*, Frontispiece opposite Index to vol. 31, 1861.

3. Richard H. Shryock, "Sylvester Graham and the Popular Health Movement, 1830–1870," *Mississippi Valley Historical Review* 18, no. 2 (1932): 174.

4. See Stephen Nissenbaum, *Sex, Diet, and Debility in Jacksonian America: Sylvester Graham and Health Reform* (Westport, Conn.: Greenwood Press, 1980), chap. 7.

5. See Sylvester Graham, "Fruits and Vegetables," *Water-Cure Journal* 11, no. 2 (February 1851): 37–39; "American Vegetarian Society," *Water-Cure Journal* 10, no. 1 (July 1850): 6 (Graham was one of several vice-presidents); and *Water-Cure Journal* 12, no. 5 (November 1851): 110–111, which contains Trall's obituary for Graham.

6. C. R. Jones, "Orson Squire Fowler, Practical Phrenologist," *Old-Time New England* 57, no. 4 (1967): 103. Fowler's belief in water cure came through personal experience—first a bruised finger, then heart trouble (p. 109). Also see Elizabeth Shafer, "Phrenology's Golden Years," *American History Illustrated* 8, no. 10 (February 1974): 36–43; Harry B. Weiss and Howard R. Kemble, *The Great American Water-Cure Craze: A History of Hydropathy in the United States* (Trenton, N.J.: Past Times Press, 1967), pp. 26, 36; and O. S. Fowler, "Hereditary Descent: Its Laws and Facts," *American Phrenological Journal* 5, nos. 9, 10, 11, 12(1843).

7. Shryock, "Sylvester Graham," pp. 175–176.

8. Mary Sargeant (Neal) Gove Nichols, *Mary Lyndon: or, Revelations of a Life: An Autobiography* (New York, 1855); John B. Blake, "Nichols, Mary Sargeant Neal Gove," in *Notable American Women 1607–1950: A Biographical Dictionary*, vol. 2, ed. James Boyer (Cambridge: Belknap Press of Harvard University Press, 1971), pp. 627–629; John B. Blake, "Mary Gove Nichols, Prophetess of Health," in *Women and Health in America*, ed. Judith Walzer Leavitt (Madison: University of Wisconsin Press, 1984), pp. 359–375.

9. Blake, "Nichols," p. 627; and Blake, "Mary Gove Nichols," p. 360. See also Chapter One.

10. Blake, "Mary Gove Nichols," p. 360.

11. Blake, "Nichols," p. 627; and Blake, "Mary Gove Nichols," p. 362. See also Chapter Two.

12. Blake,"Nichols," pp. 627–628; Blake, "Mary Gove Nichols," pp. 361–362; and Gove Nichols, *Mary Lyndon.*

13. "Mrs. Mary S. Gove," *Water-Cure Journal* 2,no. 1 (June 1846): 16; and Blake, "Mary Gove Nichols," p. 363.

14. Mary S. Gove Nichols, *Experience in Water-Cure* (New York: Fowler and Wells, 1850), p. iii.

15. See Mary Gove Nichols, "Errors in Water-Cure," *Water-Cure Journal* 10, no. 4 (October 1850): 156–157; "Maternity; and the Water-Cure of Infants," *Water-Cure Journal* 11, no. 3 (March 1851): 57–59; "The New Costume," *Water-Cure Journal* 12, no. 2 (August 1851): 20; "A Lecture on Woman's Dress," *Water-Cure Journal* 12,no. 2 (August 1851): 34–36; "Woman the Physician," *Water-Cure Journal* 12, no. 4 (October 1851): 73–75; "Letter from Mrs. Gove," *Water-Cure Journal* 14, no. 5 (November 1852): 112; and "Letter from Mrs. Gove Nichols," *Water-Cure Journal* 15, no. 1 (January 1853): 10–11.

16. See Gove Nichols, *Mary Lyndon;* Blake, "Mary Gove Nichols," p. 370; and Blake, "Nichols."

17. Blake, "Nichols," p. 68.

18. Blake, "Mary Gove Nichols," p. 365.

19. See T. L. Nichols, "A Position Defined, on Reasons for Becoming a

Water-Cure Physician," *Water-Cure Journal* 9, no. 4 (April 1850): 100–103; and T. L. Nichols, M.D., "Human Physiology the True Basis of Reform," *Water-Cure Journal* 13, no. 1 (January 1852): 1–5. See also "Illustrations of Physiology," *Water-Cure Journal* 13, nos. 2 through 5 (February–June 1852): n.p. Other articles by T. L. Nichols on physiology appeared in September, October, and November 1852.

20. Nichols, "A Position Defined," p. 102.

21. See "American Hydropathic Convention," *Water-Cure Journal* 10, no. 1 (July 1850): 14; and "American Vegetarian Society," *Water-Cure Journal* 10, no. 1 (July 1850): 6.

22. See T. L. Nichols, M.D. "Medical Education. The American Hydropathic Institute," *Water-Cure Journal* 12, no. 3 (September 1851): 65–66; and *Water-Cure Journal* 12, no. 5 (November 1851): 114, which announces the first term of the American Hydropathic Institute and its course of study.

23. Also, according to an advertisement in the Journal, Nichols opened an office at 45 White Street in New York City. See *Water-Cure Journal* 13, no. 6 (June 1852): 136.

24. While Thomas argued theoretically for changed social relations, Mary did counsel adultery if the conditions of the "true marriage" (e.g., love and mutual attraction) were present for the potential adulterers. See Blake, "Mary Gove Nichols," p. 368.

25. Harry B. Weiss and Howard R. Kemble, *Great American Water-Cure Craze*. See, especially, "The Water-Cure Giants, Doctors Shew, Nichols and Trall," pp. 74–77, esp. p. 77; originally appeared in *The New York Daily Tribune*, August 10, 1854.

26. Ibid., pp. 74–76.

27. Ibid., p. 78.

28. Ibid., p. 79; also see Blake, "Mary Gove Nichols," pp. 370–371, for information on the Nicholses' activities, both in health reform and Mary's literary efforts while in England. In 1867 they opened a water-cure house in Malvern, England, where they treated patients and taught pupils, and where Thomas established a new journal, the *Herald of Health*.

29. "The Pioneers of Health Reform," *Herald of Health* 5, no. 1 (January 1865): 17; Richard W. Schwarz, *John Harvey Kellogg, M.D.* (Nashville, Tenn.: Southern Publishing Association, 1970), pp. 22–23; and Weiss and Kemble, *Great American Water-Cure Craze*, chap. 7 and pp. 25–28. The journal's name became *Hygienic Teacher and Water-Cure Journal* in 1862.

30. See "Water-Cure in the City of New York," *Water-Cure Journal*, November 15, 1845, n.p.; and Shew's "Syosset Announcement," *Water-Cure Journal* 3, no. 7 (April 1, 1847): 112. Shew's contributions are discussed throughout this text.

31. See R. T. Trall, M.D. "Notes on Professional Travel," *Water-Cure Journal* 30, no. 5 (November 1860): 65–67.

32. See *Herald of Health* 4, no. 4 (October 1864): 113–116.

33. See *Water-Cure Journal* 21, no. 1 (January 1856): 4–5, wherein Trall describes the electrochemical baths he sanctions, with reservations. This is followed immediately by an article, "Water, *the* Remedy," in which Trall removes any doubts of a significant shift in therapeutic philosophy.

34. R. T. Trall, *Sexual Physiology: A Scientific and Popular Exposition of the Fundamental Problems in Sociology* (London: Health Promotion, 1861), Frontispiece; Schwarz, *John Harvey Kellogg, M.D.*, pp. 23–24; "Russell T. Trall. Portrait,

Character, and Biography. Phrenological Character," *Herald of Health*, 4, no. 1 (July 1864): 2; and Weiss and Kemble, *Great American Water-Cure Craze*, chap. 7.

35. For an excellent source on Jackson, Austin, and Our Home, see William Conklin, *The Jackson Health Resort* (Dansville, N.Y.: privately printed, 1971), available only at the Dansville Public Library.

36. See Harriet N. Austin, "To My Sick Sisters," *Water-Cure Journal* 17, no. 4 (April 1854): 75; "Woman's Present and Future," *Water-Cure Journal* 16, no. 3 (September 1853): 57; "Reform Dress," *Water-Cure Journal* 23, no. 1 (January 1857): 3–4; "Thoughts In Spare Minutes," *Water-Cure Journal* 23, no. 2 (February 1857): 28–29, wherein she expresses her "pro-dancing" views; "Thoughts In Spare Minutes," *Water-Cure Journal* 23, no. 5 (May 1857): 103–105, re women's rights via the duty to maintain health; and "For The Girls," *Water-Cure Journal* 29, no. 1 (January 1860): 5–6, an argument in favor of outdoor exercise in winter for girls.

37. Gerald Carson, *Cornflake Crusade* (New York: Rinehart & Company, 1957), p. 68; and Conklin, *Jackson Health Resort*.

38. Carson, *Cornflake Crusade*, pp. 68–70; and Conklin, *Jackson Health Resort*.

39. See Carson, *Cornflake Crusade*, pp. 71–83; Schwarz, *John Harvey Kellogg, M.D.*, pp. 24–25; Ronald L. Numbers, *Prophetess of Health: A Study of Ellen G. White* (New York: Harper & Row, 1976). Ronald L. Numbers and Rennie B. Schoepflin, "Ministries of Healing: Mary Baker Eddy, Ellen G. White, and the Religion of Health," in *Women and Health in America*, ed. Judith Walzer Leavitt (Madison: University of Wisconsin Press, 1984), pp. 376–389, point out that White's Adventist medical workers "helped to transform sectarian hydropathy into the hydrotherapy of scientific medicine" (pp. 387–388).

40. Numbers, *Prophetess of Health*, p. 101.

41. Ibid., pp. 110–111.

42. Ibid., p. 118. Kellogg's influence at the WHRI lasted four years until friction between Kellogg and Elder James White resulted in a "vision" that sanctioned (1878) a Medical and Surgical Sanitorium under Kellogg's direction.

43. Schwarz, *John Harvey Kellogg, M.D.*, pp. 51, 57–58.

44. Carson, *Cornflake Crusade*, pp. 107–108, 116–128. These were shipped to Canada, New Zealand, India, and Persia as well as used domestically.

45. Ibid., pp. 116–128, 143, 145–146. Kellogg maintained sole possession of the sanitorium with no legal battles; not until after their expulsion did the Kellogg brothers start the Battle Creek Toasted Corn Flake Company.

46. Numbers, *Prophetess of Health*, pp. 200–201.

47. See Dio Lewis, M.D., *Our Girls* (New York: Harper & Brothers, 1871); Joan Paul, "The Health Reformers: George Barker Winship: Boston's Strength Seekers," *Journal of Sport History* 10, no. 3 (Winter 1983): 41–57; and John R. Betts, "Mind and Body in Early American Thought," *Journal of American History* 54 (March 1968): 787–805.

48. T. Antiseli, M.D., "Physical Education. No. IV," *Water-Cure Journal* 2, no. 5 (May 1851): n.p.; R. T. Trall, M.D., "Family Gymnastics," *Water-Cure Journal* 22, no. 1 (July 1856): 1–3; W. T. Vail, M.D., "Exercise as a Remedial Measure," *Water-Cure Journal* 23, no. 5 (May 1857): 104.

49. See Charles F. Taylor, M.D., "Kinesipathy, or the Movement Cure," *Water-Cure Journal* 23, no. 3 (March 1857): 53; George H. Taylor, M.D., "The

Movement Cure," *Water-Cure Journal* 27, no. 5 (May 1859): 65–66; and Charles F. Taylor, M.D. "The Cure of Spinal Disorders by 'Movements,'" *Water-Cure Journal* 23, no. 5 (May 1857): 51.

Brian Inglis, in "Osteopathy and Chiropractic," *Fringe Medicine*, 1964, pp. 94–122, discusses the best-known bone-manipulation cures and Andres Taylor Still, the founder of American osteopathy, who mistrusted hydropathy, homeopathy, massage, and exercises because he felt the body ought to be able to take care of itself without their assistance (p. 100).

50. See Dr. William A. Alcott, "Cold Water Facts," *Water-Cure Journal* 1, no. 2 (December 1845): 21–22; Sylvester Graham, *Science of Human Life*, reprinted as "Bathing, Air, and Clothing," *Water-Cure Journal* 3, no. 1 (June 1, 1847): n.p.; Sylvester Graham, "Fruits and Vegetables," *Water-Cure Journal* 2, no. 2 (February 1851): 37–39; and W. A. Alcott, "Vegetarian Travelling," *Water-Cure Journal* 21, no. 5 (May 1856): 74.

51. R. T. Trall, M.D., "Biographical Sketch of Sylvester Graham," *Water-Cure Journal* 12, no. 6 (November 1851): 110. Also see the obituary for William A. Alcott, *Water-Cure Journal* 27, no. 5 (May 1859): 74.

52. See James C. Whorton, "'Tempest in a Flesh-Pot'; The Formulation of a Physiological Rationale for Vegetarianism," in *Sickness and Health in America: Readings in the History of Medicine and Public Health*, ed. Judith Walzer Leavitt and Ronald L. Numbers (Madison: University of Wisconsin Press, 1978), pp. 315–330, 327, esp. pp. 318–319.

53. See *Water-Cure Journal* 1, no. 6 (February 15, 1846): 88–90 (apples); *Water-Cure Journal* 1, no. 7 (March 1, 1846): 100 (Indian pudding); *Water-Cure Journal* 2, no. 7 (September 1, 1846): 107 (loafbread); *Water-Cure Journal* 2, no. 11 (November 1, 1846): n.p. (fruits); and *Water-Cure Journal* 7, no. 3 (March 1849): n.p. (potatoes as cure/preventive for scurvy).

54. See R. T. Trall, M.D., "Hydropathic Recipes," *Water-Cure Journal* 10, no. 4 (October 1850): 158–159; and "Domestic Recipes," *Herald of Health* 9, no. 3 (March 1867): 144.

55. Trall, "Hydropathic Recipes," p. 158.

56. See Dr. Andrew W. Combe, "The Physiology of Digestion," *Water-Cure Journal* 9, no. 3 (March 1850): 80; "Thorough Mastication," *Hygienic Teacher and Water-Cure Journal* 34, no. 5 (November 1862): 109–110; and "A Great National Reform," *Water-Cure Journal* 10, no. 5 (November 1850): 196.

57. Combe, "Physiology of Digestion," p. 80.

58. "A Great National Reform," *Water-Cure Journal* 10, no. 5 (November 1850): 198.

59. See R. T. Trall, M.D., "Topics of the Month. Contagious Diseases," *Water-Cure Journal* 29, no. 5 (May 1860): n.p.; J. H. Hanaford, "Vegetarianism," and S. M. Hobbs, "Diseased Meat," *Water-Cure Journal* 10, no. 2 (1850): 50.

60. See Whorton, "'Tempest in a Flesh-Pot.'"

61. T. L. Nichols, M.D., "American Vegetarian Convention," *Water-Cure Journal* 10, no. 1 (July 1850): 6.

62. Ibid., p. 5.

63. Ibid., p. 6.

64. See "Announcement of the 3rd Annual Meeting of the American Vegetarian Society in Philadelphia," *Water-Cure Journal* 12, no. 4 (October 1851): 89.

65. "Constitution of New York Vegetarian Society," *Water-Cure Journal* 14, no. 4 (November 1852): 118.

66. "Dietetic Reform Association," *Hygienic Teacher and Water-Cure Journal* 33, no. 2 (February 1862): 41–42. Whether this is the same or a different society from his earlier affiliation is unclear.

67. Carson, *Cornflake Crusade*, p. 19.

68. "Coffee as Narcotic or Poison," *Water-Cure Journal* 2, no. 9 (October 1, 1846): n.p.; "Palpitations of the Heart—Tea, Coffee and Tobacco," *Water-Cure Journal* 6, no. 1 (July 1848): 11.

69. William A. Alcott, "Effects of Coffee and Tea on Human Health," *Water-Cure Journal* 12, no. 5 (November 1851): 106–108.

70. "Tea and Coffee," *Water-Cure Journal* 28, no. 4 (October 1859): 64.

71. "Effects of Tobacco upon the Nerves," *Water-Cure Journal* 2, no. 9 (October 1, 1846): n.p.; "Tobacco; Its Action upon the Health, and Its Influences upon the Morals and Intelligence of Man," *Water-Cure Journal* 8, no. 7 (December 1849): 161–164; Thomas Laycock, "On the Diseases Resulting from the Immoderate Use of Tobacco," *Water-Cure Journal* 4, no. 1 (July 1, 1847): 216 (reprinted from the *London Medical Gazette*).

72. Laycock, "On Diseases Resulting," p. 216.

73. William Lloyd Garrison, "Anti-Tobacco Society," *Herald of Health and Journal of Physical Culture* 6, no. 2 (August 1865): 48.

74. "Petition," *Water-Cure Journal* 17, no. 1 (January 1854): 18.

75. *Water-Cure Journal* 10, no. 6 (December 1850): 245.

76. Trall was quoted in the Reverend William White Williams, "The Medical Abuses of Alcohol," *Herald of Health and Journal of Physical Culture* 6, no. 4 (October 1865): 117.

77. By the Editor, "Beecher in a Muddle," *Herald of Health and Journal of Physical Culture* 5, no. 4 (April 1865): 87–89.

78. "The Editorial Department, Topics. Horace Greeley Mistaken," *Herald of Health and Journal of Physical Culture* 10, no. 3 (September 1867): 129–130.

79. By the Editor, "A Muddled Muddlement," *Herald of Health and Journal of Physical Culture* 6, no. 5 (November 1865): 137.

80. "Topics. Drunkenness among Women," *Herald of Health and Journal of Physical Culture* 9, no. 1 (January 1867): 33–34.

81. See William F. Bynum, "Chronic Alcoholism in the First Half of the Nineteenth Century," in *Bulletin of the History of Medicine*, vol. 42 (Baltimore: Johns Hopkins University Press, 1968), pp. 160–185.

82. See Sarah Stage, *Female Complaints: Lydia Pinkham and the Business of Women's Medicine* (New York: Norton, 1979), p. 32; and Sarah Stage, "The Woman Behind the Trademark," in Leavitt, ed., *Women and Health in America*, pp. 255–269.

83. Stage, *Female Complaints*, p. 32.

84. Ibid., p. 167.

85. Ibid., p. 62. Hydropathists were not alone in their beliefs. Benjamin Rush, the prominent Philadelphia physician, was a vocal opponent of the steady consumption of alcohol and urged the use of "cold showers" in treating alcoholics. See Bynum, "Chronic Alcoholism," pp. 167–168. Other prominent allopathic physicians spoke against hard liquor but were in favor of beer and wine for "anyone who had a tendency to drink stronger alcoholic beverages to excess" (p. 174).

86. See "Drug Department: Hypodermic Syringes," *1897 Sears Roebuck Catalogue* (New York: Chelsea House, 1976). Reprinted from the 1897 original.

87. "Letter from Mrs. Spencer," *Water-Cure Journal* 1, no. 12 (May 15, 1846): 181.

88. H.C.F., "Water-Cure and the Temperance Reform versus Drugs, Tobacco, and Liquors," *Water-Cure Journal* 16, no. 4 (October 1853): 77.

89. Ibid.

90. The drawing can be found in the *Water-Cure Journal* 20, no. 3 (September 1855): 64; the ad for Trall's *Alcoholic Controversy* appeared in the *Water-Cure Journal* 21, no. 1 (January 1856): n.p.; "Temperance—What Is It?" *Herald of Health* 3, no. 4 (April 1864): 131; "National Temperance Convention," *Herald of Health and Journal of Physical Culture* 6, no. 1 (July 1865): 10–11; "Topics. re: Temperance Convention in Saratoga Springs of August 1," *Herald of Health and Journal of Physical Culture* 6, no. 3 (September 1865): 81; and L. N. Fowler, "How to Live; or, Temperance in a Nutshell," *Herald of Health and Journal of Physical Culture* 10, no. 5 (November 1867): 209–216.

91. See *Herald of Health* 3, no. 1 (January 1864): 21.

92. Ibid.

93. *Water-Cure Journal* 32, no. 1 (July 1861): 9.

94. *Water-Cure Journal* 33, no. 1 (January 1862): 1; *Water-Cure Journal* 33, no. 3 (March 1862): 57.

95. See "Soldiers' Department," *Herald of Health* 3, no. 2 (February 1864): 66–68; 3, no. 4 (April 1864): 149–151; 4, no. 2 (August 1864): 66–67; 4, no. 3 (September 1864): 104–105.

96. Noggs, "Gossip from Boston," *Water-Cure Journal* 10, no. 3 (September 1850): 124.

97. Paula Baker, "The Domestication of Politics: Women and American Political Society, 1780–1920," *American Historical Review* 89, no. 3 (June 1984): 620–647, argues that only by expanding our definition of politics to include women's *informal* voluntary action can we fully understand the complex nature of political life in nineteenth-century America.

98. Nancy F. Cott, *The Bonds of Womanhood* (New Haven: Yale University Press, 1977), pp. 197–198.

99. Mrs. R. B. Gleason, "Woman's Dress," *Water-Cure Journal* 11, no. 2 (February 1851): n.p.

100. Dr. W. E. Coale, "Woman's Dress, a Cause of Uterine Displacements," *Water-Cure Journal* 12, no. 5 (November 1851): 105–106; "Dress Reform. A Short Piece on Long Skirts," *Water-Cure Journal* 18, no. 2 (August 1854): 34; D. W. Ranney, M.D., "Tight Lacing," *Water-Cure Journal* 19, no. 3 (March 1855): 53–54; Madame Demorest, "Dress and Its Relation to Health," *Herald of Health and Journal of Physical Culture* 9, no. 1 (January 1867): 16; and M. L. Holbrook, M.D., "General Topics of the Month. Drunkenness among Women," *Herald of Health and Journal of Physical Culture* 9, no. 1 (January 1867): 33–34.

101. See "The American and French Fashions," *Water-Cure Journal* 12, no. 4 (October 1851): 96; the Hungarian bloomers appear in the *Water-Cure Journal* 13, no. 3 (March 1852): 67; "The Rocky Mountain Bloomers," *Water-Cure Journal* 13, no. 1 (January 1852): 19; Mary B. Williams, "The Bloomer and Webber Dresses. A Glance at Their Respective Merits and Advantages," *Water-Cure Journal* 12, no. 2 (August 1851): 33; and the Water-Cure bloomer appears in the *Water-Cure Journal* 16, no. 5 (November 1853): 120.

102. See Mrs. M. S. Gove Nichols, "A Lecture on Woman's Dress," *Water-Cure Journal* 12, no. 2 (August 1851): 34–36, drawing on p. 36. Regina Morantz,

"Nineteenth Century Health Reform and Women: A Program of Self-Help," in *Medicine Without Doctors: Home Health Care in American History,* ed. Guenter B. Risse, Ronald L. Numbers, and Judith Walzer Leavitt (New York: Science History Publications, 1977), pp. 82–85, also notes the persuasive impact of this particular graphic.

103. "The Fashionable Lady's Prayer," *Water-Cure Journal* 4, no. 6 (December 1846): 351. Reprinted from *Watchman of the Valley.*

104. A.S.A., "The Victim," *Water-Cure Journal* 15, no. 1 (January 1853): 16.

105. Mattie, "A Parody," *Water-Cure Journal* 15, no. 6 (June 1853): 132.

106. "Success to the Bloomers," *Water-Cure Journal* 15, no. 2 (February 1853): 40.

107. Theodosia Gilbert, "An Eye Sore," *Water-Cure Journal* 11, no. 5 (May 1851): 117.

108. Ibid.

109. M. S. Gove Nichols, "A Word to Water-Cure People," *Water-Cure Journal* 13, no. 1 (January 1852): 8.

110. A report on Jackson's 1856 speech at the National Dress Reform Convention appeared in the *Water-Cure Journal* 22, no. 2 (August 1856): 39–41. Austin's speech was reported in the "National Health Convention," in *The Sibyl—For Reforms,* vol. 4, ed. Lydia Sayer Hasbrouk (Middletown, N.Y.: January 1, 1860) pp. 676–677. Trall and J. C. Jackson were also present at the 1859 convention and spoke on related topics.

111. See *Herald of Health and Journal of Physical Culture* 3, no. 2 (February 1864): n.p.

112. Clara, "Dress Reform and Water-Cure," *Water-Cure Journal* 16, no. 5 (November 1853): 107.

113. "Dress Reform. A Southerner's Impressions," *Water-Cure Journal* 17, no. 2 (February 1854): 36.

114. "Bloomerism in New York," *Water-Cure Journal* 15, no. 5 (May 1853): 110.

115. Julia Kellogg, "Bloomers; or, Is It a Duty to Wear the New Costume?" *Water-Cure Journal* 15, no. 2 (February 1853): 34.

116. Mrs. E. Potter, "Dress Reform. Is It Duty?" *Water-Cure Journal* 15, no. 4 (April 1853): 82–83.

117. Mary V. W. Radcliff, "Dress Reform Difficulties," *The Sibyl—For Reforms* 4 (February 1, 1860): 693. Dr. Lydia Sayer Hasbrouck was the editor of this periodical published in Middletown, N.Y.

118. Mary S. Gove Nichols, "The New Costume, and Some Other Matters," *Water-Cure Journal* 12, no. 2 (August 1851): 30.

119. Ibid.

120. Mary S. Gove Nichols, "A Lecture on Woman's Dresses," *Water-Cure Journal* 12, no. 2 (August 1851): 36.

121. "Another Female Gentleman," *Herald of Health* 4, no. 5 (November 1864): 163. This item originally appeared in the *New York Evening Post.* The journal's refutation was a response to the *Post* article—no explanation was given as to how this confusion began or was resolved.

122. "An Autobiography, Chapter III," *Water-Cure Journal* 11, no. 2 (February 1851): 27.

123. Harriet N. Austin, "Thoughts in Spare Minutes," *Water-Cure Journal* 23, no. 5 (May 1857): 103. For a less sympathetic analysis of women's com-

placency and complicity with their limited role, see S. S. Socwell, "Women's Rights," *Water-Cure Journal* 32, no. 3 (September 1861): 61.

124. See *Water-Cure Journal* 15, no. 3 (March 1853): 69.

125. See *Water-Cure Journal* 15, no. 2 (February 1853): 45.

126. See *Water-Cure Journal* 13, no. 3 (March 1852): 69.

127. "Women Inventors," *Water-Cure Journal* 19, no. 6 (June 1855): 144.

128. See *Water-Cure Journal* 3, no. 10 (May 15, 1847): 159.

129. Harriet Austin, "Letter No. 2," *Water-Cure Journal* 25, no. 2 (February 1858): 19–20.

130. L. H. Bigarel, "Working Girls," *Herald of Health* 3, no. 1 (January 1864): 13.

131. M. L. Holbrook, M.D., "Topics of the Month. Working Women," *Herald of Health* 4, no. 5 (November 1864): 161.

132. R. T. Trall, "Woman as Farmer," *Herald of Health* 3, no. 3 (March 1864): 81–82, esp. p. 82.

133. Ibid.

134. Ibid.

135. Delos Dunton, "Items from 'Home of the Free,'" *Herald of Health* 3, no. 6 (June 1864): 213–214.

136. M.T.C., "A Farm for Women," *Herald of Health* 4, no. 6 (December 1864): 206.

137. "A Misfortune to Be a Woman!" *Herald of Health* 4, no. 6 (December 1864): 190.

138. Ibid., p. 191.

139. Janet Golden, "Our Bodies Our History," *Women's Review of Books* 2, no. 1 (October 1984): 18, a review of *Women and Health in America*, ed. Judith Walker Leavitt (Madison: University of Wisconsin Press, 1984).

140. "Matrimonial Correspondence," letter No. 19, *Water-Cure Journal* 17, no. 3 (March 1854): 60. Morantz, "Nineteenth Century Health Reform," pp. 87–88, discusses the journal's "Matrimonial Correspondence."

141. "Matrimonial Correspondence," letter No. 24, *Water-Cure Journal* 17, no. 3 (March 1854): 60.

142. See *Water-Cure Journal* 17, no. 6 (June 1854): n.p.

143. "Matrimony. No. 2, Irene of Massachusetts," *Water-Cure Journal* 18, no. 1 (July 1854): 17.

144. "Matrimony. No. 14," *Water-Cure Journal* 18, no. 2 (August 1854): 41.

145. "Matrimony. No. 30," *Water-Cure Journal* 18, no. 4 (October 1854): 88.

146. "Matrimony," *Water-Cure Journal* 18, no. 6 (December 1854): 134.

147. "Matrimony," *Water-Cure Journal* 19, no. 5 (May 1855): 133; and "Matrimony," *Water-Cure Journal* 21, no. 4 (April 1856): 95.

148. "Matrimony," *Water-Cure Journal* 22, no. 3 (September 1856): 71.

149. "A Wedding on Hydropathic Principles," *Water-Cure Journal* 24, no. 5 (November 1857): 107.

Chapter Five

1. Conceptualized in a 1975 path-breaking article, this "Female World of Love and Ritual" revealed an all-encompassing homosocial network that fulfilled

many of the Victorian woman's emotional/romantic and sensual needs. Characterized as relationships in which women could share sorrows, anxieties, and joys and develop inner security and self-esteem, these bonds endured for a lifetime. This female world was, essentially, a positive women's culture in which male influence was minimal and female nurturance supreme. See Carroll Smith-Rosenberg, "The Female World of Love and Ritual," *Signs* 1, no. 1 (Autumn 1975): 1–29.

2. *Sunday Telegram*, July 21, 1946, p. 63, as quoted from Brigham, *Elmira Directory for 1863–1864*. The majority of the establishments specifically advertised their interest and facilities aimed at helping the sufferers of women's diseases. See "Communication from Mrs. R. B. Gleason of the Elmira Water Cure: Symptoms of Pelvic Displacement, and Their Treatment" (this information was communicated to Catharine Beecher at her request) in *Letters to the People on Health and Happiness* (New York: Harper & Bros., 1855), pp. 7–15; Mrs. R. B. Gleason, M.D., *Hints to Patients*, pamphlet (29 pp.), Chemung County Historical Society, 1889: "Ladies are under the care of DR. RACHEL B. GLEASON and her Daughter, DR. ADELE A. GLEASON. The former has had forty years experience in treating diseases peculiar to women. The latter gives also special attention to Disease of the Eye" (pp. 3–4); Mrs. R. B. Gleason, M.D., *Talks to My Patients; a Valuable Home Book for Women: Hints on Getting Well and Keeping Well*, advertised in *Herald of Health*, July 1873, p. 44; Zippie Brooks Wales, M.D., "Nursing," *Herald of Health* 22, no. 1 (July 1873): 17–19; *Round Hill Water-Cure and Motorpathic Institute, Northampton, Mass.*, pamphlet (5 pp.), Forbes Library, Northampton, Mass. n.d.: "He [Halsted] continues to pay particular attention to WOMAN'S Diseases and Weaknesses" (p. 3); and the reader is referred to Chapter Three, note 4, which lists the cures and their advertisements, many of which refer specifically to their treatment of women's diseases.

3. Kathryn Kish Sklar, "All Hail to Pure Cold Water," in *Women and Health in America*, ed. Judith Walzer Leavitt (Madison: University of Wisconsin Press, 1984) pp. 246–254, identifies and elaborates on these unique features of water-cure establishments.

4. Ibid.

5. Ibid., p. 248.

6. Ibid., p. 251; and H. B. Weiss and H. R. Kemble, "The Forgotten Water-Cures of Brattleboro, Vermont," *Vermont History* 37 (Summer 1969): 165–176.

7. Forrest Wilson, *Crusader in Crinoline: The Life of Harriet Beecher Stowe* (Philadelphia: Lippincott, 1941), pp. 219–220.

8. Ibid., p. 221.

9. Ibid., p. 223.

10. Ibid.

11. Ibid., pp. 220–222, esp. 224.

12. Ibid., p. 228; Also see Edmund Wilson, *Patriotic Gore* (New York: Farrar, Straus and Giroux, 1962), pp 17–28.

13. Johanna Johnston, *Runaway to Heaven: The Story of Harriet Beecher Stowe* (Garden City, N.Y.: Doubleday 1963), p. 170; and Mrs. R. B. Gleason, *Hints to Patients*, pamphlet, Chemung County Historical Society, 1889, pp. 19–23. Although Harriet Beecher Stowe was not at the Elmira Cure, the list of activities between the two is somewhat similar.

14. See Harriet Beecher Stowe, "Our Houses—What Is Required to Make

Them Healthful," *Herald of Health* 6, no. 4 (October 1865): 109–111, esp. p. 111. [Extracted from the *Atlantic Monthly*.]

15. Ibid.

16. Catharine Beecher and Harriet Beecher Stowe, *An American Woman's Home: Or Principles of Domestic Service* (New York: 1869; reprint ed., New York, 1971), p. 36.

17. See "Fading Beauty of American Women," *Water-Cure Journal* 18, no. 6 (December 1854): 126, wherein mention is made of Stowe's recently published "Sunny Memories of Foreign Lands," which describes the sedentary ways and the eating habits of American women.

18. See William D. Conklin, *The Jackson Health Resort* (Dansville, N.Y.: privately printed, 1971).

19. T. L. Nichols, "Diseases of Women," *Water-Cure Journal* 11, no. 5 (May 1851): 122–124.

20. Sklar, "All Hail to Pure Cold Water," p. 252.

21. T. L. Nichols, "The Curse Removed: A Statement of Facts Respecting the Efficacy of Water-Cure in the Treatment of Uterine Diseases, and the Removal of the Pains and Perils of Pregnancy and Childbirth," *Water-Cure Journal* 10, no. 5 (November 1850): 171. Also see "Vaginal Injections," *Water-Cure Journal* 10, no. 6 (December 1850): 219.

22. Audre Lorde, *Uses of the Erotic: The Erotic as Power* (New York: Out and Out Books, 1978), argues that eroticism has been used against women to belittle them. By acknowledging the existence of and being in touch with the erotic, women become less willing to accept powerlessness, resignation, despair, self-effacement, depression and self-denial (p. 7).

23. Dr. Richard von Krafft-Ebing, *Psychopathia Sexualis* (New York: Putnam, 1965; originally published in Stuttgart, Germany, in 1882). Krafft-Ebing viewed sex between women as a result of "constitutional hypersexuality" (see pp. 22–23); later, as a result of "cerebral anomalies," that constituted a "taint." See Lillian Faderman, *Surpassing the Love of Men: Romantic Friendship and Love between Women from the Renaissance to the Present* (New York: Morrow, 1981), pp. 241 and 453n. He, along with other early sexologists, had a profoundly negative affect on labeling homoerotic love as illness and upon women's consequent self-perceptions (to be discussed more fully in the conclusion). See pp. 239–254, esp. pp. 241, 244, 248, 252, 291, 300, 314–317. Illness labeling aside, his case reports on lesbian activity are instructive as behavioral evidence.

24. Krafft-Ebing, *Psychopathia Sexualis*, pp. 444–445.

25. Ibid., p. 445. According to one historian, the wearing of masculine clothing unnerved some male observers, who could tolerate same-sex love between women if both appeared feminine and if the erotic contact between them was seen as occurring in the absence of men or as an apprenticeship to heterosexual sex, but these same men recoiled at the idea of a woman dressed like a man because it was seen "as the attempted usurpation of male prerogative by women who behaved like men." See Faderman, *Surpassing the Love of Men*, p. 17. The reader is also reminded of the hydropathic "denouncement" of the supposed cross-dresser in Chapter Four.

26. Krafft-Ebing, *Psychopathia Sexualis* p. 446. These intense feelings, however, are not necessarily interchangeable with genital and sexual intimacy, as he infers. There does seem to be evidence, however, that these particular women were sexually intimate with each other.

27. Ibid., pp. 446, 433–434.

28. Ibid., p. 434.

29. Ibid.

30. Smith-Rosenberg, "The Female World"; and Faderman, *Surpassing the Love of Men*, p. 16.

31. Leila J. Rupp, "'Imagine My Surprise': Women's Relationships in Historical Perspective," in Leavitt, ed., *Women and Health in America*, p. 94, uses the term "woman-committed women," which conveys the all-encompassing nature of the bonds. As to the difficulties in determining the precise sexual nature of these relationships, see Blanche W. Cook, "The Historical Denial of Lesbianism," *Radical History Review* 20 (1979): 60–65, wherein she responds to Anna Mary Wells's analysis of the intimacy in *Miss Marks and Miss Woolley* (Boston: Houghton Mifflin, 1978). Cook asserts that women in homosocial/sensual love relationships *were* lesbians regardless of the precise nature of their intimate sexual contact. Also see Rupp, "'Imagine My Surprise,'" pp. 90–91; and Estelle B. Freedman, "Sexuality in Nineteenth-Century America: Behavior, Ideology, and Politics," in *The Promise of American History: Progress and Prospects*, ed. Stanley I. Kutler and Stanley N. Kat (Baltimore: Johns Hopkins University Press, 1982), pp 196–215, wherein she discusses the historiographical interpretation of nineteenth-century women's (presumed) passionlessness; Faderman, *Surpassing the Love of Men*, similarly concludes that throughout the nineteenth century these relationships were not sexual.

32. Faderman, *Surpassing the Love of Men*, p. 16; see Freedman, "Sexuality," p. 200, for an analysis of Faderman.

33. See Faderman, *Surpassing the Love of Men;* and Freedman, "Sexuality," pp. 199–201, wherein she discusses historical interpretations of passionlessness. She considers the scholarship of Linda Gordon, Carl Degler, Nancy Sahli, Carroll Smith-Rosenberg, Vern Bullough and Martha Voght, and William Shade.

34. Freedman, "Sexuality," p. 200, discussing Faderman, *Surpassing the Love of Men*.

35. Rupp, "'Imagine My Surprise,'" p. 92, 90–91.

36. Faderman, *Surpassing the Love of Men*, p. 19. I, too, advocate the women defining themselves; the task of women's historians is to avoid either denying or heralding their subjects' intimate lives in terms known only to our era; we ought, however, to allow the material to speak to the homoerotic intimacy as a viable and complete form of affectional and sensual expression, rather than trivialize it as secondary to (or in mimicry of) "real" love—heterosexual love. Recognizing the totality of these relationships forces us to consider them as a viable whole, not as a surrogate anomaly.

37. Elizabeth Mavor, *The Ladies of Llangollen* (New York: Penguin, 1973), p. 122; Faderman, *Surpassing the Love of Men*, pp. 74–75, 85, 427n, 429n, 433n, 436n.

38. Mavor, *Ladies of Llangollen*, p. 166. Seward resided at a mineral (not cold-water) cure.

39. See E. S. Turner, *Taking the Cure* (Britain: Michael Joseph, 1967), pp. 119–120.

40. Margaret Farrand Thorp, *Female Persuasion: Six Strong-Minded Women* (New Haven: Yale University Press, 1949).

41. Catharine Beecher, *Letters to the People on Health and Happiness* (New York: Harper & Bros., 1855), pp. 7–15; and "Communication from Mrs. R.

B. Gleason of the Elmira Water Cure: Symptoms of Pelvic Displacement, and Their Treatment," as quoted in Nancy Cott, *Root of Bitterness* (New York: Dutton, 1972), pp. 271–276.

42. Beecher, *Letters to the People*, p. 117.

43. See Kathryn Kish Sklar, *Catharine Beecher: A Study in American Domesticity* (New York: Norton, 1976), p. 184. and Charles Stowe, *The Life of Harriet Beecher Stowe Compiled from Her Letters and Journals* (Boston: Houghton Mifflin, 1889), pp. 112–119. Also see Weiss and Kemble, "The Forgotten Water-Cures."

44. Sklar, *Catharine Beecher*, pp. 183, 187–192, 195–196.

45. Ibid., pp. 186–187.

46. Rupp, "Imagine My Surprise,'" p. 92, contends that in mid-twentieth-century homosocial relationships. "devotion to a charismatic leader" was oftentimes manifested in bonds such as these. Beecher, in the nineteenth century, seems to have exerted such an influence. Couple relationships, according to Rupp, were the other women-committed type of relationships.

47. Sklar, *Catharine Beecher*, p. 187.

48. Ibid., p. 191, as quoted in Vivian C. Hopkins, *Prodigal Puritan: A Life of Delia Bacon* (Cambridge: Harvard University Press Belknap Press, 1959), p. 125. Sklar notes that Beecher's improved health coincided with the publication of the text that discussed Bacon's thwarted courtship.

49. Sklar, *Catharine Beecher*, p. 314n.

50. Ibid., pp. 189, 192. The latter as chronicled in Hopkins, *Prodigal Puritan*.

51. Sklar, *Catharine Beecher*, pp. 195–202.

52. Ibid., p. 218.

53. Ibid., p. 206.

54. Ibid., pp. 206, 272, and 330n.

55. Catherine Beecher, *A Treatise on Domestic Economy, For the Use of Young Ladies at Home and at School* (Boston, 1841), pp. 100–103.

56. "Miss Beecher on Water-Cure," *Water-Cure Journal* 10, no. 1 (July 1850): 13–14.

57. Ibid., p. 13.

58. Ibid., p. 14.

59. Jean Strouse, *Alice James: A Biography* (Boston: Houghton Mifflin, 1980), pp. ix–x.

60. Ibid., pp. 121–122.

61. Ibid., p. 225.

62. Ibid., n.p. Henry James, Sr., eventually adhered to the writings of Swedenborg.

63. Faderman, *Surpassing the Love of Men*, pp. 195–197, discusses the James/Loring relationship, Henry James's enthusiastic support of it, and the vital role it played in both women's lives. Also see Leon Edel, ed., *The Diary of Alice James* (New York: Dodd, Mead, 1934), p. 15, wherein he describes their use of hypnosis to aid A. James.

64. Edel, ed., *Diary of Alice James*, p. 13.

65. Faderman, *Surpassing the Love of Men*, p. 196, as quoted in Gay Wilson Allen, *William James: A Biography* (New York: Viking Press, 1967), p. 227.

66. See "Worcester Hydropathic Institute," *Water-Cure Journal* 19, no. 6 (June 1855): 137.

67. Susan B. Anthony, as quoted in "Your Worcester Street," in *Worcester Telegram* (Ivan Sandrof Franklin Publishing, 1948).

68. Wells, *Miss Marks and Miss Woolley,* p. 107.

69. Ibid., pp. 107, 145–148, 157.

70. Marks's own career included heading the English Literature Department at Mount Holyoke College for twenty years, the publishing of nearly twenty books, and the founding of the well-known Laboratory Theatre, hardly an inauspicious career. See ibid.; and Faderman, *Surpassing the Love of Men,* pp. 228–229.

71. See Wells, *Miss Marks and Miss Woolley;* and Cook's review of the book, which appeared as "Historical Denial of Lesbianism," pp. 60–65.

72. Cook, "Historical Denial of Lesbianism," p. 64.

73. Faderman, *Surpassing the Love of Men,* pp. 229–230 and notes 69, 70, and 71 on p. 451; Jeannette Marks, *A Girl's Student Days and After* (New York: Fleming H. Revell, 1911), pp 36–37; and Jeannette Marks papers, unpublished correspondence with Dr. Arthur Jacobson, Williston Memorial Library, Mount Holyoke College.

74. Faderman, *Surpassing the Love of Men,* pp. 279, 290–294, 297–313, traces the effects of the early sexologists (and larger cultural factors) in helping to create this revised and extremely negative view of same-sex bonding between women in the twentieth century.

75. Sklar, *Catharine Beecher,* pp. 214–215.

76. Hattie B. L. Brown, "A Personal Experience," in Conklin, *Jackson Health Resort,* pp. 40–42, delivered at the Fiftieth Anniversary Celebration in 1908. Following her first marriage to Dr. William E. Brown, who had been the head of a sanitarium in North Adams, Massachusetts, Hattie Blake Lee remarried to Dr. James H. Jackson, who had also lost his first spouse. He died in 1928, she in 1961. Both are buried in Dansville.

Testimonial poems and letters such as Brown's, written to their mentor–physicians, were not uncommon. They reflect an appreciation, warmth, and at times, reverence that signifies the exceptionally close physician-patient relationship. See the following excerpts in the *Jackson Health Resort:* Fanny B. Johnson, "An Old-Time Patient of Father Jackson's," pp. 24–25; Dr. Edwin L. Wood, "Between Friends" (re: the impact of the cure on one of J. C. Jackson's patients and how she affected her community when she returned home); Alice Wood, "The Art of Living," p. 50 (re: the grateful testimony of a woman college student who was sick and cured at "Our Home"); and "Clara Barton Tells What 'Our Home' Did for Her," pp. 326–330. Also see "Letter from M. W. Gray, M.D., Former Physician to Springfield Water Cure Certifying the Value and Skills of Dr. E. Snell's Therapeutics," *Springfield City Directory, 1851–1852,* pp. 108–109; "Round Hill Water Cure," *Daily Hampshire Gazette,* August 24, 1847, pp. 2–3, wherein a former pupil of the Round Hill School visited the cure and wrote a letter to the *National Intelligencer* testifying to the cure he witnessed of an old rheumatic man.

77. "Clara Barton Tells," p. 326, excerpt from an address given at "Our Home" on June 2, 1880.

78. Ibid., p. 327.

79. Ibid.

80. Ibid.

81. Conklin, *Jackson Health Resort*, p. 181, as quoted in correspondence from Clara Barton to her cousin Jere Learned, July 15, 1876.

82. "Clara Barton Tells," p. 328.

83. Ibid., p. 330.

84. Ibid., p. 329.

85. The list does not include Hattie B. L. Brown or Mrs. Fanny B. Johnson who were also employees and/or residents at the Cure; they bring the total to 26. While the positions of the female personnel were not stipulated, the list is valuable nonetheless: Helen Dumuth, 29 years; Mrs. Helen D. Gregory, 27 years; Cornelia A. Palmer, 26 years; Alice Wood, 25 years; Elizabeth MacCallum, 21 years; Emma Spencer and Elizabeth Lizzie Harrison, 20 years; Caroline B. Shankland, 17 years; Katherine Maloney and Elizabeth Swartz, 15 years; Mrs. M. M. Michael, 14 years; Minnie Nolan, 13 years; Anna Morrison, 12 years; Mary Smith, Frances Kornbau, Molly Molyneux, Mary Maloney and Mary Edwards, 11 years; Mary G. Austin, Anna Miller, Mrs. Mary Root, and Margaret Gunther, 10 years. See Conklin *Jackson Health Resort*, p. 298. "Our Home" in 1861 estimated that they had treated roughly equal numbers of men and women (more closely, in a ratio of 4:3). See *Water-Cure Journal* 32, no. 1 (July 1861): 21.

86. (Elmira) *Sunday Telegram*, August 5, 1923.

Conclusion

1. Conceptual pieces that informed this section include Robert N. Bellah et al., *Habits of the Heart: Individualism and Commitment in American Life* (Berkeley: University of California Press, 1985); Christopher Lasch, *Haven in a Heartless World: The Family Besieged* (New York: Basic Books, 1977); Thorstein Veblen, *The Theory of the Leisure Class: An Economic Study of Institutions* ([1899] New York: Penguin, 1979). Kathleen Peiss, *Cheap Amusements: Working Women and Leisure in Turn-of-the-Century New York* (Philadelphia: Temple University Press, 1986); Richard W. Fox and T. J. Jackson Lears, eds., *The Culture of Consumption* (New York: Pantheon Books, 1983); and James R. McGovern, "The American Woman's Pre-World War I Freedom in Manners and Morals," in *Our American Sisters*, ed. Jean E. Friedman and William G. Shade (Boston: Allyn and Bacon, 1973), pp. 237–259. Reprinted from the *Journal of American History*, 55 (September 1968): 315–333.

2. See Adrienne Rich, "Compulsory Heterosexuality and Lesbian Existence," *Signs: Journal of Women in Culture and Society* 5, no. 4 (Summer 1980): 631–660; Lillian Faderman, *Surpassing the Love of Men: Romantic Friendship and Love between Women from the Renaissance to the Present* (New York: Morrow, 1981), esp. "The Reaction" and "The Twentieth Century"; and Judge Lindsay, Benjamin Barr, and Wainwright Evans, *The Companionate Marriage* (New York: Boni and Liveright: 1927).

3. Changing perceptions of the female character and how these had an impact on gender relations are discussed by Shelia Rothman, *Woman's Proper Place: A History of Changing Ideals and Practices, 1870 to the Present* (New York: Basic Books, 1979); Rosalind Rosenberg, "In Search of Woman's Nature, 1850-1920," *Feminist Studies* 3, nos. 1 and 2 (Fall 1975): 141–155; McGovern, "American Woman's Pre-World War I Freedom;" Agnes Repplier, "The Repeal

of Reticence," *Atlantic Monthly* 113 (March 1914), 297–304; Margaret Deland, "The Change in the Feminine Ideal," *Atlantic Monthly* 105 (March 1910).

4. See Richard von Krafft-Ebing, *Psychopathia Sexualis* (New York: Putnam, 1965); Havelock Ellis, *Studies in the Psychology of Sex: Sexual Inversion* (1897); George Chauncey, Jr., "From Sexual Inversion to Homosexuality: Medicine and the Changing Conceptualization of Female Deviance," *Salmagundi* 58/59 (Fall 1982–Winter 1983): 114–146; Lillian Faderman, "The Morbidification of Love between Women by Nineteenth-Century Sexologists," *Journal of Homosexuality* 4, no. 1 (1978): 73–90; Lillian Faderman, "The Reaction," "The Contribution of the Sexologists," "Lesbian Exoticism," and "Lesbian Evil," all in Faderman, *Surpassing The Love of Men.*

5. Estelle Freedman, "Separatism as Strategy: Female Institution Building and American Feminism, 1870–1930," *Feminist Studies* 5 (Fall 1979): 512–529, notes that this public activism was a result of the middle-class women's culture of the nineteenth century and that this "female institution building" helped mobilize women to gain political leverage in the larger society. Women's increased participation in the traditionally defined public and political realm is discussed by Mari Jo Buhle, *Women and American Socialism, 1870–1920* (Urbana: University of Illinois Press, 1983); Ellen DuBois, "The Radicalism of the Woman Suffrage Movement: Notes toward the Reconstruction of Nineteenth-Century Feminism," *Feminist Studies* 3, nos. 1 and 2 (Fall 1975): 63–72; Frank Stricker, "Cookbooks and Law Books: The Hidden History of Career Women in Twentieth-Century America," in *A Heritage of Her Own*, ed. Nancy F. Cott and Elizabeth H. Pleck, (New York: Simon & Schuster, 1979), pp. 476–498; Mary Roth Walsh, *Doctors Wanted: No Women Need Apply; Sexual Barriers in the Medical Profession, 1835–1975* (New Haven: Yale University Press, 1977); and Rosalyn Baxandall, Linda Gordon, and Susan Reverby, eds., *America's Working Women: A Documentary History — 1600 to the Present* (New York: Random House, 1976), pp. 167–222.

6. Freedman, "Separatism as Strategy," p. 524.

7. McGovern, "American Woman's Pre-World War I Freedom," notes that women's sex roles and identification shifted in the direction of more masculine norms (p. 239), women joined men as comrades, and the differences between the sexes were narrowed (p. 242). This meant a "reversal in the traditional role of women just as it describes a pronounced familiarity of the sexes" (p. 242).

8. This shift away from women-only pursuits is elaborated by Judith Walzer Leavitt, "'Science' Enters the Birthing Room: Obstetrics in America Since the Eighteenth Century," *Journal of American History* 70, no. 2 (September 1983): 281–304; Adrienne Rich, *Of Woman Born: Motherhood as Experience and Institution* (New York: Norton, 1977); Freedman, "Separatism as Strategy;" and Virginia G. Drachman, *Hospital with a Heart: Women Doctors and the Paradox of Separatism at the New England Hospital, 1862–1969* (Ithaca: Cornell University Press, 1984).

9. See Peiss, *Cheap Amusements;* Kathleen Peiss, "'Charity Girls' and City Pleasures: Historical Notes on Working-Class Sexuality, 1880–1920," in *Powers of Desire: The Politics of Sexuality*, ed. Christine Stansell and Sharon Thompson (New York: Monthly Review Press, 1983), pp. 74–87; Frederick J. Stielow, "Resorts and Vacationers on the Island of The Awakening; Grand Isle, Louisiana and the 'New' Leisure—1866–1893," lent by the author in 1982 prior to publication. (A modified version of this paper appeared as "Grand Isle, Louisiana, The New

Leisure, 1866–1893," *Louisiana History* 23, no. 3 (1982): 239–257.) John F. Kasson, *Amusing the Million: Coney Island at the Turn of the Century* (New York: Hill & Wang, 1978); Louis A. Erenberg, *Steppin' Out: New York Night Life and the Transformation of American Culture 1890–1930* (Westport, Conn.: Greenwood Press, 1981); and Lary May, *Screening Out the Past: The Birth of Mass Culture and the Motion Picture Industry* (New York: Oxford University Press, 1980).

10. Stielow, "Resorts and Vacationers," notes that the growth of a resort industry coincided with increased conspicuous consumption and conspicuous leisure.

11. Ibid., p. 22.

12. See Mrs. R. B. Gleason, M.D., *Hints to Patients,* pamphlet, 1889, which cites as activities piano, billiards, gymnastics, and dancing (p. 4); William D. Conklin, *The Jackson Health Resort* (Dansville, N.Y.: privately printed, 1971), pp. 141a–141b, describes activities held at the San or the lawn circa 1895 that included a song recital by Mrs. Shannah Cumming Jones and a grand open-air vaudeville featuring the Lilliputian Cake Walkers, Herbert W. Kidd, "The Teller of Touching and Telling Truths," and "That Naughty Little Gay Golf Ball," with Nicholas and Jansen Noyes, Sam Welsh "Just Foolishness," and "No Cake Comes Too High for Me" (originally appeared as an advertisement in *Town and Village Historian,* no date given). Conklin also notes that "The Musical Krebses" lived on the Hill and provided excellent popular music (pp. 200a–200b). Activities at the Round Hill Water-Cure and Motorpathic Institute included gymnasium, billiards, and bowling alleys. See *Round Hill Water-Cure and Motorpathic Institute,* pamphlet, Forbes Library, n.d.; charades were also a favorite at Round Hill. See also "Letters from Round Hill—No. 2. Entertainment at the Water-Cure," *Daily Hampshire Gazette,* August 27, 1861, p. 1.

13. In fact, well before competition was posed by consumer-leisure activities, an editorial filler in the Journal in 1850 sought to expand the cures' appeal. It urged the use of the establishments as summer retreats for recreation and rest, not only for sickness. See "Summer Retreats," *Water-Cure Journal* 10, no. 1 (July 1850): 29.

14. James A. Jackson, "Years of Uncertainty and Change 1910–1929," in Conklin, *Jackson Health Resort,* pp. 341–342.

15. Stielow, "Resorts and Vacationers," pp. 7–9.

16. See Jacqueline S. Wilkie, "Submerged Sensuality—Technology and Perceptions of Bathing," *Journal of Social History* 19, no. 4 (1986): 649–664; and Harold Donaldson Eberlein, "When Society First Took a Bath," in *Sickness and Health in America,* ed. Judith Walzer Leavitt and Ronald L. Numbers (Madison: University of Wisconsin Press, 1978), pp. 331–341.

17. Richard W. Schwarz, *John Harvey Kellogg, M.D.* (Nashville, Tenn.: Southern Publishing Association, 1970), p. 24.

18. Brian Inglis, "Osteopathy and Chiropractic," in his *Fringe Medicine,* Foreword by G. M. Carstairs (London: Faber & Faber, 1964), argues that mechanical devices might well harm one of the main attributes that chiropractors bring to the healing encounter—the "diagnostic knack" that so soothes patients (pp. 121–122). The applicability to hydropathic therapeutics is readily evident.

19. "Topics of the Month. Fees." *Herald of Health* 3, no. 3 (March 1864):102.

20. Harry B. Weiss and Howard R. Kemble, *The Great American Water-Cure Craze: A History of Hydropathy in the United States* (Trenton, N.J.: Past Times Press, 1967), pp. 60–68. They date the first name change at 1856.

21. See Board of Trade Review of Binghamton, N.Y., *Industries of Binghamton 1892* (Binghamton: James P. McKinney, 1892), pp. 111–112; *Elmira Star Gazette*, November 24, 1959; Adele A. Gleason, *In Memorium, 1820–1905 Rachel Brooks Gleason*, booklet, n.p., n.d. (lent by Ada Gleason Bush); Evelyn Giammichelle and Eva Taylor, "Elmira Water Cure; Silas and Rachel Gleason and Their 'Tavern for the Sick,'" *Chemung Historical Journal*, December 1966, pp. 1535–1541; Conklin, *Jackson Health Resort;* John Elderkin, "Miscellaneous, Letter from Round Hill Northampton," *Daily Hampshire Gazette*, February 15, 1870; and *New York Evening Mall*, as reprinted in *Daily Hampshire Gazette*, July 19, 1870.

22. Weiss and Kemble, *Great American Water-Cure Craze*, p. 64.

23. Simon Baruch, *The Principles and Practices of Hydropathy, A Guide to the Application of Water in Disease* (New York, 1898); and J. H. Kellogg, *Rational Hydrotherapy* (Philadelphia: F. A. Davis, 1901). Kellogg published *First Book in Physiology and Hygiene* (New York, 1885) and *Ladies' Guide in Health and Disease* (Des Moines, 1883).

24. See "Editorial Department," *Herald of Health*, April 1885, p. 107.

25. Ibid.; the entire issue spans pp. 97–119. See, especially, "How to Give Massage," from the *Homeopathic News* pp. 104–105; "Health in Workshops," p. 112; Rachel B. Gleason, "Hints to Husbands," pp. 97–101; and Jennie Chandler, "Studies in Hygiene for Women," p. 113. Numerous pieces address sanitation and pollution; see "Impure Water at Albany," p. 112; "Sewer Gas a Cause of Measles and Pneumonia," p. 111; "Construction of Healthy Houses," p. 109; "Infection from Laundries," p. 109; and "Heisch's Test for Sewage Contamination," p. 105.

26. Ibid; see, especially, Editor, "Answers to Questions: Pure Water, Weak Eyes, and Beer," ibid., p. 106.

27. Ibid.; see, especially, Advertisements, p. 119; and "Current Literature," pp. 116, 118.

28. Ibid., back page, unnumbered.

29. Ibid.

30. See R. T. Trall, "Topics of the Month," *Water-Cure Journal* 21, no. 1 (January 1856).

31. Weiss and Kemble, *Great American Water-Cure Craze*, p. 70.

32. See "Death of Dr. Shew," *Water-Cure Journal* 20, no. 5 (November 1855): 104–105; James Caleb Jackson, "Dr. Shew and His Mantle," *Water-Cure Journal* 21, no. 1 (January 1856): 2–4; J.A.R., "Dr. Shew. 'Who Shall Wear His Mantle?'" *Water-Cure Journal* 21, no. 3 (March 1856): 58; and *Water-Cure Journal* 21, no. 4 (April 1856): 79; wherein friends of hydropathy founded the Shew Monument Association to erect a statue of Shew in Greenwood Cemetery near New York. Seth Rogers, of the Worcester Water-Cure, was on this committee.

33. Inglis in "Osteopathy and Chiropractic," notes that the reaction of orthodox medicine to an unorthodox sect can determine the latter's development even more so than its own achievements and merits (p. 116); this seems to have been an operative factor for Hydropathy. For information on allopathic sentiment against water cure, see *Water-Cure Journal* 9, no. 1 (January 1850): 5–9, wherein Trall responds to charges of quackery; *Water-Cure Journal* 24, no. 4 (October 1857): 85, wherein allopaths ridiculed the Hydropathic College; *Water-Cure Journal* 26, no. 6 (December 1858): 89, which describes the unfair treatment given water-cure graduates by allopaths; *Water-Cure Journal* 28, no. 3 (Septem-

ber 1859): 41, wherein drug doctors claim hydropathy is waning; and R. S. Houghton, M.D., "The Water-Cure and Its Assailants," *Water-Cure Journal and Herald of Reforms* 9, no. 5 (May 1850): 148–150. See also Essay on Sources.

34. *Water-Cure Journal* 28 no. 4 (October 1859): 55.

35. See Trall's challenges to a debate in *Water-Cure Journal* 30, no. 4 (October 1860): 56–57; *Water-Cure Journal* 30, no. 6 (December 1860): 90; and *Water-Cure Journal* 33, no. 4 (April 1862): 81.

In 1846 the *New York Tribune* reviewed quite positively Mrs. Shew's *Water-Cure For Ladies*, an indication that early perceptions of hydropathy among the general public were not nearly so all-encompassingly hostile—or influential—as the Hydropaths' tirades against the allopaths insinuated. See "*Water-Cure For Ladies*: Notice of the Work," *Water-Cure Journal* 2, no. 7 (September 1, 1846): 111, reprinted from the *New York Tribune*.

36. See "Revolution. To Allopathic Physicians. Nos. I–VII," *Water-Cure Journal* 22, no. 4 (October 1856), through *Water-Cure Journal* 26, no. 1 (July 1858).

37. Marshall Scott Legan, "Hydropathy in America: A Nineteenth-Century Panacea," *Bulletin of the History of Medicine* 45, no. 3 (May–June 1971): 269; and Houghton, "Water-Cure and Its Assailants."

38. Rausse criticized water cure, saying hydropathists often used radical cures when patients were too weak to tolerate them. This stemmed from an inability to differentiate strengthening cures and radical cures. See J. H. Rausse, *Errors of Physicians and Others in the Practice of the Water-Cure*, trans. C. H. Meeker (New York and London, 1849). According to the Library of Congress, J. H. Rausse was a pseudonym for Heinrich F. Francke, who was a practitioner of water cure in Mecklenburg, Germany, as described in Weiss and Kemble, *Great American Water-Cure Craze*, pp. 58–59.

39. Joseph Leidy, M.D., "Valedictory Address to the Class of Medical Graduates of the University of Pennsylvania Delivered at the Public Commencement, March 27th, 1858," Philadelphia, 1858, as quoted in Weiss and Kemble, *Great American Water-Cure Craze*, p. 51.

40. In this regard, the hydropathic experience was similar to that of other nineteenth-century health reform sects. See Paul Starr, *The Social Transformation of American Medicine* (New York: Basic Books, 1982), wherein he explicates the economic and social factors involved in the ascendancy of scientific/allopathic medicine.

41. See Philip Van Inger, *The New York Academy of Medicine: Its First Hundred Years* (New York: Columbia University Press, 1949), p. 13.

42. *Transactions of the Medical Society of Pennsylvania* (1851–1854), 1:153, as quoted in Weiss and Kemble, *Great American Water-Cure Craze*, p. 52.

43. See *Herald of Health* 3, no. 5 (May 1864): 182.

44. See "Miscellany: Society of Public Health," *Water-Cure Journal* 10, no. 1 (July 1850): 27.

45. See Weiss and Kemble, *Great American Water Cure Craze*, p. 56.

46. Barbara Ehrenreich and Deirdre English, "Science and the Ascent of the Experts," in *For Her Own Good: 150 Years of the Experts' Advice to Women* (Garden City, N.Y.: Doubleday/Anchor Press, 1978), pp. 69–70; and Robert H. Wiebe, *The Search for Order: 1887–1920* (New York: Hill & Wang, 1967), pp. 116–122.

47. See "Total and Urban Population at Each Census," U.S. Bureau of the

Census, *Twelfth Census of the U.S. Taken in the Year 1900, Statistical Atlas* (Washington, D.C.: U.S. Census Office, 1903), plates 16, 17; *Statistical History of the U.S.: Colonial Times to the Present* (Stamford, Conn.: Fairfield, 1965); William E. Leuchtenburg, ed., *The Unfinished Century* (Boston: Little, Brown, 1973); and Richard M. Abrams, "Reform and Uncertainty: America Enters the Twentieth Century, 1900–1918," in *Unfinished Century*, ed. Leuchtenburg, pp. 1–111.

48. Abrams, "Reform and Uncertainty," p. 35.

49. Gerald E. Markowitz and David Karl Rosner, "Doctors in Crisis: A Study in the Use of Medical Education Reform to Establish Modern Professional Elitism in Medicine," *American Quarterly* 25 (1973): 87; and Starr, *Social Transformation*.

50. See Jonathan Dine Wirtschafter, "The Impact and Genesis of the Medical Lobby, 1898–1906," *Journal of the History of Medicine*, January 1958, pp. 15–49.

51. Constitution, *Journal of the American Medical Association* 36 (1901): 1646; as quoted in Wirtschafter, "Impact and Genesis," p. 27.

52. Wiebe, *Search for Order*, pp. 116–122.

53. Markowitz and Rosner, "Doctors in Crisis," p. 89.

54. See Carleton Chapman's "The Flexner Report by Abraham Flexner," *Daedalus* 103 (1974): 110.

55. Markowitz and Rosner, "Doctors in Crisis," pp. 96–97; and Judy Barrett Litoff, "Midwives in America, 1870–1930," Ph.D. dissertation, University of Maine, 1975, pp. 83–87, and Judy Barrett Litoff, *American Midwives: 1860 to the Present* (Westport, Conn.: Greenwood Press, 1978).

56. See Abraham Flexner, *Medical Education in the United States and Canada: A Report to the Carnegie Foundation for the Advancement of Teaching*, (New York: Carnegie Foundation, 1910; reprinted New York: Arno Press, 1972); and Chapman, "Flexner Report." The Flexner Report, with $50 million behind it to implement its findings, endorsed and endowed certain centers of medical research and not others. Sectarian and gender- and race-specific colleges were not among the chosen recipients. See Markowitz and Rosner, "Doctors in Crisis," pp. 101–102.

57. See Regina Markell Morantz, "The 'Connecting Link': The Case for the Woman Doctor in Nineteenth-Century America," in Leavitt and Numbers, eds., *Sickness and Health in America*, pp. 117–129, esp. pp. 117–118. Also see Regina Markell Morantz, *Sympathy and Science: Women Physicians in American Medicine* (New York: Oxford University Press, 1985).

58. Ibid., pp. 124–125.

59. See Schwarz, *John Harvey Kellogg, M.D.*, p. 24; and Richard H. Shryock, "Sylvester Graham and the Popular Health Movement, 1830–1870," *Mississippi Valley Historical Review* 18, no. 2 (1932): 172–183.

60. See "Death From Vaccination," *Water-Cure Journal* 1, no. 6 (February 15, 1846): 87; *Water-Cure Journal* 1, no. 8 (March 15, 1846): 125; and *Water-Cure Journal* 12, no. 6 (December 1851): 127–130, wherein Shew articulates his antivaccination position but adds that if he changes his opinion, he will report it promptly.

61. Rosenberg, "Social Class and Medical Care," p. 163; and Rich, *Of Woman Born*, pp. 156–181, for a history of the cultural reception of anesthesia in childbirth.

62. See Wiebe, *Search for Order*, pp. 114–115; and Starr, *Social Transformation*.

63. Wilbur H. Watson, "Central Tendencies in the Practice of Folk Medicine,"

in *Black Folk Medicine: The Therapeutic Significance of Faith and Trust,* ed. Wilbur H. Watson (New Brunswick, N.J.: Transaction Books, 1984), pp. 87–97.

64. Bellah et al., *Habits of the Heart,* argue that the modern-day privatized therapeutic relationship embodies the individual-centered, noncommunal values so prevalent in contemporary American society—features antithetical to a stay at a nineteenth-century cure.

65. Sigmund Freud, *An Autobiographical Study* (1886), trans. James Strachey (New York: Norton, 1952), pp. 25–26. Later, Freud lost faith in physiological treatments for nervous and mental disorders.

66. Weiss and Kemble, *Great American Water-Cure Craze,* p. 68.

67. Ibid.

68. Sidney Licht, *Medical Hydrology* (Baltimore: Waverly Press, 1963). For information on Kneipp, see Sebastian Kneipp, *My Water-Cure* (New York: Benziger, 1893).

69. Elizabeth Bolton and Diana Goodwin, *An Introduction to Pool Exercises* (London: E. and S. Livingstone, 1967); and Fred Bennett Moor et al., *Manual of Hydrotherapy and Massage* (Mountain View, Calif.: Pacific Press Publishing, 1964), p. 2.

70. See Simon Baruch, *An Epitome of Hydrotherapy for Physicians, Architects and Nurses* (Philadelphia: Saunders, 1920); Alexander Blackhall Morison, *On Cardiac Failure and Its Treatment, With Special Reference to the Use of Baths and Exercises* (London: Rebman, 1927); *Proceedings, International Congress on Rheumatism and Hydrology* (London and Oxford, 1938); *Bicentenary Congress on Chronic Rheumatism (Bath), March 25–April 2, 1938* (London: Headley, 1938); M. H. Duffield, *Exercise in Water* (Baltimore: Williams and Wilkins, 1976); and Margaret Reid Campion, *Hydrotherapy in Pediatrics* (Rockville, Md.: Aspen Systems, 1985). Numerous contemporary medical articles discuss the uses and efficacy of hydrotherapy for rheumatism, blood-pressure control, circulation, and burns. See J. A. Cosh and G. D. Kersley, "Rheumatism Treatment Centers in Britain—Bath Ancient and Modern," *Annals of Physical Medicine* 10 (November 1969): 167–174; E. Bolton, "Hydrotherapy—Another Milestone," *Physiotherapy* 51 (1965): 314–315; A. J. Swannel et al., "Changes in Arterial Blood Pressure in Patients Undergoing Routine Pool Therapy," *Physiotherapy* 62, no. 3 (March 1976): 86–88; P. Franchimont et al., "Hydrotherapy—Mechanisms and Indications," *Pharmacology Therapeutics* 20, no. 1 (1983): 79–93; C. Garreau, "Experimental Monitoring of the Effects of Hand and Foot Douches at Barbotan on Peripheral Circulation," *Phlebologie* 36, no. 3 (July–September 1983): 265–270 [English Abstract]; L. G. Leonard et al., "Chemical Burns: Effect of Prompt First Aid," *Journal of Trauma* 22, no. 5 (May 1982): 420–423; and A. Golland, "Basic Hydrotherapy," *Physiotherapy* 67, no. 9 (September 1981): 258–262.

71. See Sandra Kallio, "Body-Wraps: Quick Relief or Weighty 'Scam'?" *Wisconsin State Journal,* June 21, 1981, p. 6. This method of wrapping clients in strips of wet cloth was sold as Trim-A-Way, a weight-reduction plan that helped the client lose weight and feel rejuvenated. See also Mark Muro, "Oozing in a Clay Bath," *Boston Globe,* July 29, 1981, pp. 33, 36, which described people bathing in smooth, white, oozy clay at Gay Head and then plunging into Vineyard Sound—a favorite pursuit of those seeking relaxation and invigoration. Modern sports medicine has integrated the use of water therapy as a central part of its therapeutics as an aid to muscular exertion, an anesthetic, a sedative, and as an

energizer. See Nancy Crowell, "Almanac. Water, Water, Everywhere," *Women Sports*, April 1982, pp. 40–41. And for information on the importance of ingesting water for athletes, see Jane Brody, "Taking the Waters. A Drinking Woman's Guide," *Women Sports*, March 1982, pp. 17–21. For a contemporary look at the relaxation and renewal promised to vacationers at water resorts in America and abroad (amid sumptuous environs) through travel magazines, see Judith Babcock Wylie, "The Sybaritic American Spa," *Travel and Leisure* 15, no. 2 (February 1985): 114–119; Malachy Duffy, "The Sumptuous Style of Baden-Baden," *Travel and Leisure* 14, no. 2 (February 1984): 65–67, 76 (these waters are now advocated for stress); J. Paul Axline, "A Splashy Spa in Monte Carlo," *Travel and Leisure* (September 1985): 80–81, which describes the cuisine, available-but-not-mandatory exercise classes, herbal wraps, pools and massages; and Anita J. Slomski, "Teutonic Treatments," *American Way*, October 1, 1985, pp. 77–87; which discusses the psychological value of an away-from-home stay, the pleasures of underwater massage, and body wraps.

72. See Harold Y. Vanderpool, "The Holistic Hodgepodge: A Critical Analysis of Holistic Medicine and Health in America Today," *Journal of Family Practice* 19 (1984): 773–781; and L. Kopelman and J. Moskop, "The Holistic Health Movement: A Survey and Critique," *Journal of Medicine and Philosophy* 8 (1981): 209–235.

73. Vanderpool, "Holistic Hodgepodge"; and Eric J. Cassel, "The Nature of Suffering and the Goals of Medicine," *New England Journal of Medicine* 306, no. 11 (March 18, 1982): 639–645.

An Essay on Sources

Several primary texts speak most directly to the allopathic management of common ailments. Among those I found most helpful are the following: Benjamin Rush, *Six Introductory Lectures* (Philadelphia: M. and J. Conrad, 1801); R. Thomas, *The Modern Practice of Physic* (New York, 1811); and W. P. Dewees, *Practice of Physic Comprising Most of the Diseases Not Treated in "Diseases of Females and Diseases of Children,"* vol. 1 (Philadelphia: Carey and Lea, 1830). While numerous interpretive sources exist on this topic, I found Henry B. Shafer, *The American Medical Profession, 1783 to 1850* (New York: A.M.S. Press, 1968, originally published in 1936); William G. Rothstein, *American Physicians in the Nineteenth-Century: From Sects to Science* (Baltimore: Johns Hopkins University Press, 1972); William F. Bynum, "Chronic Alcoholism in the First Half of the Nineteenth Century," *Bulletin of the History of Medicine* 42 (1968): 160–185; and Sarah Stage, *Female Complaints: Lydia Pinkham and the Business of Women's Medicine* (New York: Norton, 1979), to be especially valuable.

Much has been written in recent years regarding the nineteenth-century medical management of women's physiology. Among the secondary works I have found most helpful in framing my interpretation of gender relations and medical care are G. Barker-Benfield, *The Horrors of the Half-Known Life: Male Attitudes toward Women and Sexuality in Nineteenth Century America* (New York: Harper & Row, 1976); J. Delaney et al., *The Curse: A Cultural History of Menstruation* (New York: Dutton, 1976); John S. and Robin M. Haller, *The Physician and Sexuality in Victorian America* (Urbana: University of Illinois Press, 1974); Barbara Ehrenreich and Deirdre English, *For Her Own Good: 150 Years of the Experts' Advice to Women* (Garden City, N.Y.: Doubleday Anchor, 1978); Regina M. Morantz, "The Lady and Her Physician," in *Clio's Consciousness Raised: New Perspectives on the History of Women*, ed. Mary

Hartman and Lois W. Banner (New York: Harper & Row, 1974), pp. 38–54; Carroll Smith-Rosenberg, "The Hysterical Woman: Sex Roles and Role Conflict in Nineteenth-Century America," *Social Research* 39, no. 4 (1972): 652–678; Carroll Smith-Rosenberg and Charles Rosenberg, "The Female Animal: Medical and Biological Views of Woman and Her Role in Nineteenth-Century America," *Journal of American History,* June 1973 to March 1974, pp. 332–357; Carroll Smith-Rosenberg, "Puberty to Menopause: The Cycle of Femininity in Nineteenth-Century America," *Clio's Consciousness Raised,* ed. Hartman and Banner," pp. 23–53; Peter Tylor, "Denied the Power to Choose the Good: Sexuality and Mental Defect in American Medical Practice, 1850–1920," *Journal of Social History* 10, no. 4 (June 1977): 472–490; Ilza Veith, *Hysteria: The History of a Disease* (Chicago and London: University of Chicago Press, 1965); Ann Douglas Wood, "The Fashionable Diseases: Women's Complaints and Their Treatment in Nineteenth-Century America," *Journal of Interdisciplinary History* 4, no. 1 (Summer 1973): 25–52, and the critique of this interpretation by Regina M. Morantz, "The Perils of Feminist History," *Journal of Interdisciplinary History* 4 (Spring 1974): 649–660.

Representative nineteenth-century texts that promoted the idea that woman's sexual organs determined her intellectual capacity and nature are Charles Meigs, *Females and Their Diseases* (Philadelphia: Lea and Blanchard, 1848); Edward H. Clarke, *Sex in Education, or a Fair Chance for the Girls* (Boston, 1873), which argued that women's physiological cyclicity rendered them unfit for education; and William Acton, *Functions and Disorders of the Reproductive Organs,* 4th ed. (London: John Churchill and Sons, 1865), which claimed that women had no sexual desires. Examples of physician-authored prescriptive literature that were most helpful include Samual Gregory, *Facts and Important Information for Young Women, on the Self-Indulgence of the Sexual Appetite, Its Destructive Effects on Health,* etc., 11th ed. (Boston,: G. Gregory 1857); Alfred G. Hall *Womanhood: Causes of Its Premature Decline,* 2nd ed. (Rochester, 1845); Frederick Hollick, *The Marriage Guide, or, Natural History of Generation* (New York, 1860); and Augustus K. Gardner, *Conjugal Sins* (New York: J. S. Redfield, 1870). Interpretive sources are Ronald G. Walters, *Primers for Prudery, Sexual Advice to Victorian America* (Urbana: University of Illinois Press, 1974); John S. Haller, "From Maidenhood to Menopause: Sex Education for Women in Victorian America," *Journal of Popular Culture* 6, no. 1 (1972): 49–69; and Carl Degler "What Ought to Be and What Was: Women's Sexuality in the Nineteenth Century," *American Historical Review* 79, no. 5 (December 1974): 1467–1491.

Among the interpretive pieces that I found of great value when delineating the impact of these medical texts upon women's roles, were Smith-Rosenberg, "Puberty to Menopause," and with Rosenberg, "The Female Animal"; Haller and Haller, *Physician and Sexuality;* and Nancy

Sahli, "Sexuality in Nineteenth and Twentieth Century America: The Sources and Their Problems," *Radical History Review* 20 (Spring/Summer 1979): 89–96.

Among the books and articles I found most valuable in understanding the philosophy of "regular" women physicians and the strained relationship between them and scientific medicine are Mary Roth Walsh, *Doctors Wanted: No Women Need Apply; Sexual Barriers in the Medical Profession, 1835–1975* (New Haven: Yale University Press, 1977); Elizabeth Blackwell, *Pioneer Work in Opening the Medical Profession to Women* (New York: Schocken, 1977); Regina Morantz and Sue Zschoche, "Professionalism, Feminism and Gender Roles: A Comparative Study of Nineteenth-Century Medical Therapeutics," *Journal of American History* 67, no. 3 (December 1980): 568–588; Martin Kaufman, "The Admission of Women to Nineteenth-Century Medical Societies," *Bulletin of the History of Medicine* 50, no. 2 (Summer 1976); 251–260; Regina Markell Morantz, "Feminism, Professionalism, And Germs: The Thought of Mary Putnam Jacobi and Elizabeth Blackwell," *American Quarterly* 34, no. 5 (Winter 1982): 459–478; and Regina Markell Morantz-Sanchez, *Sympathy and Science: Women Physicians in American Medicine* (New York: Oxford University Press, 1985). All these sources furthered my understanding of the special relationship between women hydropaths and the water-cure movement.

Representative historical texts that portray the march of medical science include H. S. Glasscheib, *The March of Medicine: The Emergence and Triumph of Modern Medicine* (New York: Putnam's 1964); George A. Bender, ed., *Great Moments in Medicine* (Detroit: Northwood Institute Press, 1966); and Frank G. Slaughter, *Immortal Magyar: Semmelweiss, Conqueror of Childbed Fever* (New York: Schuman, 1950).

The early transition from march of science to more inclusive socioeconomic causal interpretations is exemplified in Richard H. Shryock, *The Development of Modern Medicine: An Interpretation of the Social and Scientific Factors Involved* (Philadelphia: University of Pennsylvania Press, 1936). A watershed work that emphasized the contributing factors that created modern medicine is Rothstein's *American Physicians*, which postulated that allopaths were one sect competing among others. Later texts that looked at the social factors involved in medical care are Susan Reverby and David Rosner, "Beyond 'the Great Doctors,'" in *Health Care in America: Essays in Social History*, ed. Susan Reverby and David Rosner (Philadelphia: Temple University Press, 1979); Todd L. Savitt, *Medicine and Slavery: The Diseases and Health Care of Blacks in Antebellum Virginia* (Urbana: University of Illinois Press, 1978); *The Therapeutic Revolution: Essays in the Social History of American Medicine*, ed. Morris J. Vogel and Charles Rosenberg (Philadelphia: University of Pennsylvania Press, 1979); Paul Starr, *The Social Transformation of American Medicine* (New York: Basic Books, 1982); and Barbara Melosh,

"The Physician's Hand:" Work Culture and Conflict in American Nursing (Philadelphia: Temple University Press, 1982). And Harvey Green's *Fit for America: Health, Fitness, Sport, and American Society, 1830-1910* (New York: Pantheon, 1986) chronicles the social trends and cultural ideals favoring health consciousness.

The professionalization of American medicine is addressed through primary and secondary texts that analyze the low status of allopaths and the ensuing legal measures, attempts to standardize educational requirements, and voluntary associations. Most instructive among the primary sources were Presidential Address, *Transcripts of the American Medical Association* 1 (1848): 7; Paul F. Eve, *Present Position of the Medical Profession in Society* (Augusta, Ga., 1849); "To What Cause Are We to Attribute the Diminished Respectability of the Medical Profession in the Estimation of the American Public?" *Medicine and Surgical Reporter* 1 (1858): 141-143; and Edward C. Atwater, "The Medical Profession in a New Society, Rochester, New York (1811-1860)," *Bulletin of the History of Medicine* 48 (May-June 1973): 221-235. Interpretive sources that I referred to most frequently are Joseph F. Kett, *The Formation of the American Medical Profession; the Role of Institutions, 1780-1860* (New Haven: Yale University Press, 1968); Richard H. Shryock, *Medical Licensing in America, 1650-1965* (Baltimore: Johns Hopkins University Press, 1967); Starr, *Social Transformation of American Medicine;* and Martin Kaufman, *American Medical Education: The Formative Years, 1765-1910* (Westport, Conn.: Greenwood Press, 1976). These works address the myriad issues that informed medical professionalization. For an early twentieth-century discussion of the same issues, I utilized G. Markowitz and D. K. Rosner, "Doctors in Crisis: A Study of the Use of Medical Education Reform to Establish Modern Professional Elitism in Medicine," *American Quarterly* 25 (1973): 83-107. And, finally, for insights into society formation, see Philip Van Inger, *The New York Academy of Medicine: Its First Hundred Years* (New York: Columbia University Press, 1949); and James G. Burrow, *Organized Medicine in the Progressive Era: The Move toward Monopoly* (Baltimore: Johns Hopkins University Press, 1977).

A rich literature exists that illuminates nineteenth-century sectarian medicine. Among the most insightful primary sources on homeopathy, the sect, next to hydropathy, that drugged the least, are Samuel Hahnemann, *Organon of the Art of Healing* (New York: Boericks and Tafel, 1976); J. Laurie, M.D., *Homeopathic Domestic Medicine,* (New York: William Radde, 1848); J. S. Douglass, *Practical Homeopathy for the People; Adapted to the Comprehension of the Non-Professional and for Reference by the Young Practitioner, Including a Number of the Most Valuable Remedies* (Milwaukee, Wisc.: Lewis Sherman, 1894); and Edwin Lee, *Hydropathy and Homeopathy Impartially Appreciated with an Appendix of Notes Illustrative of the Influences of the Mind on the Body* (New York: Long, 1848). The strongest interpretive sources include Martin Kaufman, *Homeopathy in America: The Rise and Fall of a Medical Heresy* (Baltimore, Johns Hopkins University Press, 1971); and Harris L. Coulter, "Homeopathic Medicine," in *Ways of Health*, ed. David Sobel (New York: Harcourt Brace Jovanovich, 1979), pp. 289–310. Phrenology, whose leadership and following overlapped a great deal with hydropathy's, also has a deep extant literature, the most instructive of which is Orson Squire Fowler and Lorenzo N. Fowler, *The Illustrated Self-Instructor in Phrenology and Physiology* (New York: Fowler and Wells, 1855). More generally, the volume edited by Guenter Risse, Ronald Numbers, and Judith Leavitt, *Medicine Without Doctors: Home Health Care in American History* (New York: Science History Publications, 1977), is extremely valuable on the subject of self-help/self-doctoring. Water cure was one of several healing sects they address whose ideology was designed and suited for home-care practices.

The separate spheres of nineteenth-century women have been explored in several excellent studies. Those that most informed my research are Barbara Welter, "The Cult of True Womanhood, 1820–1860," *American Quarterly* 28 (Summer 1966): 151–174; Ronald W. Hogelund, "The Female Appendage: Feminine Life-Style in America, 1820–1860," in *Our American Sisters*, ed. Jean E. Friedman and William G. Shade (Boston: Allyn & Bacon, 1973), pp. 133–149; Carroll Smith-Rosenberg, "Beauty, the Beast and the Militant Woman: A Case Study in Sex Roles and Social Stress in Jacksonian America," *American Quarterly* 23 (1972); Gerda Lerner, "The Lady and the Mill Girl: Changes in the Status of Women in the Age of Jackson," in Friedman and Shade, eds., *Our American Sisters*, pp 82–96; Barker-Benfield, *Horrors of the Half-Known Life*, pp. 1–104; Nancy F. Cott, *The Bonds of Womanhood: "Woman's Sphere" in New England, 1780–1835* (New Haven, Conn: Yale University Press, 1977); and William R. Taylor and Christopher Lasch, "Two 'Kindred Spirits': Sorority and Family in New England, 1839–1846," *New England Quarterly* 36, no. 1 (1963): 23–41.

Separate spheres spawned a positive women's culture that included romantic friendships. Interpretive sources that I found especially illuminating include Carroll Smith-Rosenberg, "The Female World of Love and Ritual," *Signs* 1, no. 1 (Autumn 1975): 1–29; Nancy Sahli, "Smashing: Women's Relationships Before the Fall," *Chrysalis* 8 (Summer 1979): 17–27, which describes same-sex crushes and how they became suspect; Blanche Wiesen Cook, "Female Support Networks and Political Activism: Lillian Wald, Crystal Eastman, Emma Goldman," *Chrysalis*, 1977, pp. 43–62; Martha Vicinus, "Distance and Desire: English Boarding School Friendships," *Signs* 9, no. 4 (Summer 1984): 600–622, which discusses "raves"; and Lillian Faderman, "The Enshrinement of Romantic Friendship," and "The Nineteenth-Century," in *Surpassing the Love of Men: Romantic Friendship and Love between Women from the Renaissance to the Present* (New York: Morrow, 1981).

Debate has arisen as to the precise intimate nature of these relationships. This issue is ably discussed by Blanche W. Cook, "The Historical Denial of Lesbianism," *Radical History Review* 20 (1979): 60–65, wherein she responded to Anna Mary Wells's denial of the intimacy between *Miss Marks and Miss Wolley* (Boston: Houghton Mifflin, 1978); Leila J. Rupp, "'Imagine My Surprise': Women's Relationships in Historical Perspective," in *Women and Health in America*, ed. Judith Walzer Leavitt (Madison: University of Wisconsin Press, 1981): 90–102; and Estelle B. Freedman, "Sexuality in Nineteenth-Century America: Behavior, Ideology, and Politics," in *The Promise of American History: Progress and Prospects* ed. Stanley I. Kutler and Stanley N. Katz (Baltimore: Johns Hopkins University Press, 1982), pp. 196–215.

At the turn of the twentieth century, these same-sex bonds became suspect and heterosociality became the norm. I found several sources particularly helpful in understanding this transition: the lesbian history issue of *Frontiers* 4, no. 3 (1979); Adrienne Rich, "Compulsive Heterosexuality and Lesbian Existence," *Signs* 5, no. 4 (Summer 1980): 631–660; Faderman, "The Contributions of the Sexologists," "The Reaction," and "The Twentieth Century," in *Surpassing the Love of Men;* Judge Lindsay, Benjamin Barr, and Wainwright Evans, *The Companionate Marriage* (New York: Boni and Liveright, 1927); Barbara Epstein, "Family, Sexual Morality, and Popular Movements in Turn-of-the Century America," in *Powers of Desire: The Politics of Sexuality*, ed. Christine Stansell and Sharon Thompson (New York: Monthly Review Press, 1983), pp. 117–130; and Ellen Kay Trimberger, "Feminism, Men and Modern Love: Greenwich Village, 1900–1925," in Stansell and Thompson, eds., *Powers of Desire*, pp. 131–152. Three comprehensive survey essays were especially valuable in my consideration of the changing nature of same-sex bonding: Freedman, "Sexuality in Nineteenth-Century America"; Martha Vicinus, "Sexuality and Power: A Review of Current Work in the History of Sexuality," *Feminist Studies* 8 (Spring 1982): 147–151; and Nancy Sahli, "Sexuality in Nineteenth and Twentieth Century America: The Sources and Their Problems," *Radical History Review* 20 (Spring/Summer, 1979): 89–96.

Early sources on hydropathy are numerous. Several that provided both the theory of cure and specific treatments most concisely are Francis Graeter, ed., *Hydriatics: Or Manual of the Water Cure, Especially as Practiced by Vincent Priessnitz in Grafenberg, Compiled and Translated from the Writings of Charles Munde, Dr. Oertel, Dr. Bernhard Hirschel, and other Eye-Witnesses and Practitioners*, 3d ed. (New York: William Radde, 1843); Robert May Graham, M.D., *Graefenberg; or, a True Report of the Water-Cure, with an Account of Its Antiquity (1844);* John King, M.D., *Observations on Hydropathy, or, the Cold Water Cure . . . as Witnessed by the Author During His Residence at Grafenberg, Silesia, Austria* (London: Madden, 1835); John Gibbs, *Letters from Graefenberg, in the Years 1843, 1844, 1845, & 1846; with the Report . . . of the Enniscorthy*

Hydropathic Society (London: Charles Gilpin, 1847); John Balbirnie, *The Water-Cure in Consumption,* 3d ed. (London: Longman, Brown, Green, Longmans, and Roberts, 1856); Manby Gully, *The Water Cure in Chronic Disease* (New York: Wiley & Putnam, 1846); Joel Shew, *The Hydropathic Family Physician* (New York: Fowler and Wells, 1855); and Joel Shew, *Hydropathy; or, the Water-Cure: Its Principles, Modes of Treatment* (New York: Wiley and Putnam, 1845). An invaluable secondary source on hydropathy is Harry B. Weiss and Howard R. Kemble, *The Great American Water-Cure Craze: A History of Hydropathy in the United States* (Trenton, N.J.: Past Times Press, 1967).

Sources expounding the philosophy of water cure addressed issues including leading a hydropathic life, the nature of disease, the role of nature and hygiene in curing disease, and therapeutics for specific populations. Among those I found most instructive are Russell Thacher Trall, *The Hydropathic Encyclopedia* (New York: Fowler and Wells, 1852); James Caleb Jackson, *How to Treat the Sick Without Medicine* (Dansville, N.Y.: 1874); Thomas L. Nichols, *An Introduction to the Water-Cure* (New York: Fowler and Wells, 1850); and Joel Shew, M.D., *Children, Their Hydropathic Management in Health and Disease a Descriptive and Practical Work, Designed as a Guide for Families and Physicians* (New York: Fowler and Wells, 1852). Articles from the *Water-Cure Journal* were numerous and are of inestimable use on these themes. Those I relied on most frequently were: Roland S. Houghton, "Hygiene and Hydropathy," 10, no. 2 (August 1850): 33–40; Theodosia Gilbert, "Let Nature and Capacity Control," 12, no. 3 (September 1851): 56–57; "Philosophy of Water-Cure," 19, no. 1 (January 1855): 2; H.V.H., "What Is Hygeopathy?" 22, no. 5 (November 1856): 102; "What Is Disease?" 23, no. 6 (June 1857): 13–14; and "The Water-Cure Explained," 28, no. 3 (September 1859): 44.

Water-Cure Journal sources that were particularly helpful in illuminating the therapeutic and philosophical basis for the hydropathic rejection of allopathic therapeutics include E. Gervis, "Hemorrhage from Leech-Bites," 3, no. 1 (January 1847): 25–26. Reprinted from the *London Lancet:* "Swallowed a Leech," 9, no. 3 (March 1850): 89. Reprinted from the *Sunday Dispatch:* E. Potter, M.D., "Isn't It Murder?" 14, no. 5 (November 1852): 116. Also, "The Doctor's 'Occupation Gone'—A Healthy Country," 16, no. 5 (November 1853): 110; R. T. Trall, "Allopathic Midwifery," 9, no. 4 (April 1850): 121–123; and B.S., "Bleeding during Pregnancy," 22, no. 4 (October 1856): 89.

Hydropathic authors, particularly scornful of the allopathic conceptualization and management of women's physiology, stressed what they termed the "naturalness" of women's physiology. Texts and articles that I found lent particular insight into this position were Mrs. M. L. Shew, *Water-Cure for Ladies* (New York, 1844); and R. T. Trall, M.D., *Sexual Physiology: A Scientific and Popular Exposition of the Fundamental Problems in Sociology* (London: Health Promotion, Ludgate Hill, 1861).

And from the *Water-Cure Journal*, Joel Shew, M.D., "Pregnancy And Childbirth," 2, no. 5 (August 1, 1846): 72; Mrs. O.C.W., "Childbirth—A Contrast," 11, no. 4 (April 1851): 88; "Water Cure Mothers and Water-Cure Babies Have Little Need of Doctors," 16, no. 2 (August 1853): 36; Joel Shew, M.D., "Twelve Cases in Midwifery with Details of Treatment," 11, no. 3 (March 1851): 64, and 11, no. 5 (May 1851) for the second half of "Twelve Cases"; T. L. Nichols, M.D., "The Curse Removed," 10, no. 5 (November 1850): 167–173; "Bathing to Be Practiced during the Time of Menstruation—Treatment in Suppressed and Painful Menstruation," 1, no. 3 (January 1, 1846): 43–45. See also R. T. Trall, *Pathology of the Reproductive Organs; Embracing All Forms of Sexual Disorders* (Boston: B. Leverett Emerson, 1863); and Ellen H. Goodell, M.D., "The Cause of Female Diseases," *Herald of Health* 4, no. 3 (September 1864): 95–96.

Allopathic sentiment against hydropaths, conversely, was clearly articulated in the following issues of the *Water-Cure Journal:* 9, no. 1 (January 1850): 5–9, wherein Trall responds to charges of hydropathic quackery; 24, no. 4 (October 1857): 85, wherein the allopaths ridiculed the Hydropathic College; 26, no. 6 (December 1858): 89, which describes the unfair treatment given water-cure graduates by allopaths; and 28, no. 3 (September 1859): 41, wherein allopaths claim hydropathy is waning.

The titling and format of the *Water-Cure Journal* underwent several changes each of which reflects a notable philosophical shift. The *American Periodicals Index* (pp. 99–100) lists the name changes as follows (although discrepancies emerge on the actual microfilm): *Water-Cure Journal*, December 1845–December 1861; *Hygienic Teacher and Water-Cure Journal*, January–December 1862; *Herald of Health*, January 1864–December 1867 and July 1869–December 1892; *Health*, September 1900–December 1903, January 1905–December 1906, January 1907–December 1909, and January 1910–December 1913.

Index

Abortion, 58–59, 157, 195n.52, 236; hydropathic views on, 58
Activists, women at the live-in cures, 141–142, 157
Adams Nervine Asylum, Jamaica Plain, Mass., 151
Advertising, 77, 79–80, 83, 91, 103, 137–138, 142, 166, 199n.4, 215n.2
Ailments, 42, 44, 46, 51, 80; nervousness, 37
Alcohol, 42, 48, 120–123, 127, 166, 211n.85, 229; consumption, women, 122; in medication, 6–7, 121–123, 211n.85. *See also* Patent medicine
Alcoholism, therapy, 211n.86
Alcott, Bronson, 95
Alcott, William Andrus, 13, 118–119, 183n.61
Allen, Dr. Huldah, 71
Allopathic: associations, 232; instruction in, 22, 168; licensing, hydropathic views on, 101; physicians, conversion to hydropathic practice, 81; professionalization, 7; views on female physiology. *See also* Hydropathy, allopathic attitudes toward; Philosophy, allopathic; Physicians, allopathic; Physiology, sexual, female, allopathic views of
Allopathy, 29, 34–35, 43, 51, 53, 60, 65, 69, 71, 101; costs of, 89, 203n.70; education for, 7–8, 168; exclusionary tactics of, 69, 168, 224n.40, 236; hydropathic responses to, 168; hydropathic attitudes toward, 85, 103; low status of, 7; popularity of, 7, 28; sects' attitudes toward, 11–13, 15; standards in, 232; status of, 7, 232; and women's exclusion, 197n.92

American Anti-Tobacco Society, 121–122
American costume, 48, 94, 115–116, 130, 156
American Health and Temperance Association, 116
American Hydropathic Institute (N.Y.C.), 70, 72, 99, 112, 208n.22. *See also* Hygeio-Therapeutic College
American Hydropathic Society, 26, 100, 205n.123
American Hygienic and Hydropathic Association of Physicians and Surgeons, 100, 112, 206n.128. *See also* American Hydropathic Society
American Medical Association, 168, 170–171, 197n.87; legislative committee of, 170; membership in, 170
American Phrenological Journal, 14
American Physiological Society, 14
American Vegetarian Convention, 119
American Vegetarian Society, 112, 119
Anthony, Susan B., 81–82, 95, 120, 131, 152
Antisepsis, 172
Apprenticeship, hydropathic, 72, 93, 102
Arnot-Ogden Hospital, 93
Athol (Mass.) Water-Cure, 76, 102; Southard House, 95–97
Austen, Jane, 148
Austin, Dr. Harriet N., 72, 82, 94, 102, 115, 130, 133–134, 155–156, 204n.95
Autonomy, female, 68, 87, 139, 147, 157

Bacon, Delia, 149, 218n.48
Bacteriology, 172
Bandages, 39, 46, 61, 145, 148

237

Barrenness, 64, 145
Barton, Clara, 115, 155–156, 219n.76
Baruch, Simon, 165, 174
Bath: brine, 104; cabinet, 104; cold, 37; douche, 37, 63, 148, 153; electro-chemical, 104; electro-thermal, 104; eye, 39; foot, 39; half, 37, 45, 63; hand, 39; head, 39, 64, 195n.63; hip, 45, 55; plunge, 37–38, 60, 148; pouring, 37; Roman, 104; Russian, 104; shallow, 37; sitz, 37, 39, 55, 60–63, 144–145, 153; sponge, 63; sulphur, 104; tub, 104; Turkish, 96, 104; vapor, 151; warm, 62; wave, 144
Bathing, 37, 62, 236; frequent, 174; geriatric, 62; home, 36–37; as sport, 35
Baths, 21; home, 36
Battle Creek Reform Club, 116
Battle Creek (Mich.) Sanitarium, 153, 204n.96
Battle Creek Toasted Corn Flake Company, 209n.45
Beard, Dr. Ellen, 91
Bedortha, Dr. (Troy, N.Y.), 119, 205n.123
Beecher, Catharine, 81, 144, 148, 150–151, 215n.2, 218n.48
Beecher, Henry Ward, 68, 121, 143
Beecher, James, 81
Beecher, Thomas, 81, 150
Bell, John, 20, 36
Bell, Louisa, 67
Bellevue Hospital Medical School, 116
Bigarel, L. H., 134
Bigelow, Dr., 63
Bingham, Nathaniel, 94
Binghamton (N.Y.) Water Cure, 79. See also Mount Prospect Medical Institute of Binghamton and inebriate asylum (N.Y.), Mount Prospect Water Cure (Binghamton, N.Y.)
Birth control, 13, 54, 57–59
Blacks, 14, 45
Blackwell, Elizabeth, 22, 68–69, 231
Blanket pack, 37–38
Bloomer, Mrs. Amelia, 120, 131, 133
Bloomers, 66, 127, 129, 131, 137–138
Boarding houses, vegetarian, 119
Bodily balance, 6–8, 11–12, 23, 25, 29, 38, 44, 54
Bonding, female, 112, 115, 126–127, 136, 146, 153, 155, 157–158, 180n.28, 214–215n.1, 233
Bonding, heterosexual, 163
"Boston marriage," 147, 152–154, 157, 218n.63
Boston Medical and Surgical Journal, 111, 167
Boston Quarterly Review, 54
Bowels, 48, 55, 60, 62
Brattleboro (Vt.) Water-Cure, 82, 112, 143–144, 148–149
Brewster, Capt., 83
Brightside, 155. See also Dansville (N.Y.) Water Cure; Jackson Health Resort (Jackson Sanitorium); "Our Home on the Hillside"
Brisbane, Albert, 112
Brown, Dr. Agnes, L., 95
Brown, Dr. Fanny Hurd, 93
Brown, Hattie B. L., 155, 219n.76, 220n.85
Brown, Dr. William E., 219n.76
Bryant, Mollie, 67
Buffalo University School of Dentistry, 93
Bungay, C. W., 75
"Burned-Over District" (N.Y.), 76
Burns, 15, 39, 44, 47
Butler, Lady Eleanor, 147

Campbell, David, 25
Case, Dr. Mary Ann, 72
Castleton (Vt.) Medical College, 92
Central Park Water Cure (N.Y.C.), 113
Charisma, 52, 90, 92, 94, 97, 104, 115, 149, 150, 155, 218n.46, 219n.76
Charismatic healers, 31
Charity, 84, 88, 90, 107, 143
Child care, 67
Childbearing, 10, 143, 147
Childbirth, 8, 11, 59–62, 145, 236; hydropathic care in, 61
Childrearing, 143, 169
Children, 25, 34, 47, 52, 55, 57, 62, 66, 68, 83, 117, 121, 142, 166, 229, 236; education of, 183n.61; and hygiene, 67; unwanted, 58
Chiropractic medicine. See Medicine, chiropractic
Cincinnati Eclectic Medical College, 71
Civil War, attitudes toward, 124, 160, 162–163
Clairvoyance, 15, 31
Claridge, R. T., 23
Clark, Albert, 98
Clark, Dr. Nancy Talbot, 68
Clarke, Dr. Edward H., 10
Class enmity, 128
Clemens, Samuel, 81
Clemens, Mrs. Samuel, 81
Clergy, 81, 111
"Clergyman's price," 86, 90
Clientele, female (at water cures), 139, 154; solicitation of, 142, 215n.2
Clients, recreational, 30, 105, 107, 222n.13, 227n.71; present-day, 226n.71
Coale, Dr. W. E., 127
Coffee, 42, 120–121, 138
Coggswell, Dr., 72
Colfax, Schuyler, Vice-President, U.S., 81
Combe, Dr. Andrew W., 111, 118
Combe, George, 14
Communalism, 17, 21, 172, 184n.1, 220n.85, 226n.64
Community/culture, female, 142, 153, 156–158, 214–215n.1, 220n.85
Community, supportive female, 150, 154–156

Companionship, female, 142, 149, 151–152, 154, 157–158, 233
Conflicts, water-cure philosophy vs. practitioners' methods, 77, 80, 83, 102, 165, 172, 208n.33
Conklin, J. B., 113
Conklin, Dr. William D., 75
Consumerism, 171, 173
Conversion, narratives of, 21, 27, 34, 40, 44, 46–49, 69, 73, 76, 101, 106, 130, 156, 186n.18, 201n.43, 207n.6.
"Conversion" of allopathic physicians to hydropathy, 24, 34, 47. See also Physicians, allopathic, conversion to hydropathic practice
Coronaro, Luigi, 11
Corset, 14, 66, 116, 126–127
Cost-of-living, 87, 202n.58, 203n.66
Costs, comparative, hydropathic/allopathic, 90
Costs/economic accessibility, hydropathic, 16, 84
Cox, Samuel, Congressman, 81
Crisis, 23, 38, 44, 51
Criticism, allopathic, hydropathic response to, 167, 223n.33, 224n.35
Cross-class aspects, 8, 9, 11, 15–16, 24, 30, 36, 44–46, 53, 57–58, 67, 79, 83–85, 87–88, 90, 92, 107, 123, 128, 134, 157, 160, 163, 171, 179n.23, 201n.43, 205n.123
Cross-dressing, 132, 146, 213n.121
Cuba (N.Y.) Water Cure, 92
Cultural construction, 9–11, 16, 181n.34
Culture: changes in, 169; changing opportunities for, 172; consumer-oriented, 160, 220n.1; devaluation of, 162; female, 12, 162, 173, 233
Cummings, Dr. J. A., 98, 205n.114
Cures, bone manipulation in, 210n.49. See also Medicine, chiropractic
Currie, James, 20

Daily Hampshire Gazette, 78, 98, 219n.76
Daily role, women's, 2, 136, 141–142, 151, 154, 157, 162, 173, 183n.63, 213n.128, 216n.17, 221n.7, 233
Dangers of water-cure treatments, 150
Dansville Advertiser, 105
Dansville Herald, 204n.95
Dansville (N.Y.) Water Cure, 30, 52, 76, 86–88, 94, 100, 102, 105, 107, 115, 130, 145, 155–157, 163, 165, 171, 199n.4, 204n.95, 219n.76. See also Jackson Health Resort (Jackson Sanitorium); "Our Home on the Hillside"
Daughters, 66–67
Davis, Paulina Wright, 13, 82, 111, 133
Demorest, Madame, 127
Denniston, Dr. E. E., 98, 205n.123

Denniston's Water Cure (Springdale, Northampton, Mass.), 98
Dexter, Dr., 98, 205n.114
Diet, 13, 21–22, 27, 42–43, 46–48, 51–52, 55–56, 60–61, 63–64, 66, 75, 82, 90, 102–104, 106, 110–116, 118, 128, 134, 148, 153, 156, 174, 183n.57, 192n.134, 209n.45, 216n.17, 227n.71
Digestion, 118–119
Discharge, 6–7, 15, 51, 151
Disease, 6, 42; acute, 23, 63; arthritis, 174; of bowels, 37, 51, 63; brain, congestion, 49; exhaustion, 166; bronchitis, 45; cancer, 152; cancer, skin, 93; cardiac, 151–152, 174; catarrh, 78; causes of, 32; cholera, 170; colic, 63; congestion, 38; constipation, 62; contagious, 28; cutaneous eruption, 45; diarrhea, 63; diphtheria, 170; dysentery, 34; dysmenorrhea, 62, 145; dyspepsia, 42–43, 49, 63, 118, 128; earache, 15; eye, 215n.2; fever, 5, 15, 20, 23, 37–39, 43, 46–47, 67; fever, puerperal, 62; fever, scarlet, 44, 47; fever, typhoid, 170; gout, 151; headache, 34, 44, 46, 48, 82; hemorrhage, 47; hemorrhage, uterine, 63; hemorrhoids, 43, 45–46; hepatitis, 46; hereditary, 54; hookworm, 170; indigestion, 47; inflammation, 62; leukorrhea, 65–66, 145; liver, 45; locomotor disability, 174; nervous, 37, 44, 46, 49, 65, 104, 117, 206n.136, 226n.65; neuralgia, 78, 144; neurasthenia, 146, 151, 195n.63; ovaritis, 65, 145; paralysis, 105, 148–150; psora (the itch), 12; psychosomatic, 44, 64, 141, 149, 152, 230; rheumatism, 24, 37, 46, 78, 105, 174, 219n.76; scrofula, 51, 78, 84; smallpox, 170; spinal, 37, 105, 117, 146, 151; throat and lung, 78, 83; treatment of, 44; tuberculosis, 146, 170; tumors, 37; venereal, 55; women's, 2, 51, 53, 73, 142, 215n.2, 229–230, 236; women's, allopathic management of, hydropathic views on, 53; women's, hydropathic treatment, 73–74
Disorders, sexual, 126
Dispensary, 92–93
Ditch, Rosa Ann, 137
Doctrines, hygienic, 7
Domestic relations between the sexes, 166
Domestic role, men's, hydropathic views of, 68; women's, hydropathic view of, 67–68
Domestic sphere, of women, 72–73; 125–126, 230
Douglass, Frederick, 95
Doyle, Dr. Gertrude Davies, 93
Doyle, Dr. John C., 93
Dress, allopathic ladies, 127
Dress reform, 13–15, 42, 48, 53, 62, 65–66, 70, 82, 94, 102, 110–111, 115–116, 125–127, 132, 139, 156, 166, 204n.95
Drugs, 7, 12–13, 16, 22, 29, 32–35, 44, 47, 55,

66, 70, 93, 103, 106, 123, 146, 148, 165, 167, 174, 179n.20, 182n.50, 192n.134, 229, 232
Dunton, Delos, 135

Easthampton (Mass.) Water Cure, 51, 86, 95, 98, 105
Eclectic College, 92
Eclecticism, 12, 69, 91, 103, 170, 182n.49
Economic support, solicitation of male, 88
Education, allopathic, 22; general, women's, 10, 14, 148–150; hydropathic, 70, 92, 95, 99–100, 104, 165, 205n.113, 208n.22, 225n.56; hydropathic, gender ratios, 72, 91; medical, gender ratios, hydropathic views of, 71; need for, 55–56, 121; physical, 117; of public, 165. *See also* Sex education
Electrical cure. *See* Therapeutics, electrical
Elmira College, Elmira, N.Y., 93
Elmira (N.Y.) Water Cure (Gleason Sanitarium, Gleason Health Resort), 67, 72, 76–78, 80–82, 86–87, 92–94, 102–104, 107, 126, 130, 142, 165, 171, 215n.2
Emancipationist/"feminist" ideology, 18, 70, 73, 80, 126, 132, 142, 161, 198n.108, 200n.16, 212n.97, 221n.5, 233
Empiricist, 170
Enema, 48, 59, 60–62
Enslavement, female, 58
Entertainment/activities at the cures, 143–144, 163, 215n.13, 222n.12
Eroticism, same sex, 145–146, 154, 215n.1, 216n.23, 217n.31, 233
Exercise, 2, 5, 15, 21–22, 50–51, 55–56, 60, 64–65, 79, 103, 114, 116, 128–130, 148–149, 153, 173–174; in water, 173; as therapy, 5

Facilities, separate, live-in cures, 79
Faith cure, 19, 31, 76
Farmers, female, 134
Farming, hygienic, 134–135, 139
Fear, Dr. Elizabeth, 95
Fees, 84, 86–88, 90–91, 107
Female: relationships with, 9, 146–147, 149, 152, 217n.31, 218n.46, 218n.63; sphere, 2, 5, 8–9, 13–14, 18, 53, 65–66, 72, 110, 125, 132, 151, 161, 173, 180n.27, 181n.31, 182n.41, 198n.108, 212n.97, 216n.25, 233; "world," 9, 180n.28, 214n.1, 233
Female complaints. *See* Diseases, women's
Female Medical College of Pennsylvania, 71
Femininity, 126, 131–132, 204n.95, 233
Field, Dr., 97
Flexner, Abraham, 225n.56
Floyer, John, 19
Food, 45, 47, 55; preparation of, 119; recipes for, 43, 118
Forest City (N.Y.) Water Cure, 92

Fowler, Lorenzo N., 14, 25, 46, 111, 123, 205n.123, 233
Fowler, Orson Squire, 14–15, 25, 99, 110–111, 207n.6, 233
Fowler, Mrs. Orson Squire, 15
Fowlers and Wells (publishing house, N.Y.C.), 25–26, 114, 138
Franke, H. F., 151, 224n.38
Franklin Democrat, 131
Franklin Water-Cure and Physiological School (Winchester, Tenn.), 100
"Free love," 113, 166, 208
Freez, Solomon, 47
French, Dr. Martha, 77, 91
Freud, Sigmund, 173, 226n.65
Friendship, female, 1, 145–147, 155–156; romantic, 9, 147–150, 152–153, 158, 215n.1, 216n.26, 217n.31, 233
Frothingham, Rev. O. B., 67

Gadgetry, pseudo-medical, 166
Gall, Franz Joseph, 14
Garrison, William Lloyd, 96, 121
Gender consciousness, 69, 77, 91–92, 102, 132–133, 139, 142, 157–159, 161, 171–172, 181n.31, 203n.81
Gender ratios: at the cures, 2, 16, 77, 142; among hydropathic leaders, 117
Geneva (N.Y.) Medical College, 69
Georgia Citizen, 130
Germ theory of disease, 93, 171–172
Gervis, E., 33
Gibbs, John, 24
Gilbert, Theodosia, 114, 129
Gleason, Adele A., 93, 215n.2
Gleason, Rachel Brooks, 67, 72, 78, 81, 92–93, 103–105, 126, 130, 142, 166, 215n.2
Gleason, Silas O., 67, 77–78, 81, 92–93, 103–105, 130, 205n.123
Gleason Sanitarium, Gleason Health Resort. *See* Elmira (N.Y.) Water Cure
Glen Haven Water Cure, 30, 90, 92, 94, 114, 120, 129–130
Goodell, Dr. Ellen H., 66, 68
Gospel of Health, 116
Gove, Hiram, 111
Gove Nichols, Mary, 13, 36–38, 44, 54–56, 60, 62–63, 66, 70–72, 99, 111–115, 119, 130–133, 166, 193n.15, 208n.24
Graeter, Francis, 21
Grafenberg, Silesia, 21–24, 69, 114, 186
Graham, Robert May, 23
Graham, Sylvester, 54, 110–112, 118–119, 183
Graham Journal of Health and Longevity, 13
Granger, Lyman, 94
Grant, Ulysses, S., President, U.S., 81
Granula, 94, 115, 156
Gray, M. W., 205n.123, 219n.76
Greeley, Horace, 115, 120–121

Greenwood Spring Water Cure (Cuba, N.Y.), 114
Gully, Dr. James Manby, 29

Habit, reform, 29, 47, 56, 65–66
Habits, personal, 2, 11, 16–17, 22, 27, 35, 42, 48, 65–66, 74, 85, 90, 93, 153, 166, 174
Hahn, Dr. John Sigmund, 23
Hahnemann, Samuel, 12, 27, 232
Hale, Mrs. Sarah J., 14, 71
Hall, Dr. C. A., 98, 205n.114
Halsted, Dr., 99, 105, 149, 215n.2
Hayes, P. H., 64
Healers, unorthodox, efficacy of, 184–185n.2
Healing: goals of, 188n.57; hygienic, 92; male, mystical, 21, 24; natural, 18; participation in, 8, 179n.24; system of, 4–6, 17, 35, 45, 184n.1, 186n.18. See also Nature as healer
Health, 6, 66, 106, 110, 117, 165, 168–169, 174–175, 195n.69; men's 16; military, 125; public, 170–171; reform in the South, 124
Health Journal and Advocate of Physiological Reform, 111
Health Journal and Independent Magazine, 111
Health Reformer, 116
Herald of Health, 28, 85, 114, 124, 165, 215n.2, 223n.25; circulation of, 188n.45
Herald of Health (England), 208
Hero, Butler Wilmarth, 97
Hero, George Hoyt, 97
Hero, Dr. J. H., 48, 96
Hero Cough Syrup Co., 97
Herrick, Dr. Jessie, 93
Heterosexuality, 154, 216n.25, 217n.36, 221n.9
Heterosocial, 161–162, 234
Higgins, Dr., 75
Historiography, medical, 3–4, 231; hydropathic, 4–5, 235
Holbrook, Dr. M. L., 27, 71, 134, 165
Holmes, Dr. Jacob, 96
Home management, hydropathic views on, 67–68
Home self-care/doctoring. See Self-doctoring
"Home Voices: Extracts from Letters," 47
Homeopathic News, 165
Homeopaths, 43, 69–70
Homeopathy, 5, 12–13, 27, 53, 70, 103, 106, 182n.50, 210n.49, 232–233; popularity of, 8, 12, 182n.51
Homosocial, 92, 145–146, 154, 161–162, 214n.1, 217n.31, 218n.46, 228n.85, 233
Hospitals, 93; allopathic, cholera, 168; for women only, 92, 171
Houghton, N., 205n.123
Howe, Julia Ward, 82
Howe, Dr. Samuel Gridley, 82
Howells, William Dean, 95

Howes, Mercy P., 63
Hoyt, Dr. George, 96, 102, 113
Hull, Jane V., 46
Hunt, Harriet, 68
Hurd, F. Wilson, 94
Hutchinson, Dr. Clarabell M., 93
Hydropathic College and Institute (Loretta, Pa.), 100, 167
Hydropathists, 27; women as, 71–72
Hydropathy: allopathic attitudes toward, 3, 27, 167–168, 223n.33, 236; appeal of, 29, 48, 142; conversion to, 26–27; domestic practice of, 26, 47; early response to, 24; heroic, 151; interpretations of, 5, 178n.10, 179n.17; and laws, 55–56, 59, 66; popularity of, 3, 8, 15, 35, 46, 106–107, 159, 224n.35; in the South, 124; theory of, 18, 21, 23, 25, 39, 42, 95, 234. See also Self-doctoring
Hydrotherapy, 5, 173, 209n.39, 226n.71
Hygeio-Therapeutic College (Trall's), 116, 138
Hygeio-Therapeutic Cure (Trall's), 49
Hygiene, personal, 13, 36, 166, 174; sexual, 13, 110
Hygienic care, 16; doctrines of, 7; laws of, 36, 95, 109–110, 156; in living, 2, 6, 12–16, 28–29, 32, 35, 42–43, 48, 58, 60, 65, 108, 111, 114–115, 123, 171, 183n.57, 235–236; medication in, 25–26; principles of, 15, 32, 165; writings on, 11
Hygienic Teacher and Water-Cure Journal, 208n.29
Hypnotism, 5, 14–15, 69, 76, 152
Hysteria, 64–65, 145–146, 151, 230

Ideals, cultural, changing, 154, 160–161, 163, 169, 173, 175, 219n.74, 220n.1, 226n.64, 232, 234
Ideology, hydropathic, as retreat, 74, 107
Individualism, 17, 45, 173–174, 184n.1, 220n.1, 226n.64
Infirmity, female, 131, 142, 149, 151–152
Innovations, therapeutic, 106; hydropathic exclusion, 172; medical, 170, 172; scientific, 169, 172
Insane asylums, 36, 39, 149
Insanity, 64, 111, 154, 195n.63
Institutions/organizations, women only, 171
Intellect, female, 10, 14, 68, 74, 133, 136, 139, 230
Invalidism, female, 15–16
Inventors, female, 133, 139
Ithaca Chronicle, 123

Jackson, James, A., 163
Jackson, Dr. James Caleb, 1, 30, 32–33, 48, 52, 85, 92, 94, 102, 105, 114–115, 120, 130, 155–156, 201n.43, 204n.96, 213n.110, 219n.76
Jackson, Mrs. James Caleb ("Mother Jackson"), 94

Jackson, Dr. Kate J., 95
Jackson Health Resort (Jackson Sanitorium), 75, 95, 219n.76, 220n.85, 222n.12. *See also* Dansville (N.Y.) Water Cure; "Our Home on the Hillside"
Jacobi, Mary Putnam, 231
James, Alice, 151
James, Henry, 151–152, 218n.63
James, Henry, Sr., 218n.62
James, William, 151–152
Jansen, Dr., 91
Jenks, Mary, 51–52
Johnson, Fanny B., 1, 52, 88, 219n.76, 220n.85
Johnson, Howard, 48
Johnson, Nancy, 149–150
Journal of Health, Water Cure and Human Progress, 113

Kellogg, John, 99, 116
Kellogg, Mrs. John, 116
Kellogg, Dr. John Harvey, 94, 115, 117, 153, 165, 195n.63, 204n.96, 209n.42
Kellogg, Julia, 131
Kellogg, Merritt, 99
Kellogg, W. K., 117, 209n.45
King, Dr. John, 24
Kittredge, E. A., 205n.123
Kneipp (cold-water) treatment, 173
Knickerbocker (monthly), 24
Krafft-Ebing, Richard von, 145–146, 216n.23

Laboratory, clinical, 172
Ladies' Home Journal, 122
"Ladies of Llangollen," 147
Ladies Magazine, 14
Ladies Medical Missionary Society, 71
Ladies' physiological institutes, 12
Laight Street (N.Y.C.) Water Cure, 75, 77, 130
Lamson, Phoebe, 116
Lay, Horatio S., 116
Leadership, hydropathic, 166; discrediting of, 166–167
Lebanon Springs (N.Y.) Water Cure, 40, 112
Leeches, 33–34
Leffingwell, Albert J., 95
Leisure, 160, 162–163, 220n.1, 221n.9, 222n.10, 222n.13
Lesbianism, 145–147, 152–153, 161, 216n.23, 217n.31, 218n.46, 234; changing attitudes toward, 161; historical debate over, 233–234
Letter Box, 76–77, 204n.95
Lewis, Dio, 117
Licensing, hydropathic, 100–101, 164, 166, 205n.122
Licht, Dr. Sidney, 173
Life-cycle, female, physiological, 54, 230
The Lily, 71, 133
Lind, Jenny, 83

Lines, Dr. Amelia W., 72
Literature, prescriptive, 8, 230; effects of, 230–231
Literature/texts, hydropathic, 164–167
Live-in cures, 30, 82; gender ratios at, 91, 198n.2, 199n.4, 220n.85
Lonely hearts, 137–138
Longevity. *See* Water cures, longevity of
Loring, Katharine Peabody, 152
Lydia Pinkham Vegetable Compound, 122

Magnetism, 105–106
Malthusian doctrine, 59
Mann, Horace, 113
Marks, Jeannette, 153–154, 219n.70
Marriage, 9, 67–68, 92, 110, 112–113, 133, 136, 138–139, 145–146, 157, 167, 183n.63, 208n.24; companionate, 234
Massachusetts General Hospital, 63
Massachusetts Institute of Technology, 170
Massage, 37–38, 55, 114, 145, 150–151, 164, 166, 174, 210n.49, 227n.71
Masturbation, 54–55, 111, 145
"Matrimonial correspondence," 131, 136–139
May, Carrie, 40
Medical care delivery, hydropathic exclusion, 169
Medical News, 167
Medication, hygienic, 33, 165
Medicine, 4, 8, 10–11, 53, 93, 103, 167, 169, 170, 182n.41, 185n.2, 209n.39, 232; botanic, 11, 47, 69; chiropractic, 5, 210n.49; as cultural organizing tool, 169–170; domestic, 233; historiography of, 3; hydropathic rejection of, 167; goals of, 188; preventive, 35, 54, 65, 84, 174; professionalization of, 232; reasons for ascendancy, 167–173, 224n.40, 225n.56, 229, 233; sectarian, 232–233. *See also* Sports medicine
Memnonia Institute (Yellow Springs, Ohio), 113
Menopause, 8, 11
Menstruation, 8, 10–11, 46, 56–58, 62, 192n.134, 195n.52, 236
Mesmerism. *See* Hypnotism
Michigan, University of, 93, 116
Middle class, 45. *See also* Cross-class aspects
Midwifery, 25, 61. *See also* Childbearing; Childbirth
Midwives, male, 71
Miller, E. P., 39, 43, 48
Minnesota Hygeio-Therapeutic College, 100, 114
Mitchell, S. Weir, 104; and rest cure, 206n.136
Mobility, women's, 141
Moderation, 11–12, 14, 22, 30, 32, 35, 182n.42
Modern Times (community), N.Y., 113
Monroe, Sallie M., 132
Moral Reformer and Teacher on the Human Constitution, The, 13

Morphine, 122
Mortality, infant, 170
Mortimer, Mary, 150
Motherhood, scientific, 13
Mothers, as reformers/healers, 14, 66, 236
Mount Holyoke College, 153
Mount Prospect Medical Institute of Binghamton, and inebriate asylum (N.Y.), 165. See also Mount Prospect Water Cure (Binghamton, N.Y.)
Mount Prospect Water Cure (Binghamton, N.Y.), 76–77, 86, 91, 101–102, 130, 165. See also Mount Prospect Medical Institute of Binghamton, and inebriate asylum (N.Y.)
Movement therapy, 105–106, 117
Mysticism, 31, 186n.18

National Dress Reform Convention, 130
National Health Convention, 213n.110
National Intelligencer, 219n.76
National Temperance Convention, 123
Natural healers, women as, 49, 54, 66, 88, 133, 171, 185n.4
Nature as healer, 11, 13, 15–16, 18, 21, 23, 34, 59, 62, 69, 109, 123, 142, 235. See also Healing, natural
"Nature": male and/or female, 9–10, 66, 70–71, 73, 126, 133, 139, 161–162, 171, 181n.35, 221n.7, 230; changing beliefs about, 234
Nerve force, 10, 32, 104
Nervous system, 37, 120–121
Nervousness, 29, 64–65, 148–149, 151–153, 173, 195n.63
Network, domestic, female, 9; female support of, 142, 146, 149, 161, 180n.28, 233; and reform, 13–14, 16, 91, 94, 109–113, 115, 117–119, 123–124, 134, 136, 138–139, 167, 184n.69, 204n.96, 207n.6, 208n.24, 213n.110
New Jersey Hydropathic Collegiate Institute, South Orange, 100
New Malvern (Mass.) Water Cure, 96
New York City Water Cure, 130. See also Laight Street (N.Y.C.) Water Cure
New York City Water Cure Institution, 43
New York Dietetic Reform Association, 119
New York Hydropathic College, 91. See also New York Hygeio-Therapeutic College
New York Hydropathic School, 111. See also New York Hygeio-Therapeutic College
New York Hygeio-Therapeutic College, 99, 114
New York Infirmary for Women, 69
New York Observer, 24
New York Tribune, 150, 224n.35
New York Vegetarian Society, 119
Nichols, Mary Gove. See Gove Nichols, Mary
Nichols, Thomas Low, 35, 42, 61–62, 70,
99–101, 112–114, 119–120, 145, 166, 168, 206n.125, 208nn.22–24,28
North, Dr. J. H., 77, 91
Northampton Herald, 79
Northampton (Mass.) Water Cure, 80, 86, 89, 102, 200n.14
Northampton (Mass.) Water Cure Infirmary, 200n.14
Nurses, 48, 89, 95, 154, 174
Nursing, 71, 150, 215n.2, 232

Oberlin College, 92
Occupation, changes in, 169; female, 88, 134, 141, 157
Occupational groups, wages, 83, 86–87
Organizations, allopathic, 232; vegetarian, 119
Organizations, hydropathic, 205n.123, 206n.125; costs of, 101; membership in, 101
Orgasm, 57, 145
Ossoli, Margaret Fuller, 133
Osteopathy, 210n.49
"Our Home on the Hillside," 95, 115, 155. See also Dansville (N.Y.) Water Cure; Jackson Health Resort (Jackson Sanitorium)
Out-patient service, hydropathic, 42, 89

Passionlessness, 57, 147, 194n.31, 217n.31
Passions, emotional and sexual moderation of, 22, 42, 48, 55–56, 64, 110
Pasteur, Louis, 172
Patent medicine, 7, 121–122. See also Alcohol, in medication
Pathology, 172
Patient autonomy, 2, 15–17, 29, 31–32, 35, 44, 48, 52–53, 89, 101, 164
Patient passivity, 28, 33, 35, 40, 65, 152; female, 10, 74, 206n.136
Patient-machine dyad, 222n.18
Patients, types of, 53, 73, 75, 77–78, 80–83, 85, 90, 107, 115, 156–157, 163, 200n.16, 219n.76; changes in, 163
Pediatrics, 174
Pelvic displacement, 215n.2
Penfield, Harriet, 40
Pennell, Mr., 94
Perfectibility, human, 17, 159, 160
Perfection, bodily, 159, 175
Perkins, F. B., 35
Personality, water-cure physicians'. See Charisma
Petition, 121, 126
Pharmacists, 12
Philadelphia Medical Society, 168
Philanthropy, 160, 170, 225n.56
Philosophy: allopathic, 6; hydropathic, 16–17, 29–33, 35, 48, 52, 56, 59, 73, 77, 80, 90, 101–102, 106–107, 110, 114, 151, 157, 165–166, 186n.19, 208n.33, 235; hydropathic

rejection of allopathy, 235; shifts in, 172; women's, 231
Phrenological Journal, 26, 133
Phrenology, 14–15, 76, 111, 137–138, 207n.6, 233
Physical fitness, 159, 174, 191n.126
Physician, advice of, free, 84; contracts vs. fees, 85
Physician–patient relationship, 52, 184, 219n.76; allopathic, 10, 29, 32–33, 35, 65, 164, 188n.57, 197n.92, 206n.136, 229; chiropractic, 222n.18; hydropathic, 16, 18, 22, 29–32, 42, 52–53, 73, 90–92, 104, 106, 150, 159, 164, 188n.57
Physician–researcher, 170
Physicians, allopathic, 4, 231; conversion to hydropathic practice, 81, 90; hydropathic view of, 35
Physicians, hydropathic: backgrounds of, 90–92, 98–99, 101–102; husband–wife teams, 72, 92, 112; mobility of, 90; role of, 35, 52–53, 89–90, 150, 164; women who became scientific practitioners, 94
Physicians, salaried, 84; hydropathic women, allopathic attitudes toward, 68–70; status of allopathic, 170; women, hydropathic, 18, 54, 68–70, 72–75, 91–93, 102, 111–112, 117, 126, 134, 197n.92; women, scientific, 91, 171–172, 231
Physiology, sexual, 54, 74, 235; female, 8, 54, 56, 63, 68, 74; female, allopathic views of, 2, 8, 10–11, 180n.24, 181n.35, 181n.36, 182n.41, 229–230; female, hydropathic views of, 2, 5, 8, 18, 49, 53–54, 56, 235–236; female views of, 6
Pierson, F. D., 27, 33, 64, 114
Placebo, 31, 97
Plumbing, indoor, 36, 144, 163
Poe, Edgar Allan, 112
Poems, 34, 40–41, 127–129
Poison, 12, 28, 34, 51, 95, 120, 127
Politics, women's, 133, 198n.108, 212n.97, 221n.5. *See also* Social/political sphere, women's
Ponsonby, Sarah, 147
Popular Health Movement, 7
Population, theory of, 59
Potter, Dr. E., 34
Potter, Mrs. E., 131
Pregnancy, 5, 57–58, 62, 66, 111, 143, 145, 147, 157, 236; care in, 59, 62; treatment of, allopathic, 60; treatment of, hydropathic, 60–62
"Prescriptions," hydropathic, 42, 85, 235
Priessnitz, Vincent, 20–22, 27–29, 32, 50, 105, 112, 114, 150–151, 173, 186n.19, 187n.29
Pringle, Jemima, 49
"Professional Matters," 31, 45
Professionalism, hydropathic, 30, 99–101; scientific, 170

Professionalization, hydropathic, 169, 205n.123, 206n.125
Prolapsus uteri. See Uterine displacement
Proseletyzing, 26, 89, 219n.76
Prostitution, 55, 59
Psychiatry, 152
Psychotherapy, 173, 226n.64, changes in, 226n.65
Puberty, 8, 11
Pye, Julia A., 43

Quakers, 81–82, 107, 111

Race, 123–125, 137, 225n.56, 231; black, 45; mulatto, 45, 125; Negro, 45, 68, 82, 125
Radcliff, Mary V. W., 131
Randall, Alfred, 205n.114
Ranney, Dr. D. W., 127
"Reactive power," 35, 37, 43, 151
Red Cross (American National Red Cross), 93, 155
Reform, 62, 65–66, 74, 76, 91, 100, 102, 108
Reform activities, of women, 9, 181n.31; hydropathic advocacy, 42; moral, 136; religious, 76; societal, 18, 159
Rest cure, 104; S. Weir Mitchell's, 206n.136
Restaurants, vegetarian, 119
Reuben, Dr. L., 64–65, 206n.125
Revelation, personal, 21, 186n.18
Ripley, T. S., 94
Rogers, Dr. Seth, 152, 223n.32
Role: familial, women's, 9–10; of physicians', 7–8; social, of women, 9–10; social, of women, hydropathic view of, 18. *See also* Daily role, women's
Round Hill House (Round Hill House Water Cure, Round Hill Water Cure and Motor-pathic Institute, Northampton, Mass.), 78–79, 83, 98–99, 102, 105, 107, 118, 149–150, 165, 199n.4, 205n.114, 215n.2, 219n.76, 222n.12
Roxana, R., 66–67
Ruggles, Dr. David, 80, 86, 102
Rush, Dr. Benjamin, 20, 211n.85

Salvation: physical and moral, 13, 50; religious, 31
Same-sex: political activities, 133; relation-ships, changing attitudes toward, 154, 161, 216n.23, 219n.74; 233–234
Sanctuary, 141, 153–154
Sanitation, 163, 166, 223n.25; laws on, 170
Saratoga (N.Y.) Water Cure, 40
Sauna, 174
Scott, Rev. Joseph, 43
Scott, Mrs., 62
Sects, 3–7, 11, 171–172; demise of, 224n.40, 225n.56; differences in and similarities among, 15; women's participation in, as practitioners, 12, 15, 182n.49

Self-definitions, women's, 203n.81
Self-denial/control, 159-160, 216n.22
Self-determination/improvement, 12, 15-16, 29, 35-36, 45, 53-54, 65, 85, 101, 106-107, 136, 141-142, 155, 157, 159, 174-175, 191n.126
Self-doctoring, 5, 11-12, 14, 16-17, 21, 26, 29-31, 35, 39, 44-49, 52-53, 61, 63, 69, 73, 101, 106-107, 122-123, 159, 164, 166-167, 186n.18, 215n.2, 233, 235; dangers of, 96
Self-help, tradition in, 44-45
Self-realization/involvement, women's, 158
Sensuality, 145, 147, 150, 157, 161, 215n.1, 217n.31, 233
Sentiment, anti-allopathic, hydropathic, 65
"Sentimental friendship," 147
Services, municipal, 169
Seventh-Day Adventists, 86, 94, 99, 115-116, 130, 204n.96, 209nn.39, 42, 45
Severance, Jasper, 78
Seward, Anna, 148
Sex education, 230
Sexologists, 145, 161, 216n.23, 219n.74, 221n.4, 234
Sexual abstinence, 57-58, 68
Sexual intercourse, 57-58, 113, 145-147
Sexual pleasure, female, 57, 68, 147
Sexuality, 54-57, 145, 147, 216n.22, 229, 234; female, 10-11, 230; hydropathic views on female, 54-55, 57
Sherwood, Dr. H. H., 105
Shew, Joel, 24-25, 27-30, 32-33, 38, 40, 46, 60-62, 64, 67, 83-84, 101-102, 112, 114, 119, 166-167, 205n.123, 206n.125, 223n.32, 225n.60
Shew Monument Association, 223n.32
Shew, Mrs. M. L., 32, 224n.35
Sibyl—for Reforms, The, 69, 131
Sinclair, Sir John, 11
Slade, William, 148
Slavery, 14, 82, 92, 94, 96, 102, 113-114, 125; women of men, 131-132, 136
Smith, Asheton, 84
Smith, John, 20
Smollett, Tobias, 20, 21
Snell, Dr. E., 51, 78, 97-98, 105, 219n.76
Social equality, 111, 117, 131-132, 134, 136, 138-139, 163
Social ideology, hydropathic, 49, 59
Social/political sphere, women's, hydropathic view of, 66, 68, 73-74, 108, 161-162, 221n.5, 230
Social relations/equality between the sexes, 57, 70, 72, 109-110, 126, 131, 133, 163, 208n.24
Social role, women's, 16, 53, 56, 173
Social sphere/status, women, 15, 54, 72, 115, 126, 131, 203n.81
Social status, of women, 54, 56, 233
Socialism, 113

Society of Friends, 111
Society of Public Health (N.Y.C.), 168
Somo, "a health coffee," 115
Spas, 19, 28, 162-163, 173-174, 188n.52; mineral, 17, 28
Spencer, Mr., 123
Spheres of influence, of women, 66, 68, 132-133, 135-136, 139; separate, 180n.29
Spiritualism, 113
Sports medicine, 226-227n.71
Springfield (Mass.) Water-Cure, 76, 78, 86, 97, 105, 219n.76
Stanton, Elizabeth Cady, 81-82
Still, Andres Taylor, 210n.49
Stone, Mrs. Lucy, 120, 131
Storer, Dr. Horatio, 10
Stowe, Calvin, 143-144
Stowe, Harriet Beecher, 143-144, 148, 215n.13, 216n.17
Strength, female, 134, 139
Strong, Dr., 99
Stuart, Dr. Anna, 93
Stuart, Ruth McEnery, 95
Subordination of women, 11
Suffrage, women's, 81-82, 133
Surgery, modern, 172
Sweating process, 55
Swedish movement exercise, 104
Syringe, hypodermic, 122

Taylor, Baynard, 115
Tea, 42, 120-121, 138
Teams, husband–wife water-cure physicians. See Physicians, hydropathic, husband–wife teams
Temperance, 13, 15, 47-48, 53, 94, 102, 109-110, 114, 116, 120, 122-123, 137, 166
Tenth Street Water-Cure (N.Y.), 112
Testimonials, 1, 11, 23-24, 26, 34, 40, 43-47, 49-52, 61, 63-64, 66, 75-76, 80-81, 83, 95, 99, 119-120, 126, 129-130, 142, 148-150, 155-156, 158, 182n.42, 195n.63, 199n.4, 219n.76
Texts, hydropathic, early, 234-235
Thayer, Dr. Orson V., 91
Theory, hydropathic, 18, 234-235; of disease, 16, 235
Therapeutic touch, 18, 184-185n.2
Therapeutics, 55, 62, 73-74, 148; allopathic, 2, 6-7, 22-23, 33-34, 43, 46, 50-51, 60, 63, 65, 70, 122, 182n.41, 229, 235; allopathic, efficacy of, 34, 206n.136; allopathic, hydropathic views of, 33-35, 235; allopathic, sect's views of, 11, 183n.52; alternate to, 106; electrical, 98, 102-104, 116, 152, 208n.33; homeopathic, 43; hydropathic, 2, 16, 21, 23, 36, 43-44, 59, 103, 114, 153, 195n.63, 234-235; hydrotherapy, present-day, 174, 226n.71; preventive, 172;

similarities between allopathic and hydro-pathic, 7
Therapy, hydropathic, description of, 144, 148, 153
Thomson, Samuel, 11–12
Thomsonianism, 12, 53, 69
Tight lacing, 42, 66, 70, 126, 128
Tobacco, 42, 66, 120–121, 123, 135, 137–138
Trall, R. T., 24–25, 27–29, 31–33, 38, 42–43, 55–59, 62, 65, 71, 85, 89, 99–100, 111–112, 114, 116–117, 119, 123–124, 134–135, 138, 167, 205n.123, 213n.110
Trauma, 174
Truth, Sojourner, 95
Tuckey, Dr. Lloyd, 152
Turner, Ann, 84

Una, The, 133
Underground Railroad, 96, 125
U.S. Dept. of Health, 170
Unmarried women, 72, 132, 134, 139, 141–142, 147, 157
Urbanization, 160, 169
Uterine displacement, 63–64, 127, 145

Vaccination, 103, 225n.60; hydropathic views on, 172
Vail, W. T., 48, 117
Vegetarianism, 13, 15, 43, 45, 47–48, 53, 94, 103, 106, 110–112, 115–116, 118–120, 137–138, 209n.45
Vergnes, Prof. M., 106
"Vital force," 6–7, 54, 56, 58, 122
Vivisection, 103, 172

Wage differential, occupational groups, 88, 202n.62, 203n.66
Waite, Isabella, 80–81
Wales, Dr. Theron Augustus, 93
Wales, Dr. Zippie Brooks, 93, 215n.2
Walker, Dr. Alexander, 10
Wallace, Dr. J. P., 90
Warren, Josiah, 113
Water, 25; cold, 29; as conduit, 15, 19, 20–21, 23, 25, 36, 38, 60, 150, 171, 185n.5; deem-phasized, 165; drinking, 22, 46, 55, 148, 174, 227n.71; as healing agent, 17–18, 25, 35, 164–165, 185n.5, 208n.33; injections of, vaginal, 58, 60, 62, 145; medicinal use of, 17, 20, 165, 226n.71; mineral, 19, 28, 148, 188n.52, 217n.38; Native American use of, 18–19, 185n.5; as relaxant, 227n.71; religious/mystical associations, 18–19, 38, 185n.5; ritual use of, 18–19, 185n.5; supply of, 166, 223n.25; symbolism of, 18; tem-perature of, 35, 48, 96, 153
Water-Cure and Health Almanac, The, 114
Water-Cure College (Dansville, N.Y.), 100
Water-cure: dangers of, 28, 150–151, 224n.38; diagnosis and "prescription," by correspon-dence, 46, 192n.134, 201n.43; differences from and similarities to other sects, 29; efficacy of, 30–31, 39, 44–46, 52–53, 62, 67, 97, 106, 114, 141, 148, 159, 164, 167, 173, 195n.63; establishments, 24–25, 39, 76, 95, 104, 165; establishments as psychologi-cal havens, 5, 227n.71; facilities of, 75, 78–80, 82–83, 215n.2, 220n.85; facilities, recreational, 83, 98; history of, 19, 24, 187n.29; home use, 48; opponents of, 68; processes of, 39, 44, 114, 166; publications of, 186n.19; reform movement of, as women's health reform movement, 67
Water-Cure Journal, 3, 18, 24–26, 33–34, 39, 43, 46, 51, 71–72, 76–77, 83, 88, 101, 109–114, 116–119, 121, 123–126, 131, 133, 164–165, 184n.69, 186n.19; circulation of, 26, 188; cost of, 26, 83; correspondents of, 129; editors of, 27, 188; format change in, 236; name changes, 27, 236; owners of, 27; popularity of, 26
Water cures: costs of, 86–90, 107, 192n.134; economic accessibility of, 46, 83–85, 89–90, 107, 171, 201n.43; employees of, sex ratios, 157; environs of, 77–80, 107, 156, 199n.6, 227n.71; live-in, 74, 84, 156; longevity of, 76, 94, 102, 107; modifications of, 163; name changes in, 222n.20; popularity of, 46, 76, 99, 107, 142, 161, 163–164, 167, 172; present-day, 227n.71; profits from, 88; stability of, 76, 94–95, 97, 107, 220n.85; for women only, 77, 91
Waterbury, Maria, 82
Wayland, R. Milo, 138
Weed, Dr. Adaline M. W., 72, 138
Wellington, Dr., 43
Wells, S. R., 26, 119, 205n.123
Wesley, John, 20
Wesselhoeft, Dr., 148, 205n.123
West Twenty-Second Street Water-Cure (N.Y.C.), 112
Westboro (Mass.) Water Cure, 95
Western Health Reform Institute (Battle Creek, Mich.), 115–116, 209n.42
Wet-sheet wrap, 21, 37–40, 42, 44–45, 47, 55, 60, 63, 148, 153
Wheeler, Dr. Edith Flower, 93
White, Ellen G., 115–117, 209n.39
White, James, 115–116, 209n.42
Whitmarsh, Samuel, 98
Wiggin, Kate Douglas, 95
Willard, Frances, E., 95
Willis, Dr. Adeline M., 138
Willow Park (Mass.) Water Cure, 96
Willow Park Seminary, 96
Wilmarth, Dr. B., 96, 101, 206n.125
Woman's Medical College (N.Y. Infirmary for Women), 69
Woman's Medical College of Pennsylvania, 93

Women as caretakers of others, 18, 185n.4

Women, as natural healers. *See* Natural healers, women as

Women, broadened horizons of, 66

Women's Christian Temperance Union (W.C.T.U.), 116, 122

Women's rights, 10, 14, 57, 91, 94, 111–112, 115, 120, 126, 132–133, 137

Wood, A. L., 28

Wood, Alice, 219

Wood, Dr. Edwin L., 219n.76

Woodward, Dr. Samuel B., 98, 205n.113

Woolley, Mary, 153

Worcester Hydropathic Institute (Mass.), 152, 223n.32

Worcester (Mass.) State Lunatic Hospital, 98, 205n.113

Worcester (Mass.) Water Cure, 223n.32. *See also* Worcester Hydropathic Institute (Mass.)

World view/ideology, hydropathic, 5, 15–18, 29, 48, 50, 56, 106–108, 135–136, 139, 159–160, 165, 173, 184n.1

Wright, Paulina S., 54

Wyoming (N.Y.) Water Cure, 64

X ray, 172

Young, Brigham, 81